Atlas of Cutaneous Lymphomas

Joi B. Carter • Amrita Goyal
Lyn McDivitt Duncan
Editors

Atlas of Cutaneous Lymphomas

Classification and Differential Diagnosis

Springer

Editors
Joi B. Carter
Department of Dermatology
Massachusetts General Hospital
Boston, MA
USA

Lyn McDivitt Duncan
Dermatopathology Service
Massachusetts General Hospital
Boston, MA
USA

Amrita Goyal
Division of Health Sciences and Technology
Harvard Medical School
Boston, MA
USA

ISBN 978-3-319-35477-4 ISBN 978-3-319-17217-0 (eBook)
DOI 10.1007/978-3-319-17217-0

Springer Cham Heidelberg New York Dordrecht London

Softcover reprint of the hardcover 1st edition 2015

Printed on acid-free paper

Springer International Publishing AG Switzerland is part of Springer Science+Business Media (www.springer.com)

To my parents, who instilled in me their love of teaching and caring for others. To my daughters, Seija, Annika, and Kaia for bringing a joyous perspective to each day. And finally to my husband, Pete, who helps keep our lives in balance and our family on course.

Joi B.Carter, M.D.

To my parents, Nita and Nakul Goyal; grandparents, Krishan and Pushpa Raheja; aunt, Nina Raheja; siblings, Kavita and Nihkil Goyal; cousin, Meera Jain; and last, but not least, my best friend, Daniel O'Leary. This book would not have been possible without your love, encouragement, and support.

Amrita Goyal, M.D.

To my father, Robert McDivitt, the best pathologist I know and my first teacher. To my mother, who taught me the power of small steps to reach a goal. To Micki, Elias, Allie, and Sam, no longer children, they continue to bring joy and teach me about life. And finally to my husband, Frank, who inspires me to enjoy.

Lyn McDivitt Duncan, M.D.

Preface

This atlas was inspired by the Massachusetts General Hospital Cutaneous Lymphoma Conference, a multidisciplinary meeting of dermatologists, dermatopathologists, hematopathologists, medical oncologists, and radiation oncologists. We have found that the integration of clinical findings, laboratory results, and disease progression is critical for the diagnosis and treatment of patients with skin lymphoma. Using the clinical and histological images of our patients as the framework, this atlas follows the recent classification scheme for cutaneous lymphoma published by the World Health Organization (WHO) and the European Organization for Research and Treatment of Cancer (EORTC) Cutaneous Lymphoma Group.

Our intent was to produce an atlas of clinical and histological images with diagrams, tables, and text describing each entity in the current cutaneous lymphoma classification scheme. The outline of each chapter includes an introduction with synonyms, clinical features (presentation, prognosis, and treatment), laboratory findings (histopathology, immunophenotype, and molecular), differential diagnosis, and presentation of clinical cases. In addition to chapters for each diagnostic entity, we have included introduction chapters for T-cell lymphomas, B-cell lymphomas, a chapter on ancillary techniques including immunohistochemistry and molecular tests, and a glossary of terms.

We hope this resource will help clarify the conceptual framework underlying the classification of cutaneous lymphoma. More importantly, we hope to have produced a book that will serve as a helpful reference for physicians involved in the diagnosis and treatment of patients with cutaneous lymphoma.

Boston, MA, USA

Joi B. Carter, M.D.
Amrita Goyal, M.D.
Lyn McDivitt Duncan, M.D.

Acknowledgment

We acknowledge the invaluable contributions of our patients who share their stories and allow us to further understand the diversity of these diseases. This work is also inspired by the teachings of our mentors, Dr. Nancy Harris, Dr. Tom Kupper, and Dr. Martin Mihm; they have taught us many lessons including the value of shared knowledge.

Contents

Contributors

Jeffrey A. Barnes, M.D., Ph.D. Comprehensive Cutaneous Lymphoma Program, Department of Medicine, Massachusetts General Hospital Cancer Center, Boston, MA, USA

Joi B. Carter, M.D. Department of Dermatology, Massachusetts General Hospital, Harvard Medical School, Boston, MA, USA

Lyn McDivitt Duncan, M.D. Dermatopathology Service, Department of Pathology, Massachusetts General Hospital, Harvard Medical School, Boston, MA, USA

Judith A. Ferry, M.D. Hematopathology Service, Department of Pathology, Massachusetts General Hospital, Harvard Medical School, Boston, MA, USA

Amrita Goyal, M.D. Harvard-MIT Division of Health Sciences and Technology, Harvard Medical School, Boston, MA, USA

Kavita Goyal, B.S. Drexel University College of Medicine, Philadelphia, PA, USA

Nancy Lee Harris, M.D. Hematopathology Service, Department of Pathology, Massachusetts General Hospital, Harvard Medical School, Boston, MA, USA

Mai P. Hoang, M.D. Dermatopathology Service, Department of Pathology, Massachusetts General Hospital, Harvard Medical School, Boston, MA, USA

Alexandra E. Kovach, M.D. Department of Pathology, Boston Children's Hospital, Boston, MA, USA

Daniela Kroshinsky, M.D. Department of Dermatology, Massachusetts General Hospital, Harvard Medical School, Boston, MA, USA

Thomas S. Kupper, M.D. Department of Dermatology, Brigham and Women's Hospital, Harvard Medical School, Boston, MA, USA

Nicole R. LeBoeuf, M.D. Department of Dermatology, Brigham and Women's Hospital, Harvard Medical School, Boston, MA, USA

Valentina Nardi, M.D. Hematopathology Service, Department of Pathology, Massachusetts General Hospital, Harvard Medical School, Boston, MA, USA

Rosalynn M. Nazarian, M.D. Dermatopathology Service, Department of Pathology, Massachusetts General Hospital, Harvard Medical School, Boston, MA, USA

Adriano Piris, M.D. Department of Dermatology, Brigham and Women's Hospital, Harvard Medical School, Boston, MA, USA

Aliyah R. Sohani, M.D. Hematopathology Service, Department of Pathology, Massachusetts General Hospital, Harvard Medical School, Boston, MA, USA

1 Introduction and a Brief History of Cutaneous Lymphoma Classification

Amrita Goyal, Joi B. Carter, Nancy Lee Harris, and Lyn McDivitt Duncan

Over the past decade, a worldwide consortium of dermatologists, oncologists, hematopathologists, and dermatopathologists has collaborated to develop a unified classification scheme for lymphomas, including primary cutaneous lymphomas. Every year, new publications and workshops lead to a clearer understanding of the nuances of diagnosis and treatment of cutaneous lymphomas. Over the past 20 years, advances in the classification of cutaneous lymphomas have revolutionized the clinical and histopathologic approaches to diagnosis and treatment of these highly varied diseases. This chapter outlines some aims of this book and offers a brief history of cutaneous lymphoma classification.

1.1 Goals of This Book

Understanding cutaneous lymphoma can be challenging for even the most determined, for several reasons:

1. Some of these diseases share clinical presentations.
2. Some display similar histopathological features.
3. While immunophenotypic and genetic features may support a specific diagnosis, there is overlap between tumors.
4. The terminology used to describe these tumors has evolved and only in the past decade has there been a more uniform approach to classification.
5. Few textbooks offer concise descriptions of the clinical and histopathologic characteristics of these diseases in accordance with the most recent classification system. This atlas seeks to fill that gap.

This book was written with several goals in mind:

1. Assemble an atlas of cutaneous lymphomas, organized according to the most recent classification system, as designed by the World Health Organization–European Organization for Research and Treatment of Cancer (WHO-EORTC)
2. Offer flowcharts and other schemas to help organize the cutaneous lymphomas in an easy to understand format
3. Provide a concise summary of current knowledge about the clinical presentation, histopathological, immunophenotypic and genetic characteristics, prognosis, and treatment of each cutaneous lymphoma
4. Demonstrate the importance of clinical–pathologic correlation using real clinical cases, in most cases by juxtaposing both the clinical and histopathologic images from the same patients
5. Present this information at a level appropriate for students, trainees, and practitioners in dermatology and pathology.

1.2 History of the Classification of Cutaneous Lymphomas

For more than a century and a half, lymphomas arising in the skin were classified as one of three entities: mycosis fungoides, Sézary syndrome, or spread of lymphoma from a noncutaneous site. Although mycosis fungoides was first described

A. Goyal, M.D.
Harvard-MIT Division of Health Sciences and Technology, Harvard Medical School, Boston, MA, USA

J.B. Carter, M.D.
Department of Dermatology, Massachusetts General Hospital, Harvard Medical School, Boston, MA, USA

N.L. Harris, M.D.
Hematopathology Service, Department of Pathology, Massachusetts General Hospital, Harvard Medical School, Boston, MA, USA

L.M. Duncan, M.D. (✉)
Dermatopathology Service, Department of Pathology, Massachusetts General Hospital, Harvard Medical School, Boston, MA, USA
e-mail: duncan@helix.mgh.harvard.edu

J.B. Carter et al. (eds.), *Atlas of Cutaneous Lymphomas: Classification and Differential Diagnosis*, DOI 10.1007/978-3-319-17217-0_1

by Alibert [1] in 1806, and Sézary syndrome in 1938 [2], it was not until the 1970s that primary cutaneous lymphomas other than mycosis fungoides and Sézary syndrome were differentiated from cutaneous manifestations of systemic lymphoma. At that time a classification system reflecting the heterogeneity of cutaneous lymphomas began to be developed.

At the end of the last century, it became increasingly clear that a wide range of B-cell and T-cell lymphomas can occur as primary tumors in the skin, and that they have quite variable clinical outcomes: some primary cutaneous lymphomas are indolent and never disseminate to extracutaneous sites, while others disseminate widely with an aggressive clinical course. This variability in clinical outcome is one of the primary reasons that an accurate classification system is necessary.

From the 1970s to the 1990s, there were three principal classification schemes for lymphomas: Kiel [3–5], Lukes-Collins and Working Formulation [6], all based predominantly upon morphological findings and cell type [7]. In many cases diagnoses were reported using more than one scheme's terminology. However, in 1994, the International Lymphoma Study Group achieved an international consensus on the classification of lymphomas. This led to the publication of the Revised European–American Lymphoma Classification (REAL) [8]. The REAL classification incorporated morphologic, immunologic, genetic, and clinical features to identify "real" biological entities. The REAL Classification also recognized the differences between nodal and extranodal lymphomas. Shortly thereafter, the European Organization for Research and Treatment of Cancer (EORTC) Cutaneous Lymphoma Program Project Group devised a classification scheme specifically for primary cutaneous lymphoma [9]. In addition to the features used in the REAL classification scheme, the EORTC scheme incorporated the clinical presentation and biologic behavior of the lymphomas.

In 2001, the World Health Organization (WHO) International Agency for Research and Cancer published *The Pathology and Genetics of Tumours of Haematopoietic and Lymphoid Tissues*, 3rd edition [10]. Although EORTC schema for understanding the cutaneous T-cell lymphomas was largely integrated into this WHO publication, there continued to be debate about the subtypes of cutaneous B-cell lymphomas and their relationships to their nodal counterparts. Points of contention included: the use of terms "primary cutaneous" versus "extranodal," "diffuse follicular lymphoma" versus "diffuse large B-cell lymphoma," "follicle centre" versus "follicular," and the use of "leg type" in describing primary cutaneous B-cell lymphoma not arising on the leg. In 2003 and 2004, the authors of the WHO and EORTC classifications met in Lyon and Zurich to resolve these issues through review of cases and active discussion. This review included not only the histopathological, immunophenotypic, and genetic features of the tumors, but their clinical outcomes and response to therapy. These meetings resulted in the 2005 joint EORTC/WHO classification for primary cutaneous lymphoma [11].

In 2008, the 4th edition of the *WHO Classification of Tumours of Haematopoetic and Lymphoid Tissues* was published. This volume, "the blue book," integrated the primary cutaneous lymphoma classification into the broader classification of nodal and other extranodal lymphoma classification [12]. The integrated EORTC and WHO classification has become the basis for diagnosis and treatment of patients with cutaneous lymphomas. Persistent inconsistencies between the WHO/EORTC (2005) and WHO (2008) classifications include the use of the terms, primary cutaneous marginal zone lymphoma and CD4+ CD56+ hematodermic neoplasm, in the former and the terms extranodal marginal zone lymphoma of mucosa-associated lymphoid tissue (MALT lymphoma) and blastic plasmacytoid dendritic cell neoplasm in the latter. Because the WHO classification found in the "blue book" encompasses all leukemias and lymphomas, it can be cumbersome and challenging for dermatologists and dermatopathologists to dissect out the information on skin-specific diseases. Our aim is to provide a resource for diagnosis of primary cutaneous lymphomas that includes clinical and histopathological images of the diseases described in accordance with the most recent classification scheme. We refer to the classification as WHO-EORTC to recognize the important contributions of both of these groups.

1.3 Terminology

The field of cutaneous lymphomas is rife with terminological ambiguity. For example, the term "primary cutaneous" is itself controversial. It has been used by some to describe lymphoma arising in the skin without evidence of concurrent extra-cutaneous lymphoma after staging (often including both radiological and bone marrow evaluation) [9, 13]. While no longer used, early on some defined primary cutaneous lymphoma as lymphoma arising in the skin without evidence of extra-cutaneous lymphoma *for 6 months* following initial presentation [14]. In the WHO-EORTC Classification, the term "primary cutaneous lymphoma" refers to cutaneous lymphomas that present in the skin without evidence of extracutaneous disease at the time of diagnosis [11].

The majority of lymphomas are named descriptively after their cell of origin. For example, "primary cutaneous follicle centre lymphoma (pcFCL)" is a tumor composed of neoplastic BCL-6+ follicle center B cells. This biologically based, descriptive naming system carries two complications. First, names of the lymphomas are changed as new biological information is discovered. For example, what was once CD4+ CD56+ hematodermic neoplasm is now called blastic plasmacytoid dendritic cell neoplasm, because of better understanding of the cell of origin of the disease. A better understanding of the risk of progression has led some disease entities to be divided and re-defined; for example the Ketron-Goodman variant of pagetoid reticulosis is now considered to be best classified as either aggressive epidermotropic CD8+ cutaneous T-cell lymphoma or cutaneous gamma-delta T-cell lymphoma, depending on the immunophenotype. Second, given the descriptive terminology, the names of these diseases can be up to seven to eight words long, as with primary cutaneous CD4+ small-medium pleomorphic T-cell lymphoma. One student even suggested that cutaneous lymphoma may be the one case in which eponymous naming might actually make things *easier*. There has even been discord over these extensive descriptive names. For example, while some prefer "extranodal marginal zone B-cell lymphoma of mucosa-associated lymphoid tissue (MALT lymphoma)," others use the term "primary cutaneous marginal zone lymphoma (pcMZL)." The use of the term "extranodal" indicates that this tumor is biologically related to those occurring at other extranodal sites (most commonly the gastrointestinal tract); however, some argue that the use of "MALT" is inappropriate given that the skin is not mucosa.

Other terms require understanding of the specific classification criteria, for example subcutaneous panniculitis-like T-cell lymphoma (SPTCL). This lymphoma is defined as a tumor of cytotoxic T cells with an alpha-beta TCR. Although lymphomas with a gamma-delta TCR phenotype were once grouped with SPTCL and may occur predominantly in the subcutaneous fat, given evolving information about their clinical progression, these lymphoma are now classified separately as primary cutaneous gamma-delta T-cell lymphoma.

One of the aims of this book is to help clarify some of this confusion. We list synonyms at the beginning of every chapter and note shifts in terminology based on medical advances. In each chapter we have used tables and illustrations to help organize the approach to diagnosis of primary cutaneous lymphoma. Finally, we have included a glossary of terms to provide a quick reference to access the occasionally cryptic terminology.

1.4 Case-Based Approach in Primary Cutaneous Lymphomas

The diagnosis of primary cutaneous lymphomas requires the correlation of clinical and laboratory findings. At the Massachusetts General Hospital, a dedicated team of experts in Dermatology, Hematology-Oncology, Hematopathology, Dermatopathology, and Radiation Oncology diagnose and treat patients with cutaneous lymphoma. This group meets regularly to review the clinical, histopathological, immunophenotypic, and genetic features of patients with a comprehensive evaluation of the ongoing evolution of patients' disease including recurrence, dissemination, and response to therapy. As a patient's disease evolves, his or her clinical picture is revisited, underscoring the importance of clinical pathological correlation over time.

The cases presented in this atlas are derived from this experience: nearly all the cases represent patients who were diagnosed and treated at the Massachusetts General Hospital. Most chapters contain examples of complete cases of patients with primary cutaneous lymphoma including images of both clinical and histopathological findings. Juxtaposition of clinical and pathologic images from a single patient helps enhance an understanding of clinical and pathological correlations. Overall, we hope that this work is a practical tool for those who care for patients with cutaneous lymphoma.

References

1. Alibert J. Tableau du pian fongoide: description des maladies de la peau, observées à 1 Hôpital Saint-Louis et exposition des meilleurs methodes suivies pour leur traitement. Paris: Barrois L Aine et Fils; 1806.
2. Sézary A, Bouvrain J. Erythrodermie avec presence de cellules monstrueuses dans le derme et le sang circulant. Bull Soc Fr Dermatol Syphiligr. 1938;45:245–60.
3. Lennert K. Histopathology of non-Hodgkin's lymphomas: based on the Kiel classification. New York: Springer; 1981.
4. Lennert K, Feller AC. Histopathology of non-Hodgkin's lymphomas (based on the updated Kiel classification). Berlin: Springer; 1992.
5. Stansfeld AG, Diebold J, Noel H, Kapanci Y, Rilke F, Kelényi G, et al. Updated Kiel classification for lymphomas. Lancet. 1988;1:292.
6. National Cancer Institute sponsored study of classification of non-Hodgkin's lymphomas: summary and description of a working formulation for clinical usage. The non-Hodgkin's lymphomas pathologic classification project. Cancer. 1982;49:2112–35.
7. Lukes R, Collins R. Immunologic characterization of human malignant lymphomas. Cancer. 1974;34:1488.
8. Harris NL, Jaffe ES, Stein H, Banks PM, Chan JK, Cleary ML, et al. A revised European-American classification of lymphoid neoplasms: a proposal from the International Lymphoma Study Group. Blood. 1994;84:1361–92.
9. Willemze R, Kerl H, Sterry W, Berti E, Cerroni L, Chimenti S, et al. EORTC classification for primary cutaneous lymphomas: a proposal from the Cutaneous Lymphoma Study Group of the European Organization for Research and Treatment of Cancer. Blood. 1997;90:354–71.
10. Jaffe E, Harris N, Stein H, Vardiman J. World health organization: pathology and genetics of tumors of hematopoetic and lymphoid tissues. Lyon: IARC Press; 2001.
11. Willemze R, Jaffe ES, Burg G, Cerroni L, Berti E, Swerdlow SH, et al. WHO-EORTC classification for cutaneous lymphomas. Blood. 2005;105:3768–85.
12. Swerdlow SH, Campo E, Harris NL, et al., editors. WHO classification of tumours of haematopoietic and lymphoid tissues. 4th ed. Lyon: IARC; 2008. World health organization classification of tumors.
13. Bailey EM, Ferry JA, Harris NL, Mihm Jr MC, Jacobson JO, Duncan LM. Marginal zone lymphoma (low-grade B-cell lymphoma of mucosa-associated lymphoid tissue type) of skin and subcutaneous tissue: a study of 15 patients. Am J Surg Pathol. 1996;20:1011–23.
14. Kerl H, Cerroni L. Primary B-cell lymphomas of the skin. Ann Oncol. 1997;8 Suppl 2:29–32.

2 Introduction to Cutaneous Lymphomas

Amrita Goyal, Joi B. Carter, and Lyn McDivitt Duncan

The term *cutaneous lymphoma* encompasses an array of neoplasms that vary widely in their clinical presentation, prognosis, histopathology, immunohistochemistry, and molecular biology. The World Health Organization–European Organization for Research and Treatment of Cancer (WHO/EORTC) classification system recognizes 15 primary cutaneous lymphomas (Table 2.1). These lymphomas are divided into three overarching categories: T-cell lymphomas, B-cell lymphomas, and precursor neoplasms. Each chapter in this book is dedicated to one of these cutaneous lymphomas and offers a clinical and histopathologic description, differential diagnosis, and one or more clinical cases. Our intent in writing this book is to familiarize the reader with the most recent classifications of the cutaneous lymphomas, offer relevant clinical and histopathologic characteristics, and provide direction in navigating the often difficult task of distinguishing the various forms of cutaneous lymphoma.

A. Goyal, M.D.
Harvard-MIT Division of Health Sciences and Technology, Harvard Medical School, Boston, MA, USA

J.B. Carter, M.D.
Department of Dermatology, Massachusetts General Hospital, Harvard Medical School, Boston, MA, USA

L.M. Duncan, M.D. (✉)
Dermatopathology Service, Department of Pathology, Massachusetts General Hospital, Harvard Medical School, 55 Fruit Street, WRN 825, Boston, MA, USA
e-mail: duncan@helix.mgh.harvard.edu

J.B. Carter et al. (eds.), *Atlas of Cutaneous Lymphomas: Classification and Differential Diagnosis*, DOI 10.1007/978-3-319-17217-0_2

Table 2.1 WHO-EORTC classification of cutaneous lymphomas

Lymphoma	Abbreviation	Incidence (%)
T-cell lymphomas:	CTCL	77
Mycosis fungoides	MF	50
Sézary syndrome	SS	3
Adult T-cell leukemia/lymphoma	ATLL	<1
Subcutaneous panniculitis-like T-cell lymphoma	SPTCL	1
Extranodal NK/T-cell lymphoma	eNK/TCL	<1
CD30+ lymphoproliferative disorders:	CD30+ LPD	
Primary cutaneous anaplastic large cell lymphoma	pcALCL	8
Lymphomatoid papulosis	LyP	12
Provisional entities:		
CD8+ aggressive epidermotropic T-cell lymphoma	CD8+ AECTCL	<1
Primary cutaneous gamma-delta T-cell lymphoma	pcGDTCL	<1
CD4+ primary cutaneous small-medium pleomorphic T-cell lymphoma	pcSMPTCL	<1
B-cell lymphomas:	CBCL	23
Primary cutaneous marginal zone lymphoma	pcMZL	7
Primary cutaneous follicle center lymphoma	pcFCL	11
Primary cutaneous diffuse large B-cell lymphoma, leg-type	pcDLBCL	4
Intravascular large B-cell lymphoma	ivLBCL	<1
Precursor neoplasms:		
Blastic plasmacytoid dendritic cell neoplasm	BPDCN	<1

Adapted from Willemze et al. [1] and Swerdlow et al. [2]
The abbreviations used throughout this book and the incidence of each lymphoma are listed

2.1 The Skin as an Immune Organ

The skin is one of the most important organs of the immune system and plays a critical role in both the innate and adaptive immune systems. There are a variety of immune cells present in the skin, including T cells, B cells, dendritic cells, natural killer (NK) cells, neutrophils, eosinophils, mast cells, monocytes, and macrophages [3]. It is possible for any of these cell populations to become deranged and develop into a neoplasm (Fig. 2.1) [5].

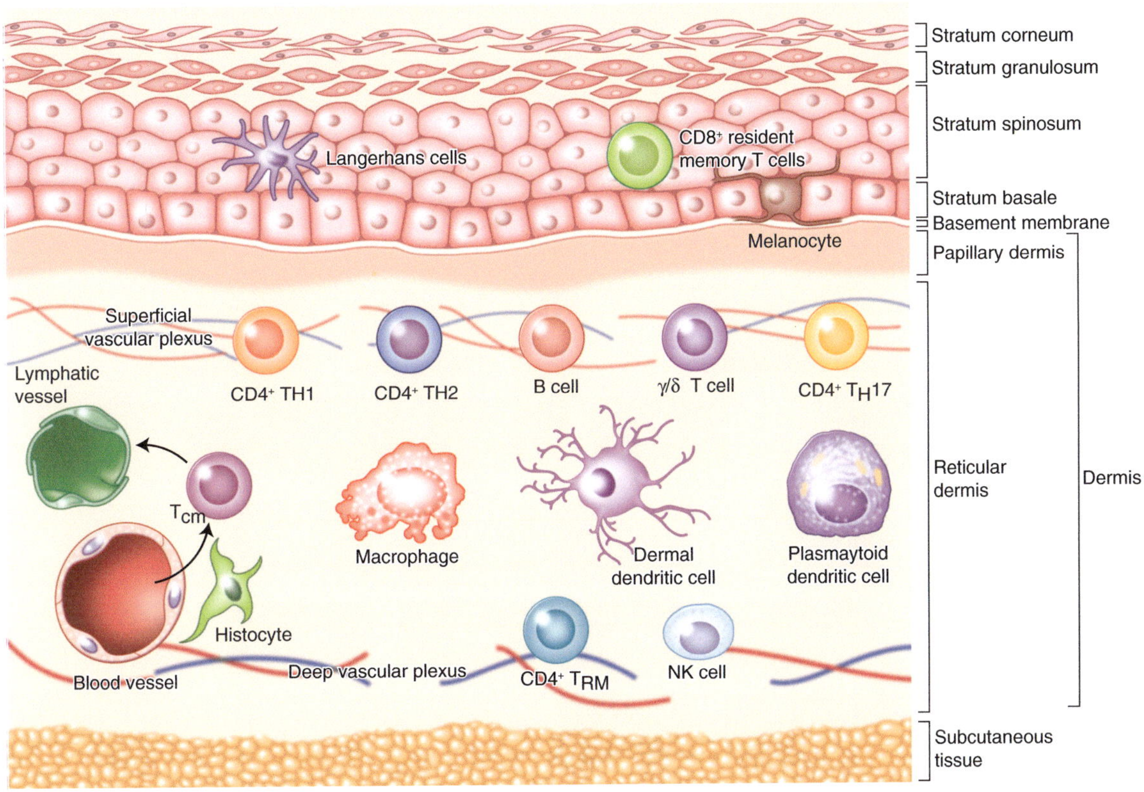

Fig. 2.1 The skin is one of the most important organs in the immune system. The epidermis is usually inhabited by CD8+ T cells and Langerhans cells. A number of cell types reside in the dermis, including CD4+ T cells of various phenotypes (including TH1, TH2, and TH17 cells), gamma/delta T cells, B cells, NK cells, mast cells, and plasmacytoid dendritic cells. Circulating memory T cells spend some time in the skin, entering via blood vessels and returning to the circulation via the lymphatics. Note the structure of the skin—the epidermis is composed of four major layers: the stratum corneum, stratum granulosum, stratum spinosum, and stratum basale. Melanocytes produce melanin and are intercalated between keratinocytes of the basal layer of the epidermis. The dermis is composed of the looser papillary and underlying denser reticular dermis. The subcutaneous fat lies beneath the dermis (Diagram adapted from Nestle et al. [4])

2.2 Classification of Cutaneous Lymphomas

Cutaneous lymphomas can be segregated into three categories: T-cell lymphomas, B-cell lymphomas, and precursor cell neoplasms. The 15 lymphomas included in the current WHO/EORTC classification schema are listed in Table 2.1 (Fig. 2.2). One schema for organizing these lymphomas is provided in the flow chart in Fig. 2.2.

The lymphomas can be further subdivided based on immunohistochemical phenotypes, as described in the flow chart in Fig. 2.3.

It is important to note that although the majority of these cutaneous lymphomas are *primary cutaneous* lymphomas clinically arising in the skin, several of these neoplasms, including Sézary syndrome, adult T-cell leukemia/lymphoma (ATLL), and intravascular large B-cell lymphoma (ivLBCL), are systemic lymphoid neoplasms. They are included in the classification of cutaneous lymphomas because of their prominent cutaneous findings.

There are many other primary cutaneous lymphomas not included in the WHO/EORTC classification system, some because they are exceedingly uncommon and some because they are not yet well defined.

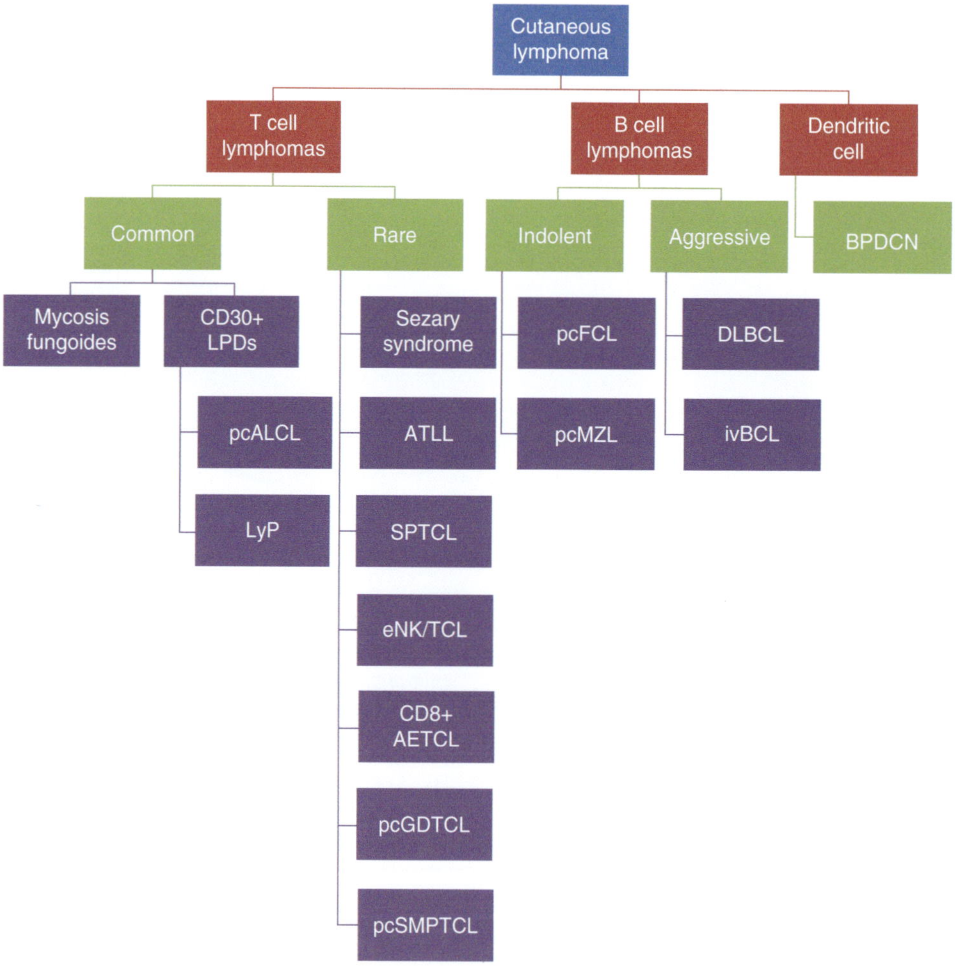

Fig. 2.2 Conceptual framework for cutaneous lymphomas. Cutaneous lymphomas can be broken down in any number of ways, but most commonly they are divided into T-cell neoplasms, B-cell neoplasms, and dendritic cell neoplasms; beyond that classification variations abound. Here, T-cell neoplasms are divided based on frequency—common versus rare. The most common lymphomas are mycosis fungoides (MF) and the CD30+ lymphoproliferative diseases (CD30+ LPDs). The rare T-cell lymphomas are a diverse group, and each one makes up less than 3 % of cases of cutaneous T-cell lymphomas. It is possible to divide the B-cell lymphomas based on prognosis, either indolent or aggressive. Finally, blastic plasmacytoid dendritic cell neoplasm (BPCDN) is the only dendritic cell neoplasm that bears lymphoid markers. *ATLL* adult T-cell leukemia/lymphoma, *DLBCL* diffuse large B-cell lymphoma, leg type, *CD8+ AECTCL* CD8+ aggressive epidermotropic cutaneous T-cell lymphoma, *eNK/TCL* extranodal NK/T-cell lymphoma, *LyP* lymphomatoid papulosis, *ivLBVL* intravascular large B-cell lymphoma, *pcALCL* primary cutaneous anaplastic large cell lymphoma, *pcFCL* primary cutaneous follicle center lymphoma, *pcGDTCL* primary cutaneous gamma/delta T-cell lymphoma, *pcMZL* primary cutaneous marginal zone lymphoma, *pcSMPTCL* primary cutaneous small-medium pleomorphic T-cell lymphoma, *SPTCL* subcutaneous panniculitis-like T-cell lymphoma

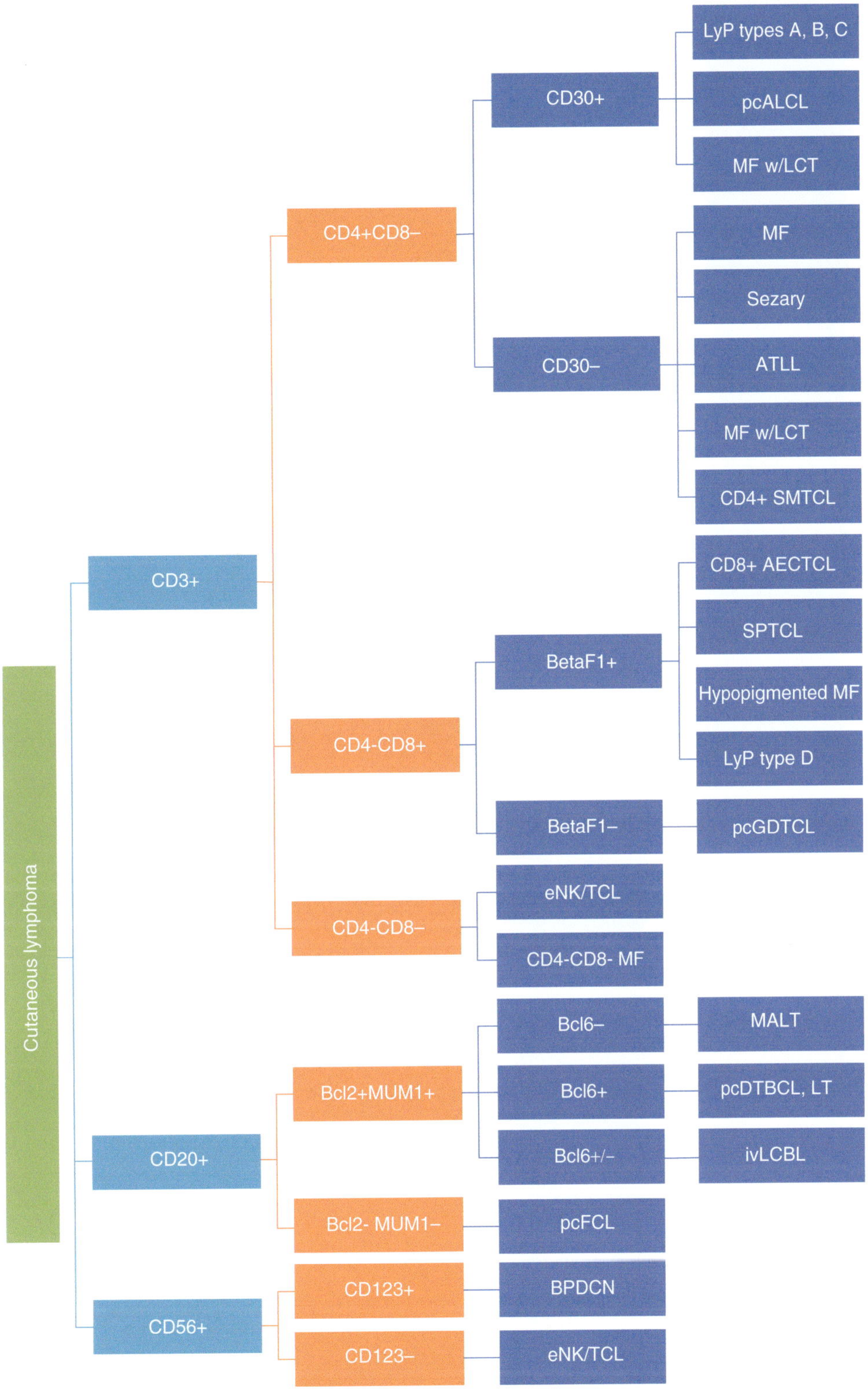

Fig. 2.3 Immunohistochemical flow chart of cutaneous lymphomas. Cutaneous lymphomas can be segregated by cell of origin (T cell, B cell, NK/T cell) or by dendritic cell. CD3+ T cells can be further subdivided based on immunohistochemical markers, including CD4, CD8, and CD30. B-cell lymphomas all stain positively for CD20; useful immunohistochemical stains for further evaluation include Bcl2, Bcl6, and MUM1. While this flow chart describes the archetypical staining patterns for each lymphoma, individual cases may vary. *ATLL* adult T-cell leukemia/lymphoma, *CD8+ AECTCL* CD8+ aggressive epidermotropic cutaneous T-cell lymphoma, *DLBCL* diffuse large B-cell lymphoma, leg type, *eNK/TCL* extranodal NK/T-cell lymphoma, *ivLBVL* intravascular large B-cell lymphoma, *LCT* large cell transformation, *LyP* lymphomatoid papulosis, *MF* mycosis fungoides, *pcALCL* primary cutaneous anaplastic large cell lymphoma, *pcFCL* primary cutaneous follicle center lymphoma, *pcGDTCL* primary cutaneous gamma/delta T-cell lymphoma, *pcMZL* primary cutaneous marginal zone lymphoma, *pcSMPTCL* primary cutaneous small-medium pleomorphic T-cell lymphoma, *SPTCL* subcutaneous panniculitis-like T-cell lymphoma, *SS* Sézary syndrome

2.3 T-Cell Lymphomas

The most recent WHO/EORTC classification recognizes ten cutaneous T-cell lymphomas, three of which are considered provisional entities (see Table 2.1) [1, 2]. T-cell lymphomas account for 75 % of cutaneous lymphomas; the incidence of each lymphoma is listed in Table 2.1 (Table 2.1 and Fig. 2.4). Further discussion of the classification of T-cell lymphomas is found in Chap. 4, followed by a discussion of each lymphoma in Chaps. 5, 6, 7, 8, 9, 10, 11, 12, 13, and 14.

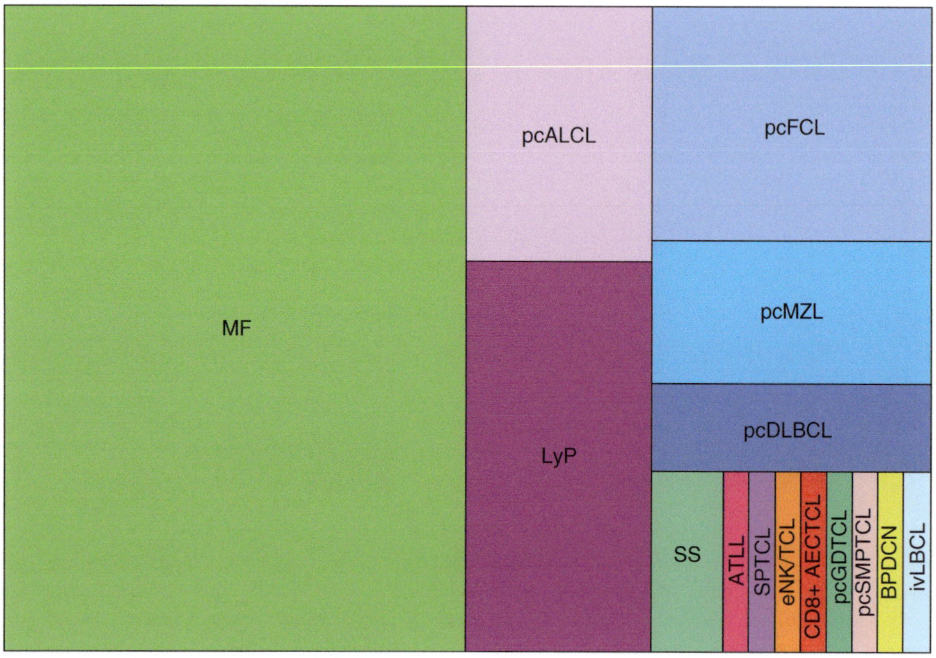

Fig. 2.4 Relative incidence of primary cutaneous lymphomas. This chart offers a visual representation of the relative frequencies of the cutaneous lymphomas in the WHO-EORTC classification scheme. The area of the chart dedicated to a given lymphoma is proportionate to its frequency. T-cell lymphomas account for 75 % of all cutaneous lymphomas. MF itself makes up 50 % of all cutaneous lymphomas. See Table 2.1 for frequencies of lymphomas. *ATLL* adult T-cell leukemia/lymphoma, *CD8+ AECTCL* CD8+ aggressive epidermotropic cutaneous T-cell lymphoma, *eNK/TCL* extranodal NK/T-cell lymphoma, *MF* mycosis fungoides, *pcALCL* primary cutaneous anaplastic large cell lymphoma, *pcGDTCL* primary cutaneous gamma/delta T-cell lymphoma, *pcSMPTCL* primary cutaneous small-medium pleomorphic T-cell lymphoma, *SPTCL* subcutaneous panniculitis-like T-cell lymphoma, *SS* Sézary syndrome

2.4 B-Cell Lymphomas

Four B-cell lymphomas are included in the WHO/EORTC classification scheme (see Table 2.1) [1, 2]. An introduction to B-cell lymphomas is included in Chap. 15. Lymphomas derived from B cells constitute 25 % of cutaneous lymphomas (see Table 2.1, Fig. 2.4). Each individual B-cell lymphoma will be addressed in Chaps. 16, 17, 18 and 19.

2.5 Precursor Neoplasms

A single precursor neoplasm is included in the WHO/EORTC classification: blastic plasmacytoid dendritic cell neoplasm [1, 2]. Although it accounts for a tiny fraction of cutaneous lymphomas (see Table 2.1 and Fig. 2.4), it has a dire prognosis, and accurate diagnosis of the neoplasm is of the utmost importance. This rare but deadly lymphoma is addressed in Chaps. 20 and 21.

References

1. Willemze R, Jaffe ES, Burg G, Cerroni L, Berti E, Swerdlow SH, et al. WHO-EORTC classification for cutaneous lymphomas. Blood. 2005;105:3768–85.
2. Swerdlow SH, Campo E, Harris NL, Jaffe ES, Pileri SA, Stein H, et al., editors. WHO classification of tumors of haematopoietic and lymphoid tissues. 4th ed. Lyon: International Agency for Research On Cancer; 2008.
3. Heath WR, Carbone FR. The skin-resident and migratory immune system in steady state and memory: innate lymphocytes, dendritic cells and T cells. Nat Immunol. 2013;14:978–85.
4. Nestle FO, Di Meglio P, Qin J-Z, Nickoloff BJ. Skin immune sentinels in health and disease. Nat Rev Immunol. 2009;9:679–91.
5. Clark RA. Skin-resident T cells: the ups and downs of on site immunity. J Invest Dermatol. 2010;130:362–70. Nature Publishing Group.

Immunohistochemistry and Molecular Techniques

3

Amrita Goyal, Kavita Goyal, Valentina Nardi, Mai P. Hoang, Joi B. Carter, and Lyn McDivitt Duncan

Immunohistochemistry (IHC), clonality analysis, and other molecular techniques are indispensable tools in the diagnosis of cutaneous lymphomas. Without the ability to identify cell surface and intracellular markers and to assess if a population is clonal, it would be impossible to accurately diagnose most lymphomas. This chapter offers a brief introduction to the use of immunohistochemistry and other molecular techniques in diagnosing cutaneous lymphomas.

3.1 Immunohistochemistry

Immunohistochemistry, the use of antibodies for specific detection of an epitope or antigen in a tissue, has its roots in the early 1940s, when Coons and associates used immunofluorescence to detect antigens in frozen tissue sections [1]. This was followed in the 1960s by the development of peroxidase-labeled antibodies by Mason and coworkers and by Nakane, which permitted the application of IHC to formalin-fixed paraffin-embedded tissue [2, 3]. In spite of its long history, IHC was not well accepted by the medical community until the 1990s [4, 5]. Since then, it has become a staple of diagnostic pathology.

IHC is critical in the diagnosis of morphologically ambiguous neoplasms, discriminating benign and malignant proliferations, subtyping of malignancies, characterizing the primary sites of metastatic tumors, and identifying prognostic and therapeutic indicators [6]. Thus, accurate diagnosis of many neoplasms would be impossible without IHC.

Although the practice and interpretation of IHC staining can be complex, the fundamental basis is straightforward. IHC uses two sets of antibodies: (1) a primary antibody that recognizes and binds to the epitope of interest, and (2) a secondary antibody that recognizes and binds to the Fc portion of the primary antibody, either conjugated to a linker molecule capable of recruiting reporter molecules or bound directly to a reporter molecule. The primary antibody binds to the protein of interest, while the secondary antibody facilitates visualization of the antigen-antibody complex formation by microscopy [7].

The primary antibodies used for IHC may be produced by injecting animals (typically a mouse, rat, or rabbit but occasionally a donkey, chicken, or cow) with the protein or peptide of interest. After the animal generates an immune response, antibodies are isolated from its blood. Polyclonal antibodies are a heterogeneous mixture of antibodies binding to various epitopes. Monoclonal antibodies are generated in vitro and represent a clonal production of a single antibody type that binds specifically to one epitope. Secondary antibodies are generated by injecting a second species with the Fc portion of the immunoglobulin from the first species; antibodies resulting from the immune response are isolated from the blood or ascites fluid. The secondary antibodies are then chemically conjugated to a linker or reporter.

A. Goyal, M.D.
Harvard-MIT Division of Health Sciences and Technology, Harvard Medical School, Boston, MA, USA

K. Goyal, B.S.
Drexel University College of Medicine, Philadelphia, PA, USA

V. Nardi, M.D.
Hematopathology Service, Department of Pathology, Massachusetts General Hospital, Harvard Medical School, Boston, MA, USA

J.B. Carter, M.D.
Department of Dermatology, Massachusetts General Hospital, Harvard Medical School, Boston, MA, USA

M.P. Hoang, M.D. • L.M. Duncan, M.D. (✉)
Dermatopathology Service, Department of Pathology, Massachusetts General Hospital, Harvard Medical School, Boston, MA, USA
e-mail: duncan@helix.mgh.harvard.edu

J.B. Carter et al. (eds.), *Atlas of Cutaneous Lymphomas: Classification and Differential Diagnosis*,
DOI 10.1007/978-3-319-17217-0_3

Immunohistochemical staining of tissue sections requires the permeabilization of the cells using protease, heat, microwave, or other antigen retrieval techniques. The tissue sections are then incubated with a solution containing primary antibody against the specific human target protein antigen. Once bound, the antigen-antibody complexes are detected using a labeled secondary antibody that recognizes the Fc component of the primary antibody. The label is then identified using one of many possible amplification techniques (most often via chromogenic or fluorescence methods) and ultimately visualized using microscopy. Pathologists analyze the pattern of staining to identify the tissue elements bearing the antigen of interest.

There are now thousands of antibodies available on the market for IHC. Several dozen of these are commonly used in IHC analysis of lymphoid and hematologic malignancies. A selection of key antibodies is presented in Table 3.1.

Table 3.1 Immunohistochemical markers frequently used in the analysis of cutaneous lymphoid proliferations

Marker	Cell type	Subcellular location	Function	Notably positive disorders	Notably negative disorders
CD1a	Langerhans cells, dermal dendritic cells, T cells [8]	Cell membrane	Transmembrane glycoprotein related to MHC that forms heterodimers with beta-2 microglobulin. Mediates lipid antigen presentation [8–10]	Langerhans cell histiocytosis[a]	Decreased in CBCL [8]
CD2[b]	T cells, NK cells [11]	Cell membrane	Also known as E rosette receptor. Mediates cell adhesion and signal transduction [11]	All CTCL	All CBCL
CD3[b]	T cells	Cell membrane	Binds TCR	Nearly all CTCL	All CBCL
CD4	Class II MHC-restricted T cells, monocytes, macrophages [12]	Cell membrane	Interacts with HLA class II and defines helper-inducer subset of T cells [13]	Most CTCL	eNK/TCL pcGDTCL SPTCL CD8+AECTCL All CBCL
CD5[b]	Most thymocytes and immature peripheral T cells [13]; IgM-producing B cells [12]	Cell membrane	Signal transduction molecule, binds to CD72 [12, 13]	Most CTCL CLL/SLL Mantle cell lymphoma Hairy cell leukemia	pcFCL pcDLBCL
CD7[b] *Note*: Most frequently lost T-subset marker that may be lost on any CTCL and reactive dermatoses [13]	All CD8+ T cells, most CD4+ T cells, most NK cells	Cell membrane	Member of the immunoglobulin family and plays important role in early lymphoid development [14]	Most CTCL AML [13]	Some MF Some Sézary syndrome Some ATLL All CBCL Rare reactive dermatoses
CD8	Class I MHC-restricted cytotoxic T cells [13]	Cell membrane	Transmembrane glycoprotein, binds MHC I and is a coreceptor for TCR [15]	pcGDTCL SPTCL CD8+AECTCL Rarely MF LyP type D Indolent CD8+ lymphoid proliferation of the ear	Most CTCL CBCL eNK/TCL
CD10	Immature and some mature B cells, lymphoid progenitors, granulocytes [13] Note: also known as CALLA	Cell membrane and cytoplasm	Zinc metallopeptidase in early lymphoid progenitors and normal germinal centers. With Bcl6 is a marker of germinal center origin [13]	pcFCL AITL[a]	Most pcMZL
CD15	Myeloid cells and eosinophils, activated B and T cells; variable staining on monocytes and basophils [16] Note: Also called Lewis X or LeuM1	Cell membrane	Carbohydrate (not a protein). Functions as adhesion molecule, mediates phagocytosis and chemotaxis [16]	pcALCL (40 % cases) [17] Nodal LyP [18] Reed-Sternberg cells [19]	LyP type A LyP type C
CD19	Earliest marker of B cell differentiation; present on most B cells except plasma cells [13]	Cell membrane *Note*: No antibody available for use with paraffin-embedded tissue [13]	Forms coreceptor complex with CD21 and CD81; signals from complex synergize with those from B-cell antigen receptor complex [12]	All CBCL	All CTCL

(continued)

Table 3.1 (continued)

Marker	Cell type	Subcellular location	Function	Notably positive disorders	Notably negative disorders
CD20	B cells from late-pre B-cell stage on; lost on plasma cells [13]	Cell membrane (cytoplasmic side)	Calcium ion channel involved in B cell activation and/or regulation [12]	All CBCL	All CTCL Plasma cells
CD21	Follicular dendritic cells [12]	Cell membrane	Regulator of complement activation; receptor for complement component C3d. Forms B-cell coreceptor complex with CD19 and CD81. EBV receptor [12]	pcMZL[c] pcFCL[c]	
CD23	Follicular dendritic cells, Activated B cells, monocytes, macrophages [12]	Cell membrane	c-Type lectin, weakly binds IgE and mediates cytokine release from monocytes, induced by IL-4 [12]	pcMZL[c] pcFCL[c]	
CD25	Activated T and B cells, regulatory T cells, activated macrophages [12]	Cell membrane	IL-2 receptor α chain; associates with IL-2Rβ (CD122) and IL-2Rγ (CD132) to form IL-2 receptor, which binds IL-2 [12]	ATLL Advanced stage MF	Early MF
CD26	Non-lineage antigen. Activated T, B, NK cells, macrophages, and some epithelial cells [20]	Cell membrane	Dipeptidyl peptidase-4 (DPP4). Has serine exopeptidase activity and functions in signal transduction [20, 21]	Few Sézary syndrome (circulating cells)	Most Sézary syndrome (circulating cells) ATLL
CD27	T cells	Cell membrane	Member of TNF-receptor superfamily; binds to CD70. Mediates activation of NF-kappaB and MAP pathways [22]. Causes apoptosis by binding to Siva [23]	Sézary syndrome	eNK/TCL
CD30	Activated T cells (likely T_H2 subset) [24]	Cell membranous or perinuclear dot-like [13]	Member of TNF-receptor superfamily. Mediates activation of NF-kappaB and MAP pathways. Marker/regulator of T_H2 T cells [24, 25]	ALCL LyP type A, C, D MF with LCT	LyP type B
CD34	Hematopoietic progenitors, vascular endothelium, embryonic fibroblasts	Cell membrane	Function unknown but potentially involved in leukocyte adhesion and homing	Myeloid leukemia[a]	CTCL CBCL Lymphocytic leukemia
CD45	All lymphoid cells CD45RB—all white cells CD45RA—B cells CD45RO—myeloid and T cells [13]	Cell membrane	Membrane protein tyrosine phosphatase. RA, RB, RC, and RO isoforms based on alternate mRNA splicing [13]	All CTCL All CBCL	
CD56	NK cells	Cell membrane	Also known as neural adhesion molecule	eNK/TCL BPDCN	Most CTCLs All CBCLs Hydroa vacciniforme-like lymphoma
CD57	NK cells, some T cells	Golgi apparatus membrane	Carbohydrate epitope containing a sulfoglucuronyl residue present in several adhesion molecules. Also known as human natural killer-1 (HNK-1) [26]	eNK/TCL	Most CTCLs All CBCLs BPDCN

CD68	Blood monocytes and tissue macrophages, including histiocytes and giant cells	Lysosomal and cell membranes	Glycoprotein, binds to low density lipoprotein (LDL) [27]	BPDCN (50 % of cases)	
CD79a	B cells	Cell membrane and/or cytoplasm	Associated with immunoglobulin molecule	All CBCL	All CTCL
CD117	Mast cells, some hematopoietic stem cells, melanocytes	Type III receptor tyrosine kinase	Also known as KIT	Myeloid leukemias[a]	
CD123	Plasmacytoid dendritic cells, some myeloid progenitor cells	Transmembrane receptor	Interleukin-3 (IL-3) receptor alpha chain	BPCDN	Most CTCLs, eNK/TCL All CBCL
CD138	Plasma cells, mature epithelial cells	Extracellular matrix receptor	Also known as syndecan-1; important in cell-cell adhesion and cell-matrix adhesion	Multiple myeloma Plasma cells in CBCL	
CD163	Exclusive to monocyte-macrophage lineage	Transmembrane glycoprotein	Endocytosis of hemoglobin-haptoglobin complexes	Langerhans cell histiocytosis	
ALK	Neurons during development, NOT in lymphocytes [28]	Cell membrane	Receptor tyrosine kinase in the insulin receptor superfamily t(2:5); translocations are often oncogenic [28]	Some sALCL	pcALCL LyP Some sALCL
Bcl2	Postgerminal center B cells	Cytoplasm	Antiapoptotic	pcDLBCL pcMZL	pcFCL
Bcl6	Germinal center B cells	Nuclear	Transcription regulation	pcFCL pcDLBCL (dim)	pcMZL
EBER[d]	EBV-infected cells	Nucleus	Most abundant RNAs in infected cells. Possible role in oncogenesis [29]	eNK/TCL HVLL Ulcerated methotrexate-associated LPD Lymphomatoid granulomatosis[d]	pcGDTCL
EMA	Neoplastic epithelial cells, some plasma cells	Cell membrane and cytoplasm	Glycoprotein isolated from milk-fat globule membranes	Some sALCL Some Hodgkin's lymphoma	cALCL Some ALCL
Granzyme B	Cytotoxic T cells and NK cells	Cytotoxic T cells and NK cells	Serine protease. Induces apoptosis of target cells via caspase cascade [30]	CD8+ AECTCL SPTCL pcGDTCL	Most CTCL All CBCL
IgG4	Plasma cells	Cell membrane	Immunoglobulin G4	pcMZL[31]	
IgM	Plasma cells	Cell membrane	Immunoglobulin M	DLBCL, leg type	pcFCL
Kappa light chain	B cells and plasma cells	Cell membrane and cytoplasm	Small subunit of immunoglobulin/antibody	Monotypic cytoplasmic in pcMZL	CTCL
Ki-67	All replicating cells	Nuclear	Nuclear protein involved cell proliferation [13]	pcDLBCL BPDCN (1/3 cases) Reactive germinal centers	
Lambda light chain	B cells and plasma cells	Cell membrane and cytoplasm	Small subunit of immunoglobulin/antibody	Monotypic cytoplasmic in pcMZL	CTCL

(continued)

Table 3.1 (continued)

Marker	Cell type	Subcellular location	Function	Notably positive disorders	Notably negative disorders
LMP-1	EBV-infected cells	Cell membrane	EBV latent membrane protein-1. Viral protein that regulates human gene expression [13]	eNK/TCL	pcGDTCL
Mum1/IRF4	Postgerminal B cells	Nucleus	Transcription factor, expressed in last step of germinal center B cells and postgerminal center B cells	pcDLBCL	pcFCL
Myeloperoxidase (MPO)	Neutrophils	Lysosomal azurophilic granules	Peroxidase enzyme	Myeloid leukemia[a]	BPDCN eNK/TCL
Pax5	Immature B cells	Transcription factor	Encodes B cell lineage-specific activator protein for lineage commitment and development	All CBCL	All CTCL
PD-1	Activated follicular helper T-cells	Cell membrane	Ig-related transmembrane protein involved in TCR signaling; inhibitory [32]	Some MF Most SS pcSMPTCL MF-like drug reaction AITL	Most MF
Perforin	Cytotoxic T cells and NK cells	Cytolytic granules	Permits transfer of cytolytic enzymes to target cells by creating transmembrane tubules [33]	CD8+ AECTCL SPTCL pcGDTCL	Most CTCL All CBCL
TCL-1	Precursor B and T cells, absent in mature lymphocytes [34]	Endoplasmic reticulum [35]	Coactivator of cell-survival kinase AKT [36, 37]	BPDCN	
TCR beta	Alpha/beta T cells	Cell membrane	Beta chain of TCR	Most CTCLs SPTCL	pcGDTCL
TCR gamma	Gamma/delta T cells	Cell membrane	Gamma chain of TCR	pcGDTCL	Most CTCLs SPTCL
TdT	Early T and B lymphoblasts	Nuclear	Also known as terminal deoxynucleotidyl transferase. DNA polymerase involved in Ig and TCR rearrangement [13]	BPDCN (some cases) Lymphoblastic leukemia/ lymphoma[a]	CTCL CBCL
TIA-1	Cytotoxic T cells and NK cells	Cytolytic granules	RNA-binding protein with nucleolytic activity; induces apoptosis of target cells [38, 39]	CD8+ AECTCL SPTCL pcGDTCL	Most CTCL All CBCL

Immunohistochemical staining listed is of the tumor cells themselves unless otherwise noted. Cell types noted are not comprehensive but are the most relevant

AITL angioimmunoblastic T-cell lymphoma, *ALK* anaplastic lymphoma receptor tyrosine kinase, *ALCL* anaplastic large cell lymphoma, *BPDCN* blastic plasmacytoid dendritic cell neoplasm, *CALLA* common acute lymphoblastic leukemia antigen, *CD8+ AECTCL* CD8+ aggressive epidermotropic T-cell lymphoma, *CD* cluster of differentiation, *CLA* cutaneous lymphocyte-associated antigen, *CLL/SLL* chronic lymphocytic leukemia/small lymphocytic leukemia, *CTCL* cutaneous T-cell lymphoma, *EBER* Epstein-Barr virus-encoded small RNAs, *EBV* Epstein-Barr virus, *EMA* epithelial membrane antigen, *eNK/TCL* extranodal NK/T-cell lymphoma, *HLA* human leukocyte antigen, *HVLL* Hydroa vacciniforme-like lymphoma, *Ig* immunoglobulin, *ivLBCL* intravascular large B-cell lymphoma, *LCT* large cell transformation, *LyP* lymphomatoid papulosis, *MF* mycosis fungoides, *MUM1/IRF4* multiple myeloma 1/interferon regulatory factor protein 4, *NK cell* natural killer cell, *Pax-5* paired box 5, *pcALCL* primary cutaneous anaplastic large cell lymphoma, *pcDLBCL* primary cutaneous diffuse large B-cell lymphoma, *pcFCL* primary cutaneous follicle center lymphoma, *pcGDTCL* primary cutaneous gamma/delta T-cell lymphoma, *pcMZL* primary cutaneous marginal zone lymphoma, *PD-1* programmed death-1, *sALCL* systemic anaplastic large cell lymphoma, *SPTCL* subcutaneous panniculitis-like T-cell lymphoma, *TCL1* T-cell leukemia/lymphoma 1, *TCR* T-cell receptor, *TdT* terminal deoxynucleotidyl transferase, *TIA-1* T-cell-restricted intracellular antigen 1

[a]Secondarily involves the skin

[b]Pan-T-cell antigen. Antigen loss possible in any of the T-cell lymphomas

[c]CD21 and CD23 stain follicular dendritic cells in a meshwork or network that invests the lymphocytes

[d]Performed via in situ hybridization

3.2 Clonality

To protect against the innumerable pathogens encountered by the body every day, the adaptive immune system requires a wide array of antigen receptors, particularly T-cell receptors (TCRs) and immunoglobulins (Igs). The generation of a diverse complement of TCRs and Ig molecules during lymphocyte development occurs via rearrangement of the antigen receptor genes. This process is facilitated by the presence of many variable (V), diverse (D), and joining (J) segments within the genome for each gene. Rearrangements of these segments yields an estimated 3×10^6 possible unique TCR molecules and 2×10^6 possible immunoglobulin genes [40].

Clonality studies depend on the fact that as a consequence of gene rearrangement, every T and B cell has a unique antigen receptor (TCR and Ig, respectively) on its surface, akin to a fingerprint. If a lymphoid cell undergoes malignant transformation and proliferation, all of its progeny will carry the same TCR or Ig. The antigen receptor gene rearrangement can thus be used as a specific marker for that clonal proliferation of cells. Therefore, an abundance of a particular Ig or TCR gene rearrangement in a lymphoid population suggests the presence of a clonal population. Likewise, the presence of the same antigen receptor gene rearrangement at two tissue sites suggests the presence of the same clonal population.

Historically, clonality analysis was based on Southern blot techniques. Today, polymerase chain reaction (PCR) amplification of segments within rearranged genes followed by capillary gel electrophoresis is the mainstay of gene rearrangement analysis. As a consequence of gene rearrangement during lymphocyte development, the lengths and sequence content of the amplified PCR products will differ between clones. The prevalence of single or multiple antigen receptor rearrangements allows differentiation among monoclonal, oligoclonal, and polyclonal cell populations. Gene rearrangement analysis for a monoclonal (also referred to as clonal) population will show a predominant or single fragment of a distinct size on capillary electrophoresis, a so-called "peak" (Fig. 3.1a). If a polyclonal population is sampled, the distribution of sizes of amplified DNA fragments from the gene segments and the resultant peaks on gel electrophoresis are expected to follow a normal (Gaussian) distribution (Fig. 3.1c, d, f). Finally, oligoclonal samples show a few dominant peaks representing the presence of a handful of different cells or cell populations with different antigen receptor gene rearrangement (Fig. 3.1e). As previously alluded to, the specific length of clonal PCR products can be used to assess whether samples from physically and/or temporally distinct sites show the same clonal antigen receptor rearrangement or "clone" (see Fig. 3.1b, c).

B-cell clonality is assessed by examining the gene rearrangement status of the Ig heavy chain (*IGH*) or less frequently the kappa light chain (*IGK*) and lambda light chain (*IGL*) genes. *IGH* rearrangement studies are performed via PCR amplification with fluorescently-labeled forward primers. Forward primers are directed to the conserved framework regions 1, 2, and 3 (FRI-V_H, FRII-V_H, and FRIII-V_H) and reverse primers to the joining region (*JH*) of the *IGH* gene [40].

Analysis of T-cell clonality is similar to that of B-cell clonality, although the interpretation of the results of capillary electrophoresis can be more challenging in the former. In T cells, clonality studies are based on PCR amplification of the TCR gamma (TCRγ) chain [41–43] or less often of the TCR beta (TCRβ) chain. The frequent use of TCRγ chain rearrangement analysis may seem paradoxical given that 95 % of T cells have an αβ TCR and only 5 % have a γδ TCR. The explanation for this lies in T-cell development. During lymphocyte development, the four TCR chains (δ, γ, β, and α) undergo rearrangement. The TCRδ and TCRγ genes rearrange first, and if successful, generate a γδ TCR. However, if either gene product is nonfunctional, TCRβ and TCRα rearrangement occurs, yielding an αβ TCR; in that case, TCRδ is deleted and TCRγ is silenced [12]. Although most mature T cells no longer express TCRγ, they still retain the uniquely rearranged TCRγ gene [42, 44]. TCRγ has a simpler structure than TCRα or TCRβ and requires fewer sets of PCR primers, thus making it an excellent subject for clonality studies [42, 45]. Primers used typically target the V segments (Vγ1-8, Vγ9, Vγ10, and Vγ11) and the J segments (Jγ1, Jγ2). The example presented in Fig. 3.1 is also applicable to TCR rearrangements. TCRγ rearrangement analysis has a sensitivity of approximately 85 %; false negatives may occur for many reasons, including that the primers cannot cover all possible TCRγ gene rearrangements or because the cells have not undergone TCRγ gene rearrangement.

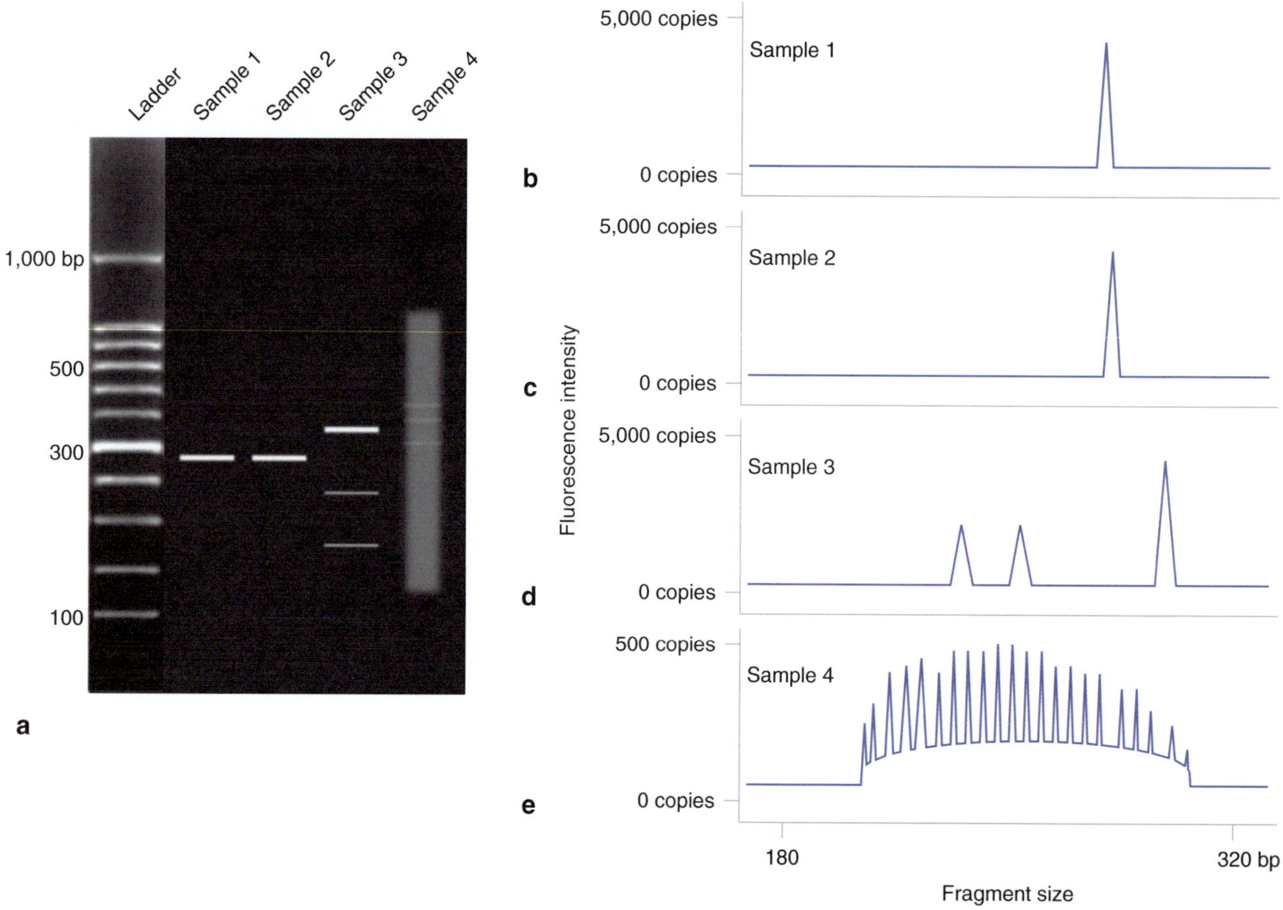

Fig. 3.1 PCR-based clonality analysis. To assess clonality, samples of DNA from the cells of interest undergo PCR amplification with primers targeted at the IgH or TCR gamma loci. (**a**) These PCR products are subject to gel electrophoresis, which separates segments of DNA on the basis of length, i.e., smaller DNA segments traveling faster than longer ones (and therefore lower on the gel). A control "ladder" is run along with the samples to allow measurement of the size of the fragments. Here, samples from 4 biopsies from a single patient are run, samples 1 through 4. Samples 1 and 2 both show a single prominent band of the same size. Sample 3 shows several bands, whereas sample 4 shows a smear and a handful of poorly defined bands. The electrophoresis results can then be visualized in parts (**b**) through (**e**) as peaks. (**b**) PCR results from sample 1 show a single peak, suggesting a clonal origin for this population of cells. (**c**) Likewise for sample 2; note that this demonstrates the same peak size as in sample 1, suggesting that these two samples coming from different lesions contain cells of the same clonal origin. (**d**) Unlike samples 1 and 2, sample 3 shows several dominant peaks corresponding to the multiple bands seen on the gel. This suggests an oligoclonal sample. (**e**) Finally, in sample 4, there is no single dominant peak but rather numerous small ones (note the low fluorescence intensity on the Y axis), corresponding with the smear seen on the gel that is consistent with a polyclonal population of cells

References

1. Coons AH, Creech HJ, Jones RN. Immunological properties of an antibody containing a fluorescent group. Exp Biol Med. 1941;47:200–2.
2. Mason TE, Phiefer RF, Spicer SS, Swallow RA, Dreskin RB. An immunoglobulin-enzyme bridge method for localizing tissue antigens. J Histochem Cytochem. 1969;17:563–9.
3. Nakane PK. Simultaneous localization of multiple tissue antigens using the peroxidase-labelled antibody method: a study on pituitary glands of the rat. J Histochem Cytochem. 1968;16:557–60.
4. Leong AS. Diagnostic immunohistochemistry–problems and solutions. Pathology. 1992;24:1–4.
5. Taylor CR. An exaltation of experts: concerted efforts in the standardization of immunohistochemistry. Hum Pathol. 1994;25:2–11.
6. de Matos LL, Trufelli DC, de Matos MGL, da Silva Pinhal MA. Immunohistochemistry as an important tool in biomarker detection and clinical practice. Biomark Insights. 2010;5:9–20.
7. Murphy KM, Travers P, Walport M. Janeway's immunobiology. 7th ed. New York: Garland Science; 2007.
8. Pigozzi B. Expression of the CD1a molecule in B-and T-lymphoproliferative skin conditions. Oncol Rep. 2006;15:347–51.
9. Martin LH, Calabi F, Milstein C. Isolation of CD1 genes: a family of major histocompatibility complex-related differentiation antigens. Proc Natl Acad Sci U S A. 1986;83:9154–8.
10. Schiefner A, Wilson IA. Presentation of lipid antigens by CD1 glycoproteins. Curr Pharm Des. 2009;15:3311–7.
11. Yang J, Ye Y, Carroll A, Yang W, Lee H. Structural biology of the cell adhesion protein CD2: alternatively folded states and structure-function relation. Curr Protein Pept Sci. 2001;2:1–17.

12. Abbas AK, Lichtman AH, Pillai S. Cellular and molecular immunology. 7th ed. Philadelphia: Saunders Elsevier; 2007.
13. Gocke CD. Immunology of non-Hodgkin lymphoma. In: Dabbs D, editor. Diagnostic immunohistochemistry. 2nd ed. Philadelphia: Churchill Livingstone Elsevier; 2006. p. 137–61.
14. Aandahl EM, Sandberg JK, Beckerman KP, Taskén K, Moretto WJ, Nixon DF. CD7 is a differentiation marker that identifies multiple CD8 T cell effector subsets. J Immunol. 2003;170:2349–55.
15. Gao GF, Jakobsen BK. Molecular interactions of coreceptor CD8 and MHC class I: the molecular basis for functional coordination with the T-cell receptor. Immunol Today. 2000;21:630–6.
16. Nakayama F, Nishihara S, Iwasaki H, Kudo T, Okubo R, Kaneko M, et al. CD15 expression in mature granulocytes is determined by alpha 1,3-fucosyltransferase IX but in promyelocytes and monocytes by alpha 1,3-fucosyltransferase IV. J Biol Chem. 2001;276:16100–6.
17. Benner MF, Jansen PM, Meijer CJLM, Willemze R. Diagnostic and prognostic evaluation of phenotypic markers TRAF1, MUM1, BCL2 and CD15 in cutaneous CD30-positive lymphoproliferative disorders. Br J Dermatol. 2009;161:121–7.
18. Eberle FC, Song JY, Xi L, Raffeld M, Harris NL, Wilson WH, et al. Nodal involvement by cutaneous CD30-positive T-cell lymphoma mimicking classical Hodgkin lymphoma. Am J Surg Pathol. 2012;36:716–25.
19. Crocker J, Skilbeck N, Brown G, Bunce C. Presence of 3-fucosyl-N-acetyllactosamine shown by monoclonal antibody AGF 4.48 in Reed-Sternberg cells. J Clin Pathol. 1986;39:564–8.
20. Boonacker EP, Wierenga EA, Smits HH, Van Noorden CJF. CD26/DPPIV signal transduction function, but not proteolytic activity, is directly related to its expression level on human Th1 and Th2 cell lines as detected with living cell cytochemistry. J Histochem Cytochem. 2002;50:1169–77.
21. Chen X. Biochemical properties of recombinant prolyl dipeptidases DPP-IV and DPP8. Adv Exp Med Biol. 2006;575:27–32.
22. Yamamoto H, Kishimoto T, Minamoto S. NF-kappaB activation in CD27 signaling: involvement of TNF receptor-associated factors in its signaling and identification of functional region of CD27. J Immunol. 1998;161:4753–9.
23. Prasad KV, Ao Z, Yoon Y, Wu MX, Rizk M, Jacquot S, et al. CD27, a member of the tumor necrosis factor receptor family, induces apoptosis and binds to Siva, a proapoptotic protein. Proc Natl Acad Sci U S A. 1997;94:6346–51.
24. Tarkowski M. Expression and a role of CD30 in regulation of T-cell activity. Curr Opin Hematol. 2003;10:267–71.
25. Schneider C, Hübinger G. Pleiotropic signal transduction mediated by human CD30: a member of the tumor necrosis factor receptor (TNFR) family. Leuk Lymphoma. 2002;43:1355–66.
26. Mitsumoto Y, Oka S, Sakuma H, Inazawa J, Kawasaki T. Cloning and chromosomal mapping of human glucuronyltransferase involved in biosynthesis of the HNK-1 carbohydrate epitope. Genomics. 2000;65:166–73.
27. Holness CL, Simmons DL. Molecular cloning of CD68, a human macrophage marker related to lysosomal glycoproteins. Blood. 1993;81:1607–13.
28. Chiarle R, Voena C, Ambrogio C, Piva R, Inghirami G. The anaplastic lymphoma kinase in the pathogenesis of cancer. Nat Rev Cancer. 2008;8:11–23.
29. Takada K, Nanbo A. The role of EBERs in oncogenesis. Semin Cancer Biol. 2001;11:461–7.
30. Lord SJ, Rajotte RV, Korbutt GS, Bleackley RC. Granzyme B: a natural born killer. Immunol Rev. 2003;193:31–8.
31. Brenner I, Roth S, Puppe B, Wobser M, Rosenwald A, Geissinger E. Primary cutaneous marginal zone lymphomas with plasmacytic differentiation show frequent IgG4 expression. Mod Pathol. 2013;26:1568–76.
32. Riella LV, Paterson AM, Sharpe AH, Chandraker A. Role of the PD-1 pathway in the immune response. Am J Transplant. 2012;12:2575–87.
33. Thiery J, Keefe D, Boulant S, Boucrot E, Walch M, Martinvalet D, et al. Perforin pores in the endosomal membrane trigger the release of endocytosed granzyme B into the cytosol of target cells. Nat Immunol. 2011;12:770–7.
34. Weng J, Rawal S, Chu F, Park HJ, Sharma R, Delgado DA, et al. TCL1: a shared tumor-associated antigen for immunotherapy against B-cell lymphomas. Blood. 2012;120:1613–23.
35. Fu TB, Virgilio L, Narducci MG, Facchiano A, Russo G, Croce CM. Characterization and localization of the TCL-1 oncogene product. Cancer Res. 1994;54:6297–301.
36. Laine J, Künstle G, Obata T, Sha M, Noguchi M. The protooncogene TCL1 is an Akt kinase coactivator. Mol Cell. 2000;6:395–407.
37. Noguchi M, Ropars V, Roumestand C, Suizu F. Proto-oncogene TCL1: more than just a coactivator for Akt. FASEB J. 2007;21:2273–84.
38. Förch P, Puig O, Kedersha N, Martínez C, Granneman S, Séraphin B, et al. The apoptosis-promoting factor TIA-1 is a regulator of alternative pre-mRNA splicing. Mol Cell. 2000;6:1089–98.
39. Förch P, Valcárcel J. Molecular mechanisms of gene expression regulation by the apoptosis-promoting protein TIA-1. Apoptosis. 2001;6:463–8.
40. Van Dongen JJM, Langerak AW, Brüggemann M, Evans PAS, Hummel M, Lavender FL, et al. Design and standardization of PCR primers and protocols for detection of clonal immunoglobulin and T-cell receptor gene recombinations in suspect lymphoproliferations: report of the BIOMED-2 Concerted Action BMH4-CT98-3936. Leukemia. 2003;17:2257–317.
41. Wood GS, Tung RM, Heaffner AC, Crooks CF, Liao S, Orozco R, et al. Detection of clonal T-cell receptor gamma gene rearrangements in early mycosis fungoides/Sezary syndrome by polymerase chain reaction and denaturing gradient gel electrophoresis (PCR/DGGE). J Invest Dermatol. 1994;103:34–41.
42. Wood GS. T-cell receptor and immunoglobulin gene rearrangements in diagnosing skin disease. Arch Dermatol. 2001;137:1503–6.
43. Dippel E, Assaf C, Hummel M, Schrag HJ, Stein H, Goerdt S, et al. Clonal T-cell receptor gamma-chain gene rearrangement by PCR-based GeneScan analysis in advanced cutaneous T-cell lymphoma: a critical evaluation. J Pathol. 1999;188:146–54.
44. Theodorou I, Raphaël M, Bigorgne C, Fourcade C, Lahet C, Cochet G, et al. Recombination pattern of the TCR gamma locus in human peripheral T-cell lymphomas. J Pathol. 1994;174:233–42.
45. Zhu D, Kadin ME, Samoszuk M. Detection of clonal T-cell receptor-gamma gene rearrangement by PCR/temporal temperature gradient gel electrophoresis. Am J Clin Pathol. 2001;116:527–34.

4 Introduction to the T-Cell Lymphomas

Amrita Goyal, Joi B. Carter, and Lyn McDivitt Duncan

The human skin contains a vast array of T cells, including cytotoxic, helper, memory, and regulatory subsets. Each of these cell types has different functional, proliferative, and migratory capacities. The diversity of cutaneous T-cell lymphomas (CTCL) reflects the multiplicity of T-cell subsets [1, 2]. The WHO/EORTC classification recognizes 15 cutaneous lymphomas, 10 of which are T-cell lymphomas. Their incidence and various organizational schemas for understanding CTCL are offered in this chapter. Each of the lymphomas is addressed individually in subsequent chapters.

4.1 Classification and Incidence of Cutaneous T-Cell Lymphomas

Cutaneous T-cell lymphomas (CTCL) constitute 75 % of all cutaneous lymphomas [3]. The term "cutaneous T-cell lymphoma" is a general one, encompassing 10 formally recognized entities (Table 4.1, Fig. 4.1) and innumerable others yet to be identified and classified. Note that three of these are currently considered provisional entities (see Table 4.1).

Table 4.1 CTCL incidence

Lymphoma	Frequency (among TCLs)
Cutaneous T-cell lymphomas	%
Mycosis fungoides (MF)	65
Sézary syndrome (SS)	4
Adult T-cell leukemia/lymphoma (ATLL)	<1
Subcutaneous panniculitis–like T-cell lymphoma (SPTCL)	1
Extranodal NK/T-cell lymphoma (eNK/TCL)	<1
CD30+ lymphoproliferative disorders (CD30+ LPD)	
Primary cutaneous anaplastic large cell lymphoma (pcALCL)	10
Lymphomatoid papulosis (LyP)	16
Provisional entities	
CD8+ aggressive epidermotropic T-cell lymphoma (CD8+ AECTCL)	<1
Primary cutaneous gamma-delta T-cell lymphoma (pcGDTCL)	<1
Primary cutaneous small-medium pleomorphic T-cell lymphoma (pcSMPTCL)	<1

Data from Willemze et al. [3]

Mycosis fungoides is by far the most common CTCL, followed by the primary cutaneous CD30+ lymphoproliferative disorders, lymphomatoid papulosis (LyP), and primary cutaneous anaplastic large cell lymphoma (pcALCL)

A. Goyal, M.D.
Harvard-MIT Division of Health Sciences and Technology, Harvard Medical School, Boston, MA, USA

J.B. Carter, M.D.
Department of Dermatology, Massachusetts General Hospital, Harvard Medical School, Boston, MA, USA

L.M. Duncan, M.D. (✉)
Dermatopathology Service, Department of Pathology, Massachusetts General Hospital, Harvard Medical School, Boston, MA, USA
e-mail: duncan@helix.mgh.harvard.edu

J.B. Carter et al. (eds.), *Atlas of Cutaneous Lymphomas: Classification and Differential Diagnosis*, DOI 10.1007/978-3-319-17217-0_4

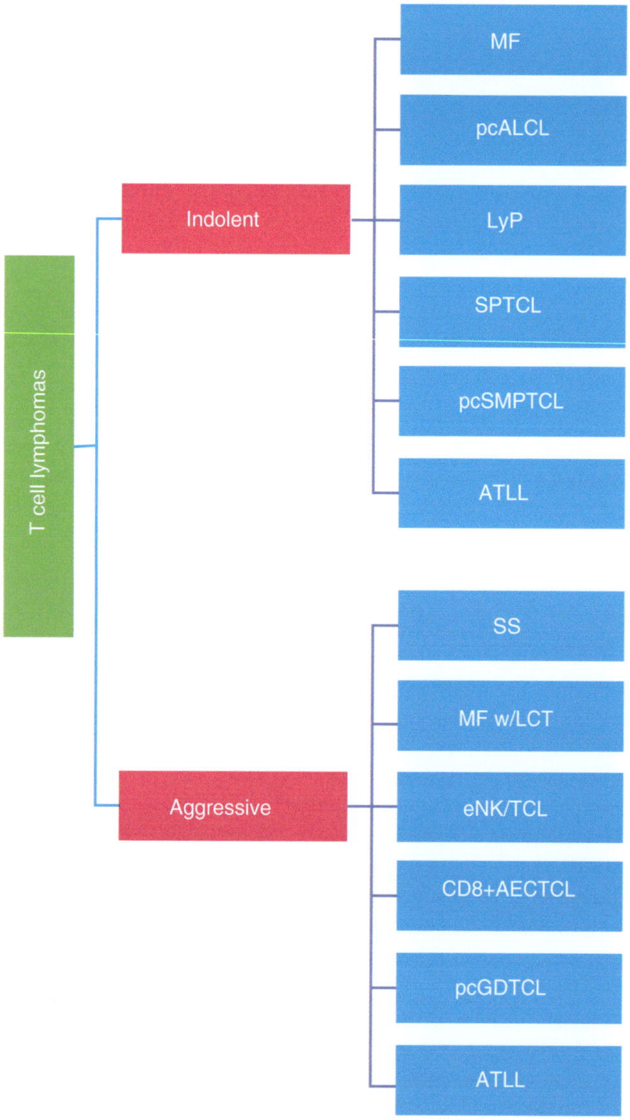

Fig. 4.1 T-cell lymphomas by prognosis. Although the prognoses of the T-cell lymphomas range widely, they can be divided into two general categories: indolent and aggressive. For more information, see Table 4.3. *ATLL* adult T-cell leukemia/lymphoma, *CD8+ AECTCL* CD8+ aggressive epidermotropic cutaneous T-cell lymphoma, *eNK/TCL* extranodal NK/T-cell lymphoma, *MF* mycosis fungoides, *pcALCL* primary cutaneous anaplastic large cell lymphoma, *pcGDTCL* primary cutaneous gamma/delta T-cell lymphoma, *pcSMPTCL* primary cutaneous small-medium pleomorphic T-cell lymphoma, *SPTCL* subcutaneous panniculitis–like T-cell lymphoma, *SS* Sézary syndrome

4.2 Clinical Presentation and Prognosis of Cutaneous T-Cell Lymphomas

The clinical presentation of CTCL varies widely, ranging from the patches and plaques of mycosis fungoides (MF), to the recurrent crops of papules of lymphomatoid papulosis (LyP), to the ulceronecrotic nodules of extranodal NK/T-cell lymphoma (eNK/TCL). These diseases have a range of prognoses, from the indolent MF to the extremely aggressive Sézary syndrome. These clinical characteristics are summarized in Table 4.2 and described in detail in subsequent chapters. Figure 4.1 offers a categorization of CTCLs by prognosis.

Table 4.2 Clinical presentation and prognosis of CTCLs

Lymphoma	Gender	Age (years)	Clinical presentation	Prognosis	5-year survival	Median survival
MF	M>F, 2:1	50s	Patch—plaque—tumor progression in bathing-suit distribution	Excellent	Varies by subtype, 75–98 %	Varies by stage (1–35.5 years)
SS	M>F, 2:1	60s	Diffuse erythroderma	Poor	10–33 %	3 years
ATLL	F=M	50s	Erythematous papules, nodules ± ulceration	Poor	Acute: <5 % Chronic: 30 % Smoldering: 60 %	12 months
SPTCL	F>M, 2:1	30s	Single/multiple violaceous subcutaneous nodules/plaques	Excellent	85–90 %	NA
eNK/TCL	M>F, 2–3:1	40s	Ulcerated nodules	Poor	30–50 %	6–30 months
pcALCL	F>M, 2:1	60s	Solitary or localized nodule/tumor	Excellent	90 %	NA
LyP	M>F, 3:1	40s	Crops of recurrent, self-resolving papules and nodules	Excellent	100 %	NA
CD8+ AECTCL	M>F	Adults	Disseminated eruptive papule, nodules, tumors with ulceration and necrosis; especially found on palms, soles, and mucosa	Poor	18 %	23–32 months
pcGDTCL	M=F	40s	Variable: patches/plaques, subcutaneous tumors, epidermal necrosis/ulceration	Poor	NA	15 months
pcSMPTCL	M=F	50s	Solitary erythematous nodule	Excellent	>90 %	NA

ATLL adult T-cell leukemia/lymphoma, *CD8+ AECTCL* CD8+ aggressive epidermotropic cutaneous T-cell lymphoma, *eNK/TCL* extranodal NK/T-cell lymphoma, *MF* mycosis fungoides, *NA* not available, *pcALCL* primary cutaneous anaplastic large cell lymphoma, *pcGDTCL* primary cutaneous gamma/delta T-cell lymphoma, *pcSMPTCL* primary cutaneous small-medium pleomorphic T-cell lymphoma, *SS* Sézary syndrome

4.3 Algorithms for Understanding Cutaneous T-Cell Lymphomas

The diagnosis of CTCL is based upon clinical and laboratory findings. When faced with a new possible case of CTCL, the laboratory work-up is approached by assessing the histopathologic findings and immunophenotype of the infiltrating cells. Suggested schema for organizing the cutaneous lymphomas histopathologically and immunohistochemically are presented in Figs. 4.2 and 4.3, respectively. As in all of medicine, clinical-pathologic correlation is required to reach an accurate diagnosis.

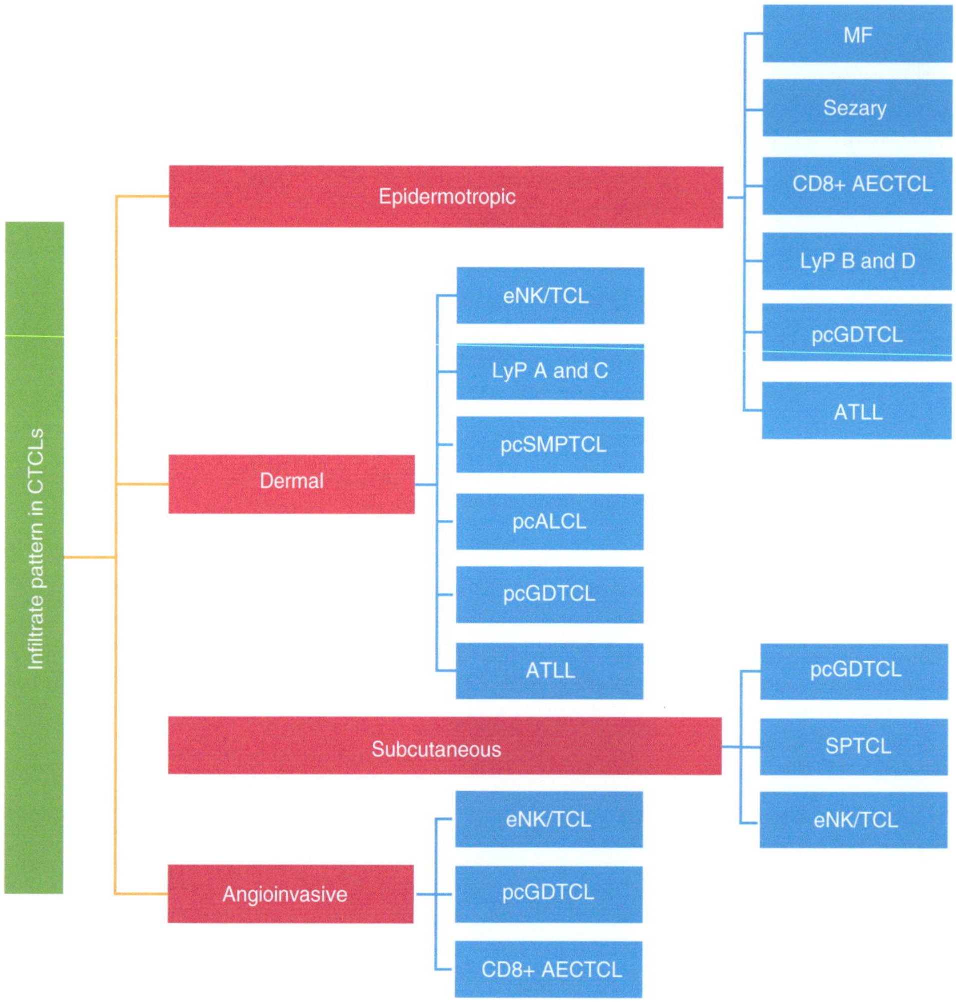

Fig. 4.2 Histopathologic pattern in CTCL. Cutaneous lymphoma can present with multiple histologic patterns, varying from patient to patient or even within the same biopsy sample. For example, eNK/TCL can manifest with epidermotropism, dermal involvement, infiltration of the subcutaneous infiltrate, and angioinvasion. Histopathology must be combined with immunohistochemistry and clinical correlation in the diagnosis. *ATLL* adult T-cell leukemia/lymphoma, *CD8+ AECTCL* CD8+ aggressive epidermotropic cutaneous T-cell lymphoma, *eNK/TCL* extranodal NK/T-cell lymphoma, *LyP* Lymphomatoid papulosis, *MF* mycosis fungoides, *pcALCL* primary cutaneous anaplastic large cell lymphoma, *pcGDTCL* primary cutaneous gamma/delta T-cell lymphoma, *pcSMPTCL* primary cutaneous small-medium pleomorphic T-cell lymphoma, *SPTCL* subcutaneous panniculitis–like T-cell lymphoma

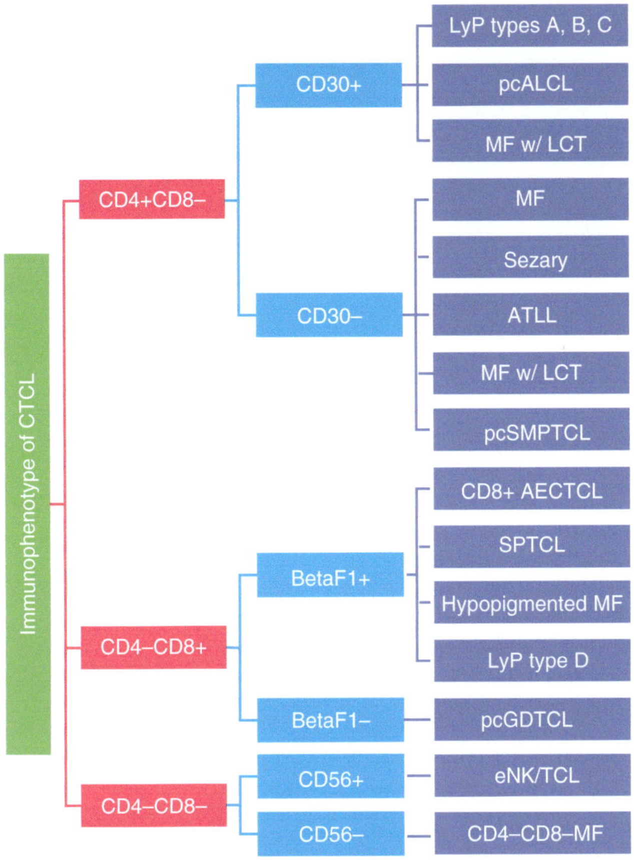

Fig. 4.3 CTCLs by immunohistochemistry. Immunohistochemistry is required for accurate diagnosis of all cutaneous lymphomas. Of note, eNK/TCL can have an NK or T-cell phenotype; hence NK cells are included here with the other CTCLs. *ATLL* adult T-cell leukemia/lymphoma, *CD8+ AECTCL* CD8+ aggressive epidermotropic cutaneous T-cell lymphoma, *eNK/TCL* extranodal NK/T-cell lymphoma, *LyP* Lymphomatoid papulosis, *MF* mycosis fungoides, *pcALCL* primary cutaneous anaplastic large cell lymphoma, *pcGDTCL* primary cutaneous gamma/delta T-cell lymphoma, *pcSMPTCL* primary cutaneous small-medium pleomorphic T-cell lymphoma, *SPTCL* subcutaneous panniculitis–like T-cell lymphoma

4.3.1 Histopathology

By definition, all cutaneous lymphomas are composed of lymphocytic infiltrates involving some component of the skin. The overarching pattern of infiltration can be divided into four major categories: epidermotropic, dermal, subcutaneous, and/or angioinvasive, based on the location of the infiltrate (see Fig. 4.2). Some lymphomas may demonstrate one or more of these patterns, but this can serve as a reasonable diagnostic starting point.

The histologic findings often correlate with the clinical manifestations. Erythematous patches of MF and adult T-cell leukemia/lymphoma (ATLL) correlate with an epidermotropic infiltrate. Subcutaneous panniculitis–like T-cell lymphoma (SPTCL) on the other hand primarily impacts the subcutis and clinically presents with subcutaneous nodules. Highly angiodestructive and invasive lymphomas, like eNK/TCL often demonstrate cutaneous ulceration and necrosis.

4.3.2 Immunohistochemistry

The vast array of CTCL reflects the varied roles that T cells play in the biology of the skin. At this time the relationships between the cutaneous lymphomas and their normal counterparts are poorly understood, and much work remains to be done in this field. Each lymphoma and its purported normal counterparts and important immunohistochemical characteristics are listed in Table 4.3.

Immunohistochemistry is an invaluable tool in our diagnostic arsenal; it would in fact be impossible to diagnose cutaneous lymphomas accurately without detection of numerous immunologic markers (Fig. 4.3). See Chap. 3 for more detailed information on the specific antigens listed.

Table 4.3 Immunohistochemical phenotypes and molecular findings

	Cell of origin	Normal counterpart	CD3	CD4	CD8	CD30	CD56	CD2/CD5/CD7Pan T-cell markers	Cytotoxic markers	Clonal TCR rearrangement	Other
MF	T cell	Mature skin-homing CD4+ T-cell, TH1	+	+	– (rare +)	– (often + with LCT)	–	CD2±, CD5±, CD7± (loss w/progression)	–	+	CD25–
Sézary syndrome	T cell	Mature epidermotropic skin homing CD4+ T cells, TH2	+	+	–	–	–	CD2+, CD5+ CD7–	–	+	CD26– CD27+
ATLL	T cell	Peripheral CD4+ T cell	+	+	–	– (rare +)	–	CD2+, CD5+ CD7–	–	+	FoxP3 ± HTLV-1+ CD25+
SPTCL	Cytotoxic T cell	Mature cytotoxic α/β T cell	+	–	+	±	–	CD2+, CD5±, CD7±	+	+	Beta F1+
eNK/TCL	NK or cytotoxic T cell	Activated NK cell or cytotoxic T cell	cCD3+ sCD3–	–	–	– (rare +)	+	CD2+, CD5+ CD7±	+	–	EBV+
pcALCL	T cell	Transformed/activated skin-homing T cell	+	+	–	+	–	CD2±, CD5±	–	+	ALK–
LyP type A, C	T cell	Activated skin-homing T cell	+	+	–	+	–	CD2±, CD5±	–	+	ALK– CD15–
LyP type B	T cell	Activated skin-homing T cell	+	+	–	–	–	CD2±, CD5±	–	+	ALK–
LyP type D	T cell	Activated skin-homing T cell	+	–	+	+	–	CD2±, CD5±	+	+	ALK– BetaF1+
CD8+ AECTCL	Cytotoxic T cell	Skin-homing CD8+ cytotoxic α/β T cell	+	–	+	–	–	CD2±, CD5, CD7±	+	+	BetaF1+
pcGDTCL	Cytotoxic T cell	Mature, activated cytotoxic γ/δ T cell	+	–	±	±	+	CD2+ CD5– CD7±	+	+	BetaF1– TCRgamma+ (may not be detectable)
pcSMPTCL	T cell	Skin-homing CD4+ T cell	+	+	–	–	–	± pan-T-cell markers	–	+	

Immunohistochemistry is necessary for accurately identifying cutaneous lymphomas. Some key immunohistochemical characteristics are listed here for comparison. Although most cases fall into these patterns, there is tremendous variation in immunophenotype even in established diagnostic categories

ALK anaplastic lymphoma kinase, *ATLL* adult T-cell leukemia/lymphoma, *cCD3* cytoplasmic CD3, *sCD3* surface CD3, *CD8+ AECTCL* CD8+ aggressive epidermotropic cutaneous T-cell lymphoma, *EBV* Epstein-Barr virus, *eNK/TCL* extranodal NK/T-cell lymphoma, *HTLV* human T-cell leukemia virus, *LCT* large cell transformation, *LyP* Lymphomatoid papulosis, *MF* mycosis fungoides, *pcALCL* primary cutaneous anaplastic large cell lymphoma, *pcGDTCL* primary cutaneous gamma/delta T-cell lymphoma, *pcSMPTCL* primary cutaneous small-medium pleomorphic T-cell lymphoma, *SPTCL* subcutaneous panniculitis-like T-cell lymphoma, *TCR* T-cell receptor

References

1. Clark R. Regulation gone wrong: a subset of Sézary patients have malignant regulatory T cells. J Invest Dermatol. 2009;129: 2747–50.
2. Clark R. Skin-resident T, cells: the ups and downs of on site immunity. J Invest Dermatol. 2010;130:362–70.
3. Willemze R, Jaffe ES, Burg G, Cerroni L, Berti E, Swerdlow SH, et al. WHO-EORTC classification for cutaneous lymphomas. Blood. 2005;105:3768–85.

5 Mycosis Fungoides

Amrita Goyal, Kavita Goyal, Joi B. Carter, Jeffrey A. Barnes, Rosalynn M. Nazarian, Mai P. Hoang, Adriano Piris, Thomas Kupper, and Lyn McDivitt Duncan

Mycosis fungoides (MF) is a CD4+ primary cutaneous T-cell lymphoma with a good prognosis. Patients with MF classicly present with pink-to-erythematous patches, well-demarcated plaques, and/or tumors on sun-protected areas, including the flanks, breasts, inner thighs, groin, and buttocks. Cutaneous biopsies of classic MF demonstrate characteristic epidermotropism, "tagging" of atypical T cells along the dermoepidermal junction, and Pautrier microabscesses. There are a number of subtypes of MF with varied presentations, including folliculotropic MF, pagetoid reticulosis, granulomatous slack skin, poikilodermatous MF, and hypopigmented MF. This chapter will discuss the clinical presentation, prognosis, treatment, histopathology, immunohistochemistry, and molecular biology of several of the subtypes of MF. It closes with five clinical cases, each representing a different subtype of MF.

5.1 Clinical

5.1.1 Clinical Presentation

Mycosis fungoides (MF) is a rare, indolent, CD4+ T-cell lymphoma [1]. In the United States, MF is the most common of the cutaneous lymphomas, comprising 54–65% of all cutaneous T-cell lymphomas (CTCLs) and 40–50% of cutaneous lymphomas overall [2–3]. It is critical to note that the terms MF and CTCL are *not* synonymous, even though they are often used as such. MF is a *subtype* of CTCL, and although MF is the most common CTCL, there are at least 10 other types.

Patients with MF have a median age of 57 [1], but pediatric cases have been reported [4]. There is a trend of increasing risk of disease progression with increasing age [5]. Men are affected twice as often as women [1, 5]. Rates

A. Goyal, M.D.
Harvard-MIT Division of Health Sciences and Technology, Harvard Medical School, Boston, MA, USA

K. Goyal, B.S.
Drexel University College of Medicine, Philadelphia, PA, USA

J.B. Carter, M.D.
Department of Dermatology, Massachusetts General Hospital, Harvard Medical School, Boston, MA, USA

J.A. Barnes, M.D., Ph.D.
Comprehensive Cutaneous Lymphoma Program, Massachusetts General Hospital Cancer Center, Boston, MA, USA

R.M. Nazarian, M.D.
Dermatopathology Unit, Pathology Service, Massachusetts General Hospital, Harvard Medical School, Boston, MA, USA

M.P. Hoang, M.D.
Dermatopathology Service, Department of Pathology, Massachusetts General Hospital, Harvard Medical School, Boston, MA, USA

A. Piris, M.D.
Department of Dermatology, Brigham and Women's Hospital, Harvard Medical School, Boston, MA, USA

T. Kupper, M.D.
Department of Dermatology, Brigham and Women's Hospital, Harvard Medical School, Boston, MA, USA

L.M. Duncan, M.D. (✉)
Dermatopathology Service, Department of Pathology, Massachusetts General Hospital, Harvard Medical School, Boston, MA, USA
e-mail: duncan@helix.mgh.harvard.edu

J.B. Carter et al. (eds.), *Atlas of Cutaneous Lymphomas: Classification and Differential Diagnosis*, DOI 10.1007/978-3-319-17217-0_5

of CTCL in general (including MF) are highest in African Americans, followed by non-Hispanic Caucasians, and last by Asians and Hispanics, at ten cases, eight cases, five cases, and five cases per million person years per ethnic group, respectively [2].

MF classicly progresses through patch, plaque, and tumor stages, although patients may manifest multiple stages at any given time. Patients with patch stage MF typically present with a history of years of having salmon-colored, slightly scaling patches long misdiagnosed as psoriasis or eczema (Figs. 5.1 and 5.2) [6]. Over the course of years, the lesions may evolve into the indurated, irregularly shaped plaques of plaque stage MF (Fig. 5.2c, d). These are distributed asymmetrically in a bathing suit or photo-protected distribution, including the breasts, inner arms, flanks, buttocks, and upper thighs [1, 6, 7]. Colors of the lesions can vary from reddish-brown to violaceous to orange [6]. There may be accompanying epidermal atrophy resulting in "cigarette paper" wrinkling (Fig. 5.2a). Other lesions may be poikilodermatous with a delicate reticulate pattern of erythema, hyperpigmentation, hypopigmentation, and telangiectasias (Fig. 5.2f) [6]. The final step in progression is the tumor stage, in which nodules or tumors of neoplastic cells are present. Ulceration may or may not be present (Fig. 5.3) [6–8].

Although rare, it is possible for MF to undergo large-cell transformation (LCT) (Fig. 5.4); transformed MF impacts 4.7 % of MF patients and follows a very aggressive clinical course [1, 9]. Visceral or lymph node involvement can occur late in the disease. Patients can also develop erythroderma reminiscent of Sézary syndrome but lack the blood involvement that defines Sézary syndrome [1]. Of note, lymphadenopathy may occur secondary to either dermatopathic change or nodal involvement of the lymphoma [1, 10, 11].

In the past some considered large-plaque and small-plaque parapsoriasis to be part of the MF family. These terms have largely fallen out of favor. Large-plaque parapsoriasis, increasingly considered patch-stage MF, has lesions greater than 6 cm and typically presents in the same bathing suit distribution as MF. Poikiloderma and atrophy are often present. The entity previously termed large-plaque parapsoriasis evolves into MF in 7.5–14 % of patients, and the majority of clinicians are moving toward terming this entity patch stage MF or in nondiagnostic cases an evolving T-cell dyscrasia [7].

The lesions of small-plaque parapsoriasis (also called digitate dermatosis) are 2–6 cm long with 10–20 digitate or fingerlike extensions and typically occur on the trunk. These lesions lack poikilodermatous changes or atrophy, and biopsies show nonspecific inflammatory changes. Small-plaque parapsoriasis has little to no potential to evolve into MF, and it is no longer considered part of the MF spectrum by many clinicians [7].

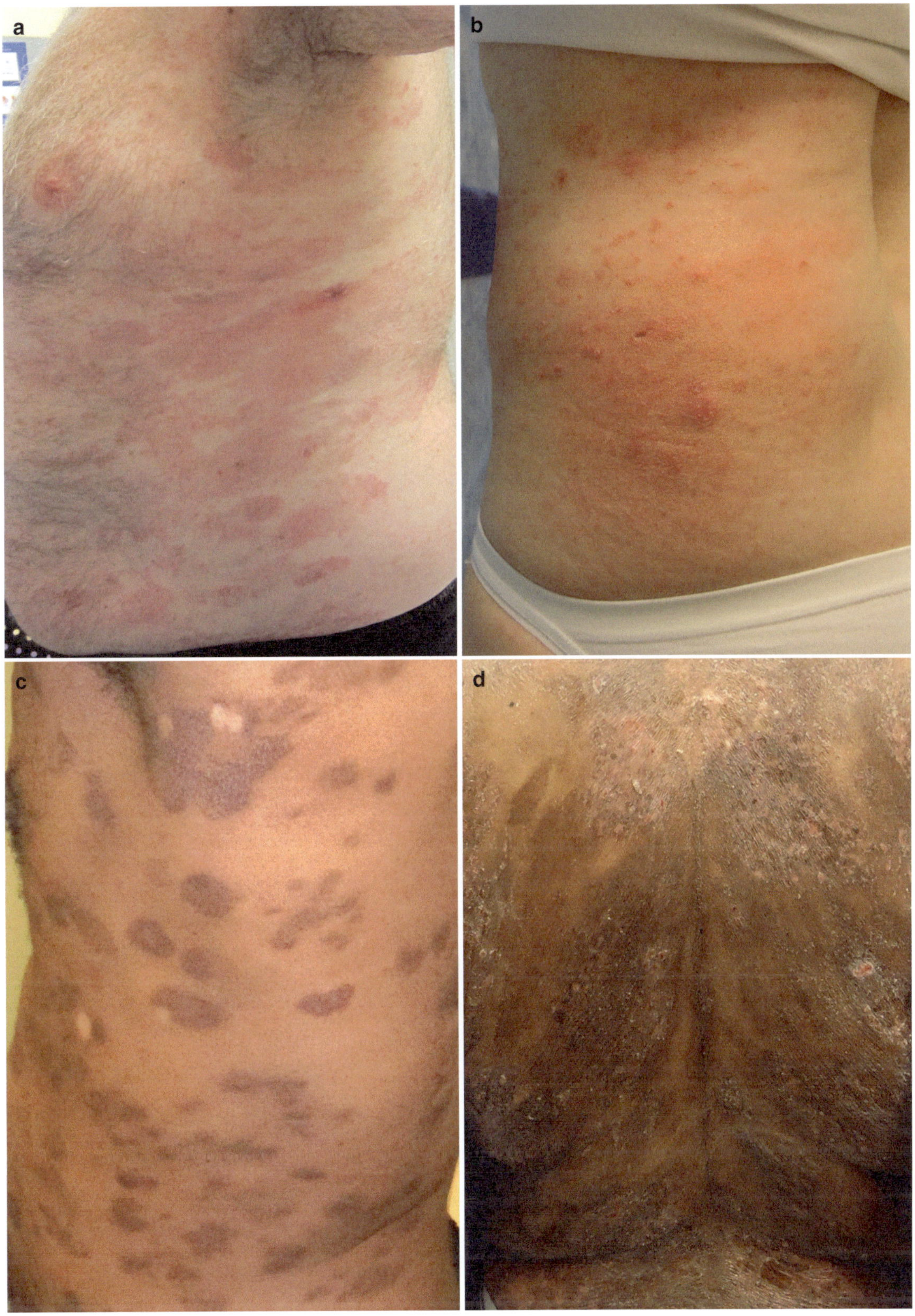

Fig. 5.1 Patch and plaque stage mycosis fungoides (MF), clinical photographs. (**a**) Large, pink-to-red, scaly patches and thin plaques on the flank and axilla of a 56-year-old man with patch/plaque MF. Similar lesions are present on the back, buttocks, and thighs (*patient featured in clinical case* 5.1). (**b**) Numerous pink, minimally scaly macules, papules, and patches on the flank of a 57-year-old woman with patch/plaque MF currently undergoing treatment with nitrogen mustard. (**c**) Scaly brown patches and plaques on the flank of a 57-year-old man with patch/plaque MF. (**d**) Innumerable hypopigmented and hyperpigmented patches and thin plaques with overlying scale and areas of xerosis, on the back of a 41-year-old woman with CD8+ MF. Similar patches and plaques are present over nearly 100 % of body surface area

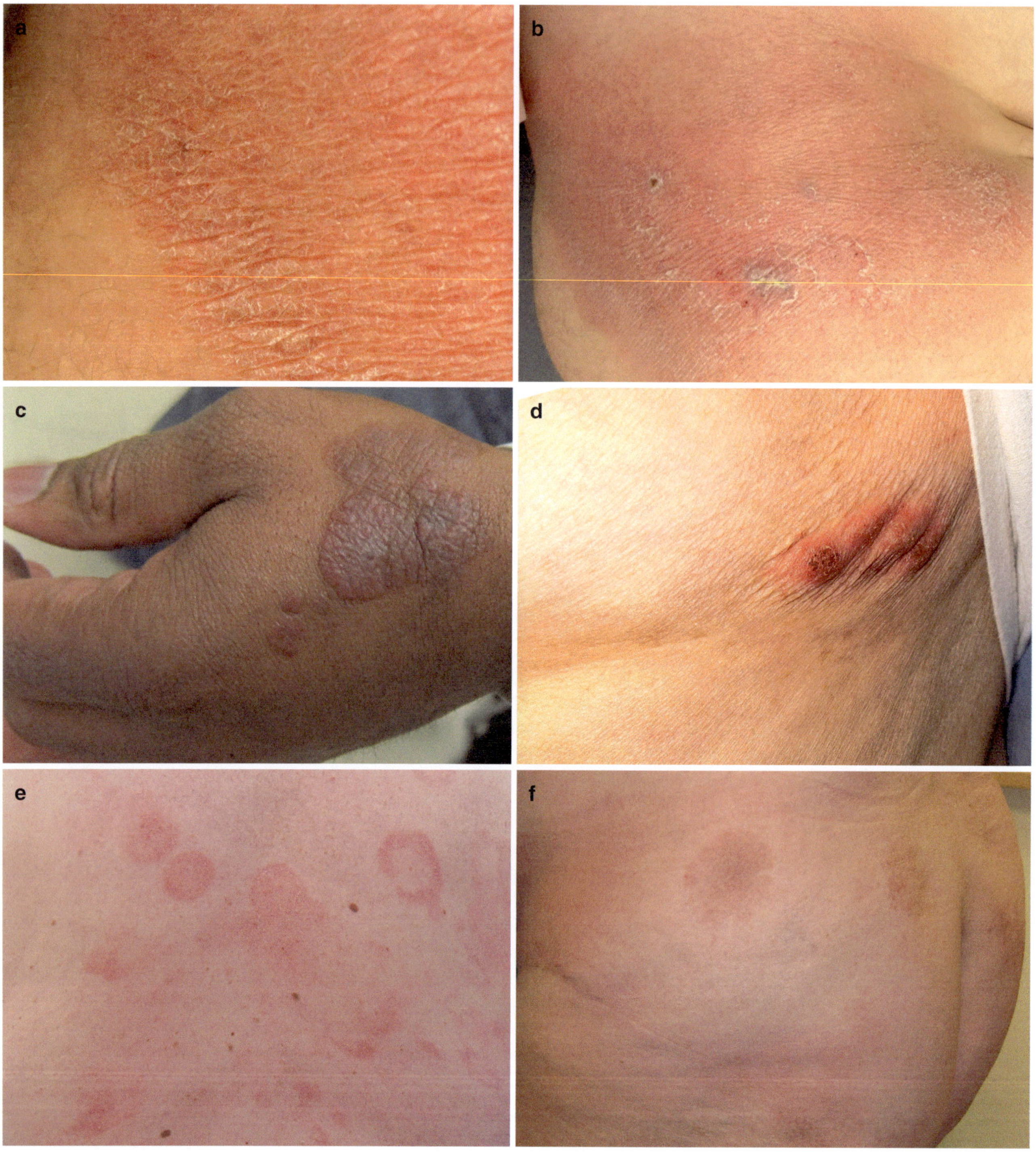

Fig. 5.2 Patch and plaque stage MF, clinical photographs. (**a**) Epidermal atrophy accompanying the atypical T-cell infiltrate results in a "cigarette paper" appearance. (**b**) Erythematous patch with areas of erosion and scale, on the anterolateral thigh of a 40-year-old man. (**c**) Indurated pink-brown plaques on the hand of a 54-year-old man. (**d**) Erythematous, indurated plaque on the chest wall of a 90-year-old man. (**e**), Numerous 1–3 cm pink annular patches and plaques on the back of a 61-year-old man. (**f**) On the buttocks of a 66-year-old woman are several annular patches with areas of atrophy, hypopigmentation, hyperpigmentation, and telangiectasias, lending a poikilodermatous appearance

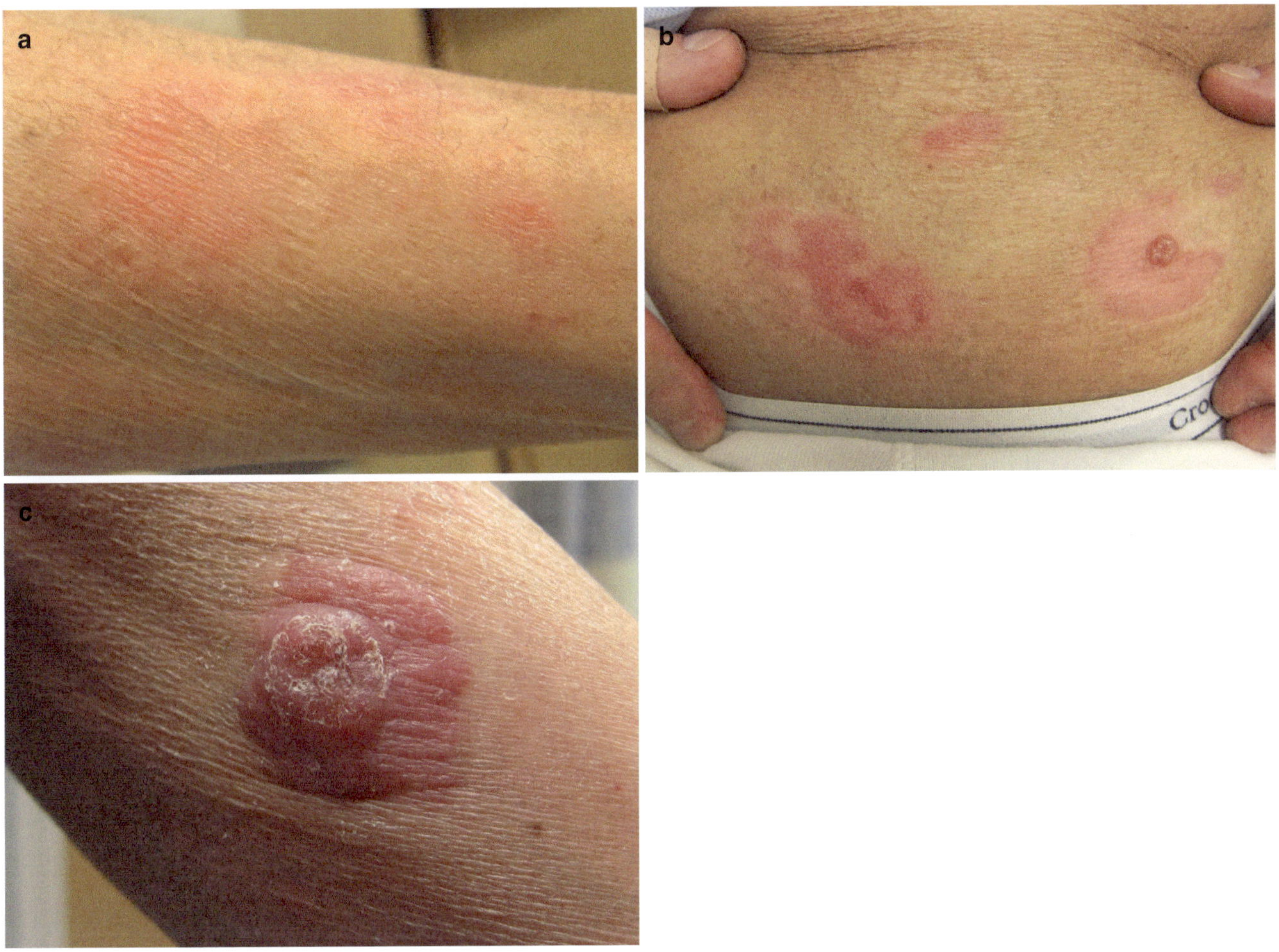

Fig. 5.3 Patch–plaque–tumor progression in MF, clinical photographs. A 64-year-old man with concurrent patches, plaques, and tumors of MF. (**a**) Scattered, pink, scaly patches on the arm. (**b**) Thin, bright pink to erythematous plaques on the lower abdomen. (**c**) Thick plaque with an overlying 3-cm tumor on the upper arm

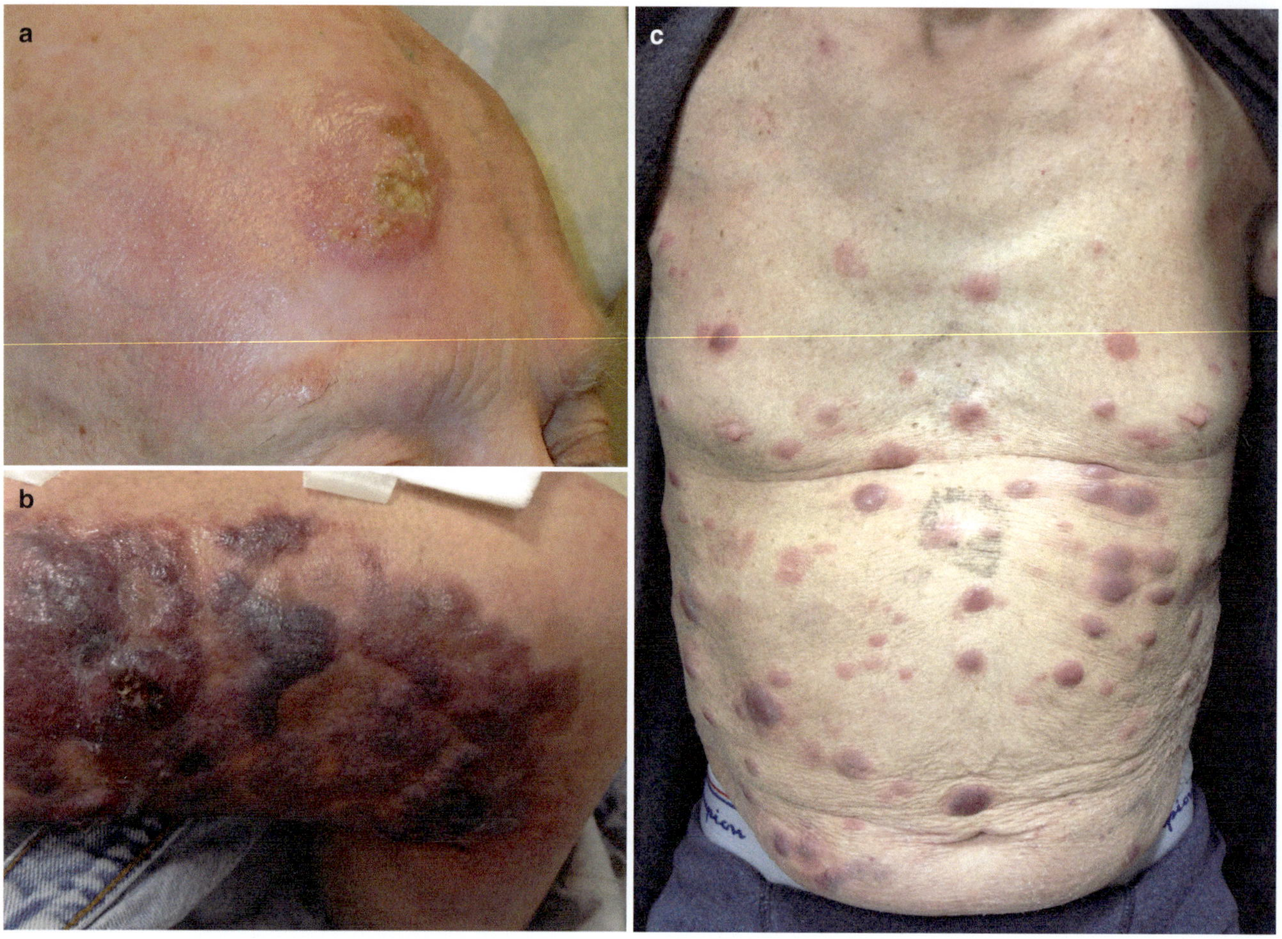

Fig. 5.4 MF with large cell transformation (LCT), clinical photographs. A 70-year-old man with MF with LCT (*patient featured in clinical case* 5.2). (**a**) Smooth, dome-shaped, skin-colored papule in the right eyebrow and 3 cm nodule with overlying crust on right forehead. (**b**) Innumerable 2–5 cm violaceous-to-black nodules coalescing into plaques on the left inner thigh. (**c**) Numerous 2–3 cm violaceous nodules scattered across the abdomen and chest

5.1.2 Prognosis and Treatment

MF generally has an excellent prognosis, with an overall 5-year disease-specific survival of almost 95 % [2]. African American patients have a slightly worse prognosis than other ethnic groups, with a 5-year mean survival of 85 % [2]. Staging guidelines for MF were revised in 2007 (Table 5.1) [12]. Although the majority of patients present with stage IA or IB disease, a higher clinical stage at diagnosis correlates with a shorter estimated survival time (Table 5.2) [10].

Large-cell transformation (LCT) has a particularly poor prognosis, with mean survival ranging from 2 to 36 months and a 5-year overall survival rate of 33 % [13]. Patients with CD30+ LCT fare somewhat better than those with CD30– transformation [13].

Negative prognostic factors of MF include increasing age, LCT, the presence of dermatopathic lymphadenopathy, and increased LDH [10]. Patients with more advanced disease at diagnosis are more likely to experience further disease progression [5]. Positive prognostic indicators include poikilodermatous or hypopigmented subtypes [10].

Although a wide array of treatment options is available, treatment is rarely curative. In early stage disease, initial therapy is typically skin directed; options include topical steroids, nitrogen mustard, topical retinoids, phototherapy, and radiation therapy. More advanced stage disease often requires systemic therapies such as bexarotene, interferon alpha, extracorporeal photopheresis, targeted therapies, single or multiagent chemotherapy, and finally bone marrow transplant [14–16]. Treatment regimens vary from patient to patient, depending on clinical presentation and subtype of MF.

Table 5.1 Staging criteria in mycosis fungoides (MF)

Stage	Skin	Nodal	Visceral	Blood	TNMB
I					
IA	**Limited patches, papules, and/or plaques on <10 % BSA (T1)**	No involvement (N_0)	No involvement (M_0)	No significant involvement (B_0) *or* Low tumor blood burden (B_1)	$T_1N_0M_0B_{0-1}$
IB	**Generalized patches, papules, and/or plaques on ≥10 % BSA (T2)**	No involvement (N_0)	No involvement (M_0)	No significant involvement (B_0) *or* Low tumor blood burden (B_1)	$T_2N_0M_0B_{0-1}$
II					
IIA	Any extent of patches or plaques (T_{1-2})	**Clinically evident dermatopathic lymphadenopathy (N1) or Early involvement by MF (N2)**	No involvement (M_0)	No significant involvement (B_0) *or* Low tumor blood burden (B_1)	$T_2N_{1-2}M_0B_{0-1}$
IIB	**One or more tumors (≥1.5 cm diameter (T3)**	Up to early lymph node involvement (N_{0-2})	No involvement (M_0)	No significant involvement (B_0) *or* Low tumor blood burden (B_1)	$T_3N_{0-2}M_0B_{0-1}$
III					
IIIA	**Erythema ≥80 % BSA (T_4)**	Up to early lymph node involvement (N_{0-2})	No involvement (M_0)	**No significant involvement (B0)**	$T_4N_{0-2}M_0B_0$
IIIB	**Erythema ≥80 % BSA (T_4)**	Up to early lymph node involvement (N_{0-2})	No involvement (M_0)	**Low tumor blood burden (B1)**	$T_4N_{0-2}M_0B_1$
IV					
IVA1	Any degree of involvement (T_{1-4})	Up to early lymph node involvement (N_{0-2})	No involvement (M_0)	**High tumor blood burden, >1,000 Sézary cells with positive TCR Clone (B2)**	$T_{1-4}N_{0-2}M_0B_2$
IVA2	Any degree of involvement (T_{1-4})	**Partial or complete nodal effacement by MF (N3)**	No involvement (M_0)	Any degree of involvement (B_{0-2})	$T_{1-4}N_3M_0B_{0-2}$
IVB	Any degree of involvement (T_{1-4})	Any degree of involvement (N_{0-3})	**Visceral involvement (M1)**	Any degree of involvement (B_{0-2})	$T_{1-4}N_{0-3}M_1B_{0-2}$

Data from Olsen et al. [12]
Key elements of the clinical or pathologic presentation differentiating each stage are in boldface
BSA body surface area, *MF* myosis fungoides

Table 5.2 Incidence of types of MF and disease specific survival (DSS)

	% of cases of MF	5-year DSS %
Classic MF	63.2	95
Folliculotropic MF	12.6	77
Poikilodermatous MF	11.2	92
MF with LyP	4.9	98
MF with LCT	4.7	65
Hypopigmented MF	3.4	98

Adapted from Agar et al. [10]

5.2 Pathology

5.2.1 Histopathology

The histopathology of classic MF differs based on the stage of the lesion (patch, plaque, tumor, or LCT). The other variants of MF also have different histopathologic characteristics.

5.2.1.1 Patch Stage

Cutaneous biopsies of early MF are characterized by a superficial bandlike or lichenoid infiltrate of atypical T-cells with marked epidermotropism (Fig. 5.5) [1]. The neoplastic T cells are small to medium and have cerebriform, hyperconvoluted nuclei with conspicuous peripheral chromatin margination [1]. The atypical cells are generally arrayed along the basal layer of the epidermis either linearly or singly; the pattern of single atypical cells along the basal layer is referred to as tagging of the dermo-epidermal junction (Fig. 5.6). The atypical lymphocytes also percolate through the epidermis and may form intraepidermal aggregates, termed "Pautrier microabscesses," usually without surrounding epidermal spongiosis (Fig. 5.7). The superficial papillary dermis may display a delicate fibrosis that leads to artifactual halo-like clearing around the dermal atypical lymphocytes. Eosinophils, histiocytes, and non-neoplastic lymphocytes may also be present.

Additional findings may include a normal to slightly acanthotic epidermis, epidermal atrophy, mild hyperkeratosis, or focal parakeratosis. Basal cell hydropic change and individual necrotic keratinocytes are very occasionally present. Red cell extravasation and pigment incontinence are common. Overall, the presence of epidermotropism, Pautrier microabscesses, and tagging are the most characteristic findings [1, 11]. Epidermotropism is most common in patch and plague stage MF and may be absent in tumor stage disease (Table 5.3).

Table 5.3 Helpful characteristics in the pathologic diagnosis of mycosis fungoides

Helpful biopsy findings in patch/plaque MF
Atypical lymphocytes with cerebriform nuclei
Lymphocytes tagging along the dermoepidermal junction forming a "string of pearls"–type configuration of lymphocytes
Pautrier microabscesses
Cerebriform cells within the epidermis, epidermotropism
Enlarged lymphocytes with surrounding halos
Epidermal lymphocytes larger than dermal lymphocytes
Lichenoid infiltrate associated with wiry bundles of collagen in the papillary dermis
Helpful biopsy findings in tumor MF
Dense diffuse/nodular dermal infiltrate of atypical cerebriform cells
<25 % Large cells
Epidermotropism, when present
Ulceration
Prominent mitotic activity, often atypical
Helpful biopsy findings in MF with large-cell transformation
>25 % Large cells
Epidermotropism, when present
Prominent mitotic activity, often atypical
CD30+ tumor cells (found in 1/3 of cases)

5.2.1.2 Plaque Stage

Biopsies of plaque stage MF demonstrate more pronounced epidermal involvement by the neoplastic T cells, including prominent epidermotropism, tagging, and Pautrier microabscesses [1, 11]. The neoplastic infiltrate is typically superficial and bandlike, although the atypical T cells are usually present singly or in clusters in the epidermis. In rare cases they can replace nearly the entire epidermis. There may be overlying mild acanthosis, compact hyperkeratosis, or patchy parakeratosis, although significant epidermal hyperplasia or scale crust is not usually seen. Other possible findings include pigment incontinence, edema, fibrosis of the papillary dermis, and proliferation of postcapillary venules. Eosinophils, plasma cells, macrophages, and dendritic cells may rarely be present [17].

5.2.1.3 Tumor Stage

Tumor stage MF is characterized by a dense, diffuse, or nodular dermal infiltrate composed of sheets of atypical T cells, in some cases extending into the subcutis [1, 17]. Ulceration is common. Epidermotropism may be present or absent [1]. In tumor stage MF cells can range in size from small to large

[1]. By definition large cells must make up less than 25 % of the infiltrate; a higher proportion would be considered LCT. Mitotic figures are readily apparent and often atypical.

5.2.1.4 Large-Cell Transformation

When LCT of MF occurs, it is characterized by the presence of more than 25 % large T cells in the dermal infiltrate on cutaneous biopsy [1]. The large cells may have prominent vesicular or hyperchromatic nuclei with conspicuous nucleoli; nuclear pleomorphism is common. Large cells not only have large nuclei but also may have apparent cytoplasm. There is typically prominent mitotic activity, and atypical mitoses are not uncommon. In one third of cases the transformed cells will be positive for CD30; the remaining two thirds are CD30-negative (Fig. 5.8) [9].

During any stage of the disease patients may develop dermatopathic lymphadenopathy, which is manifested histopathologically as lymph nodes with paracortical hyperplasia comprised of interdigitating dendritic cells, histiocytes, melanophages, and small reactive T cells; dermatopathic lymphadenopathy does not represent lymphomatous involvement of the node [1].

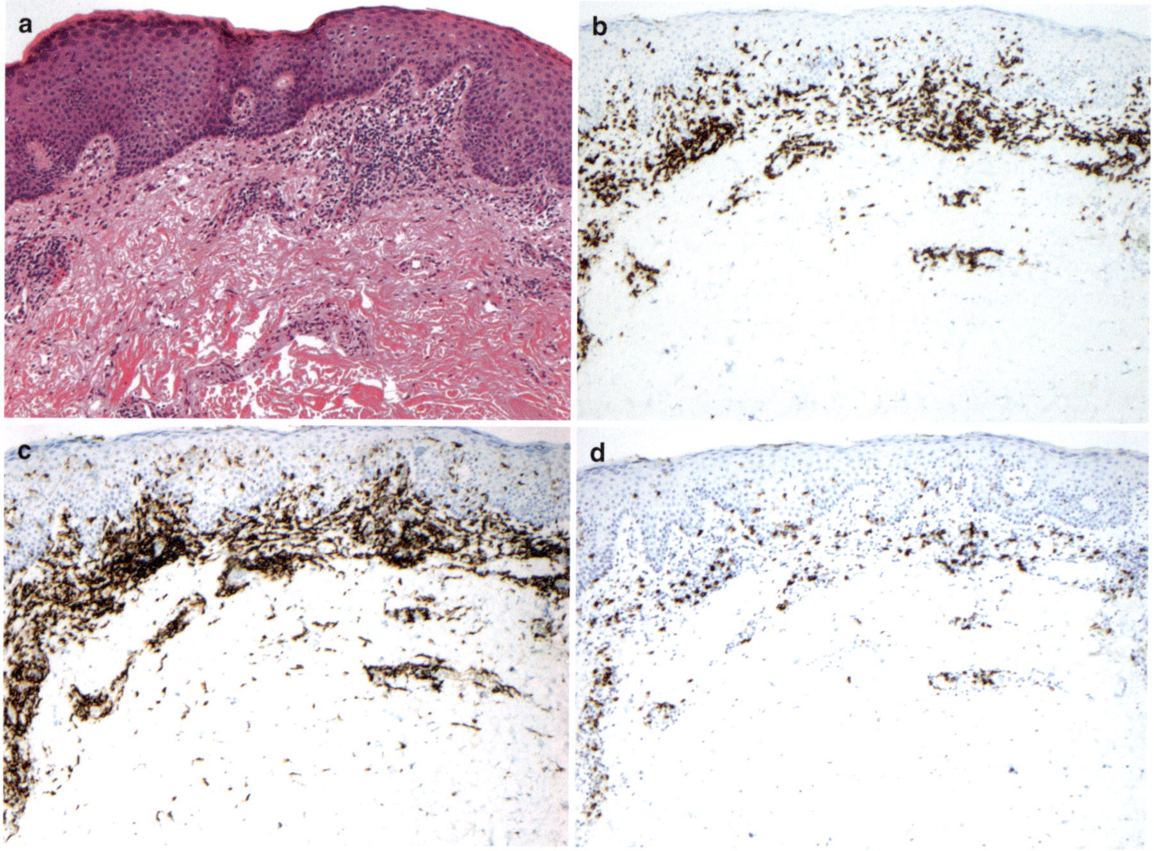

Fig. 5.5 Classic MF, histopathology and immunohistochemistry (*patient featured in clinical case* 5.1). (**a**) An epidermotropic infiltrate of atypical T cells with tagging of neoplastic cells along the dermal–epidermal junction (DEJ) (H&E, 10×). (**b**) Many of the lymphocytes cells express CD3 (CD3, 10×). (**c**) Numerous CD4+ T cells infiltrate the epidermis and superficial dermis, with tagging along the DEJ; some of these cells lack expression of CD3 (CD4, 10×). (**d**) Scattered CD8+ cytotoxic T cells are present in the lymphocytic infiltrate (CD8, 10×)

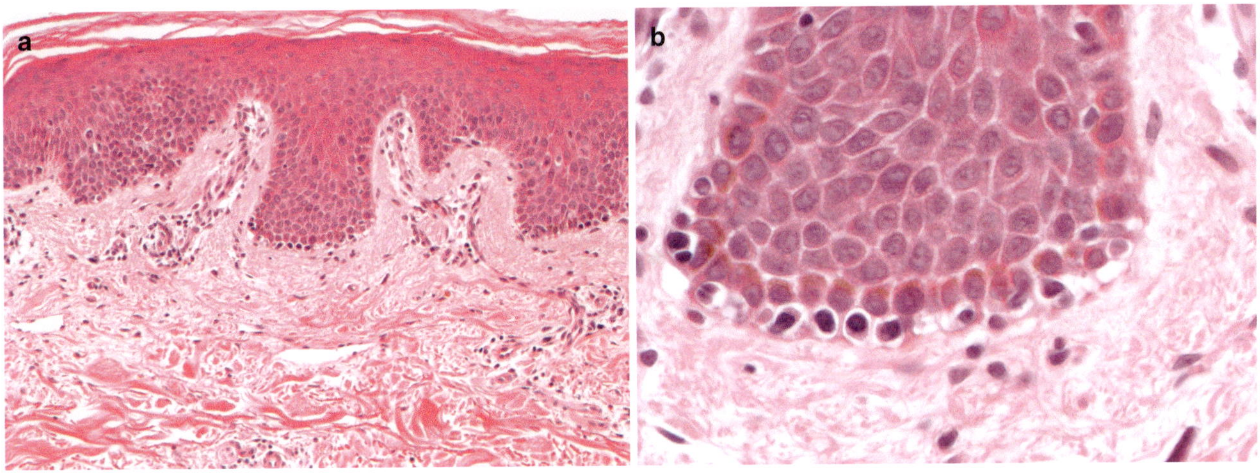

Fig. 5.6 Tagging of the DEJ and the string-of-pearls sign in MF. (**a**) Atypical lymphocytes are present along the DEJ and in the epidermis. When the cells are present singly, it is called "tagging" (H&E, 10×). (**b**) When atypical cells are present along the DEJ in series they resemble beads on a string, yielding the so-called "string-of-pearls" sign (H&E, 60×)

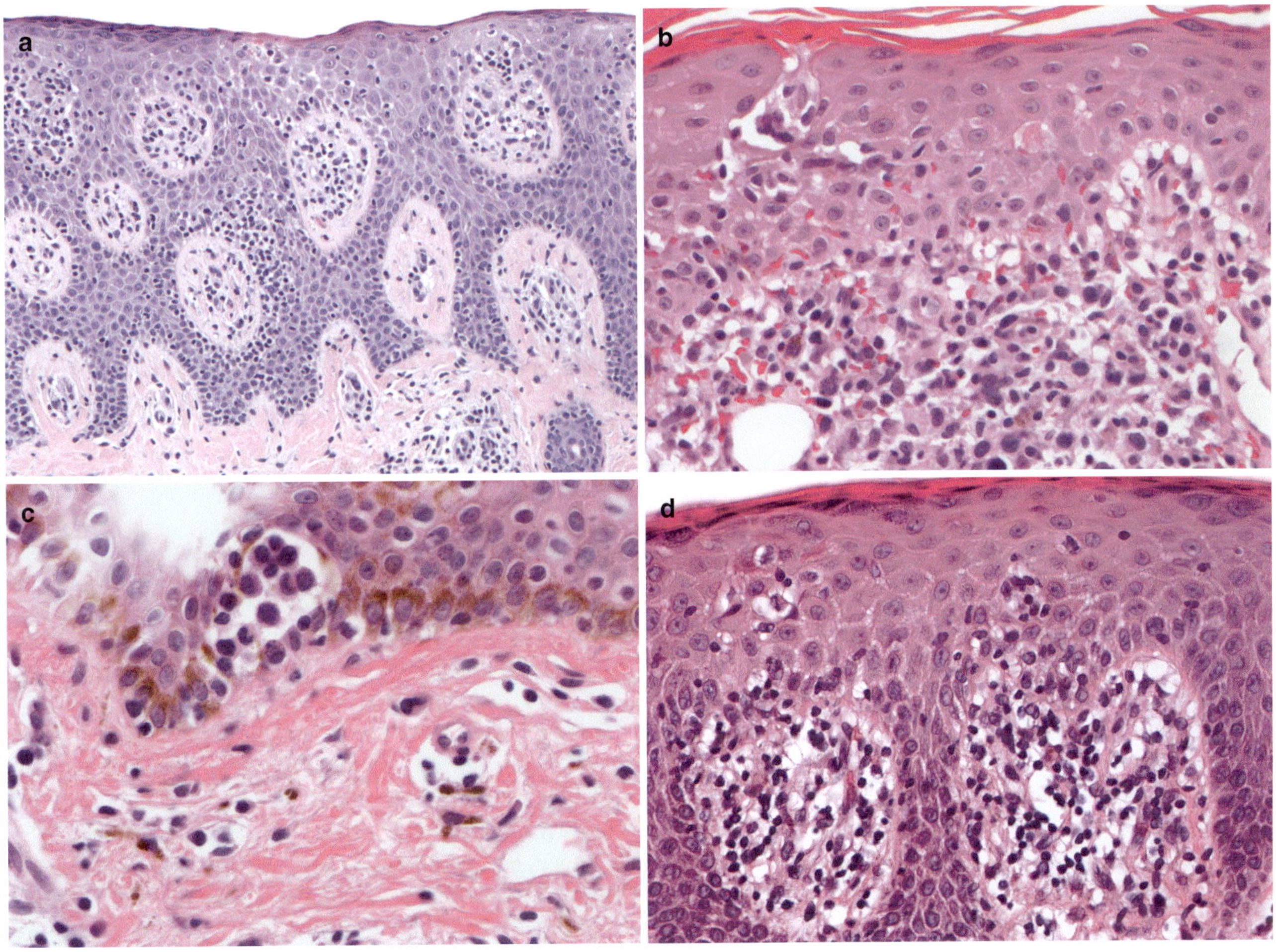

Fig. 5.7 Several examples of Pautrier's microabscesses. (**a**) Numerous Pautrier's microabscesses in the epidermis of a biopsy of a patient with patch/plaque stage MF (H&E, 10×). (**b**) A Pautrier's microabscess in the epidermis of a patient with patch/plaque stage MF (H&E, 20×). (**c**) A Pautrier's microabscess in the epidermis of a patient with exfoliative MF (H&E, 40×). (**d**) Two Pautrier's microabscesses in the epidermis of a patient with patch/plaque stage MF (H&E, 40×)

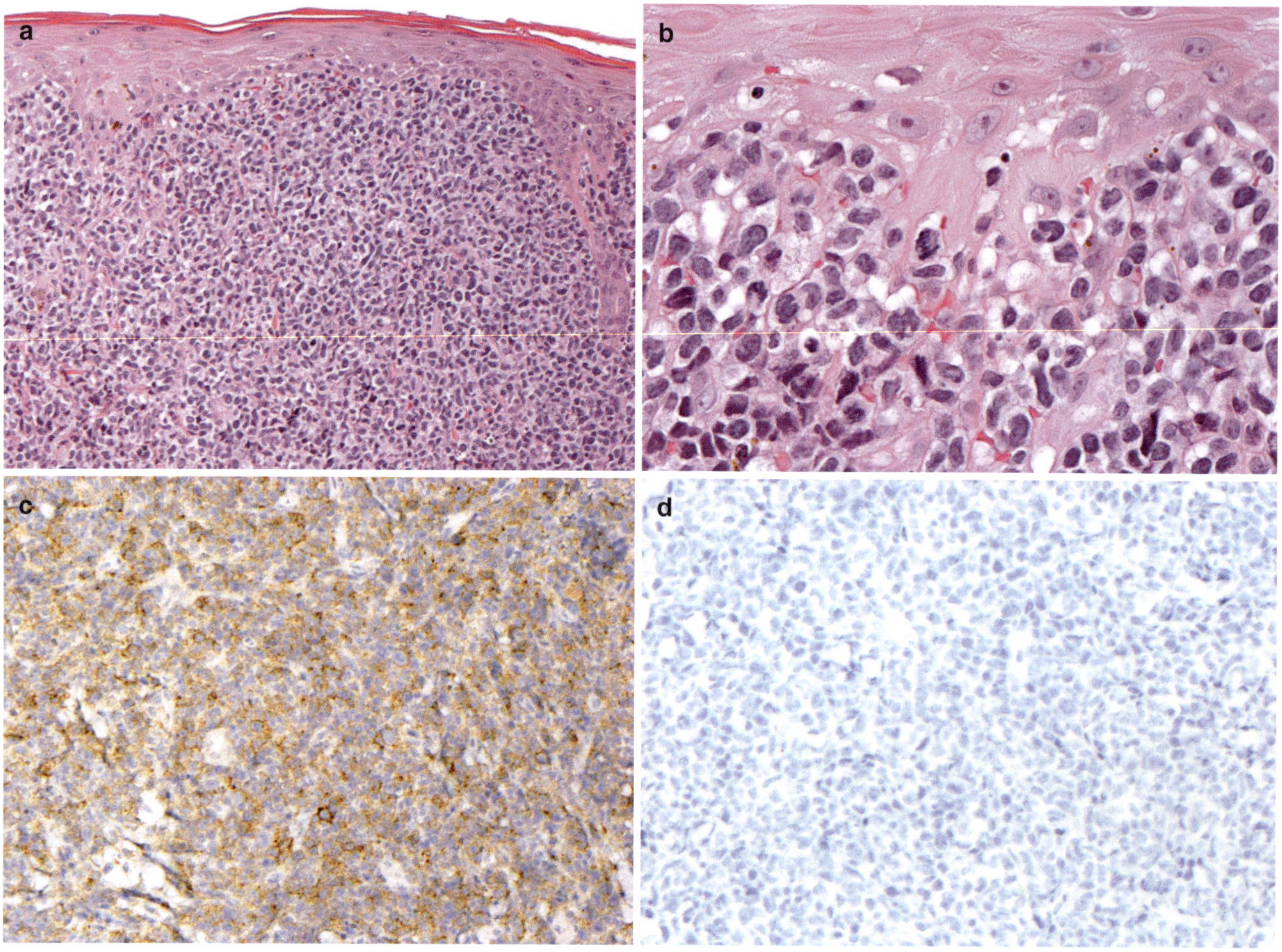

Fig. 5.8 Large-cell transformation of MF (*patient featured in clinical case* 5.2). (**a**) A dense, diffuse dermal infiltrate of sheets of neoplastic T cells, >25 % of which are large. Epidermotropism is retained in this example (H&E, 4×). (**b**) The neoplastic T cells are very large with irregularly shaped, crenellated, heterochromatic nuclei. Blastic cells have prominent nucleoli (H&E, 60×). (**c**) The majority of the large atypical cells express CD30 (CD30, 20×). (**d**) The large atypical cells are Alk negative, (Alk, 20×)

5.2.2 Immunophenotype and Molecular Findings

The neoplastic CD4+ T cells of MF often stain positively for CD2, CD3, CD4, CD5, TCRbeta, and CD45RO. In the vast majority of cases of MF, the neoplastic T cells are CD4+ CD8−; only rarely is MF composed of CD8+ CD4− T cells [1]. Neoplastic cells may show loss of pan–T-cell antigens including CD2 and CD5, a helpful diagnostic finding (*see* Fig. 5.3b–d) [1, 11]. CD7 is lost in one third of cases. However, because CD7 is frequently lost in reactive cutaneous T-cell infiltrates, it is not a useful marker of neoplastic T cells in the skin [1]. CD25 is rarely present [17]. As the disease progresses, loss of CD2, CD3, and CD5 becomes more common (Table 5.4) [17].

Cells typically express CLA, a cell surface antigen involved in homing of lymphocytes to the skin. Cytotoxic granules are rarely seen early in disease progression but may be present in neoplastic cells of advanced lesions [1].

Clonal rearrangement of the TCR is nearly always detected [1]. A concomitant loss of TCR diversity in the blood may contribute to deficiencies in immunity [11]. Of note, the presence of the same TCR clone in multiple biopsies is correlated with a worse prognosis [18].

The genetics underlying MF are poorly understood [19]. Complex karyotypes are usually present, including recurrent loss of 1p, 17p, 10q, 13a, and 19 and gains of 4q, 17q, and 18 [19–25]. Constitutive activation of STAT3, CDKN2A/p16^{INK4a}, and PTEN has also been implicated in disease progression [1, 24]. There is some evidence that microsatellite instability may play a role in the underlying pathobiology of MF [26].

Table 5.4 Common immunohistochemical findings in MF

Positive markers	Negative markers
CD2[a]	CD8
CD3[a]	CD7 (1/3 cases)
CD5[a]	CD25
CD7 (2/3 cases)	CD56
TCR-beta	TCR-gamma
CD45RO	

Although these are generally true, there are always exceptions. Notable exceptions include hypopigmented MF, which is often CD8+
[a]Often lost with disease progression

5.3 Subtypes of MF

Numerous subtypes of MF have been described. These include classic, erythrodermic, follicular, syringotropic, bullous, granulomatous, poikilodermatous, hypopigmented, hyperpigmented, unilesional (Pagetoid reticulosis), palmoplantar, hyperkeratotic, vegetating, ichthyosiform, pigmented purpura-like, and pustular, among others [17]. Notably, the only subtypes of MF explicitly mentioned in the WHO guidelines are folliculotropic MF, pagetoid reticulosis, and granulomatous slack skin [1]. Here, we will discuss the clinical presentation and histopathology of those three entities as well as hypopigmented, poikilodermatous, syringotropic, and granulomatous variants of MF (Table 5.5).

Table 5.5 Summary of clinical presentations and pathology of selected subtypes of MF

	Clinical presentation	Pathology
Classic	Patch-plaque-tumor progression	Epidermotropic infiltrate of neoplastic cells with "tagging" of the dermoepidermal junction and Pautrier microabscesses. Typically CD4+
Folliculotropic	Grouped follicular papules on the head and neck, alopecia, erythematous patches and plaques, and severe pruritus	Dense, perifollicular neoplastic infiltrate of neoplastic cells. Mucinous degeneration of hair follicles (follicular mucinosis)
Pagetoid Reticulosis	Single patch or plaque, <5 % BSA	Same as classic MF. May be CD4+ CD8– or CD4– CD8+. Often CD30+
Granulomatous slack skin	Bulky hanging skin folds in axillae and groin	Diffuse or band-like dense granulomatous infiltrate with cerebriform cells. Multinucleate giant cells with 20–30 nuclei, phagocytosed lymphocytes, and/or degenerated elastic fibers. Subtle/absent epidermotropism
Hypopigmented	Hypopigmented, slightly pruritic, scaly patches with irregular borders	Same as classic MF. Often CD4-CD8+
Syringotropic	Red-brown patches, slightly infiltrated scaly plaques, small skin colored to erythematous papules, alopecia, and anhidrosis	Dense perieccrine infiltrate of small cerebriform cells, hyperplasia of eccrine apparatus
Poikilodermatous	Patches of alternating hyperpigmentation, hypopigmentation, atrophy, and telangiectasias	Same as plaque or patch stage MF
Granulomatous	Patches and plaques, some with skin atrophy	Diffuse or nodular perivascular or periadnexal lymphocytic infiltrate. Granulomas present in a sarcoid-like pattern

BSA body surface area

5.3.1 Folliculotropic MF

Folliculotropic MF (also called pilotropic or folliculocentric MF) accounts for approximately 13 % of cases of MF [10]. Most often presenting as grouped follicular papules on the head and neck (Figs. 5.9 and 5.10) [1, 17], folliculotopic MF may be accompanied by alopecia, acneiform lesions, mucinorrhea, comedo-like plugs, epidermal cysts, follicular hyperkeratosis, erythematous patches and plaques, and severe pruritus [17, 27, 28]. This form of MF is four to five times more common in men than in women [17]. Folliculotropic MF has a worse prognosis than classic MF, with a 5-year disease-specific survival of 70–80 % (*see* Table 5.2) [1, 10, 29].

Cutaneous biopsy of folliculotropic MF demonstrates a dense, perifollicular and intrafollicular neoplastic infiltrate of small-to-medium CD4+ cerebriform T cells with sparing of the epidermis and interfollicular dermis (Fig. 5.11) [1, 27]. The majority of cases demonstrate mucinous degeneration of hair follicles (follicular mucinosis) (Fig. 5.12), but this is not necessary for diagnosis [1, 27]. Mucinous degeneration can range in severity from focal mucin to complete destruction of the hair follicle and formation of mucin lakes. The mucin stains positively as hyaluronic acid with colloidal iron (Fig. 5.12b), alcian blue, or toluidine blue stains [17]. Pautrier microabscesses may be present in the follicular epithelium [17]. Because infiltration of eccrine ducts may also occur, some consider folliculotropic MF and syringotropic MF to be forms of the overarching entity of adnexotropic MF [17].

5.3.2 Pagetoid Reticulosis

Pagetoid reticulosis is an exceedingly rare form of MF characterized by a single patch or plaque. These lesions usually occur on acral sites but may occasionally be present in a bathing-suit distribution. By definition, the lesions of pagetoid reticulosis cover less than 5 % of body surface area [1, 17]. Pagetoid reticulosis is indolent; extracutaneous spread has never been reported [1]. Of note, most consider pagetoid reticulosis to be synonymous with unilesional MF, whereas others consider these to be distinct entities [30].

The patches and plaques of pagetoid reticulosis are composed of a prominent epidermotropic intraepidermal proliferation of medium-to-large, hyperchromatic, cerebriform T cells, usually with more "pagetoid" distribution of the epi-

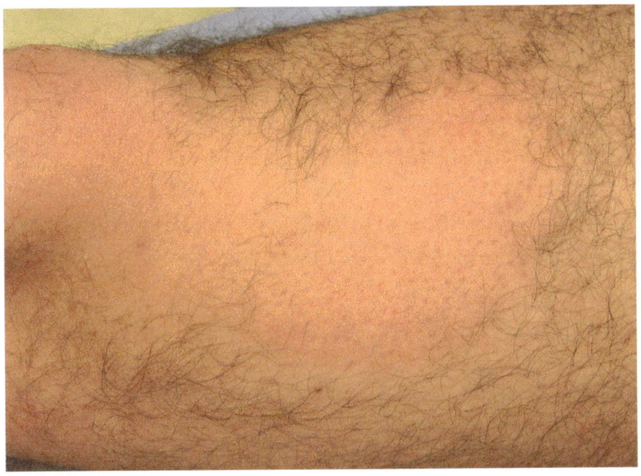

Fig. 5.9 Folliculotropic MF, clinical images. Area of alopecia and faint erythema on the anterior thigh of a 25-year-old man with folliculotropic MF

dermotropic cells than is seen in classic MF (Fig. 5.13). However, usually the pagetoid reticulosis is histopathologically indistinguishable from classic MF and requires clinicopathologic correlation for the diagnosis [1, 17]. The tumor cells may have helper (CD4+ CD8−) or cytotoxic (CD8+ CD4−) immunophenotypes and are often CD30+ [1].

Pagetoid reticulosis was once considered to have two subtypes: Woringer-Kolopp (localized pagetoid reticulosis) and Ketron-Goodman disease (disseminated pagetoid reticulosis) [1, 30, 31]. These are now believed to be distinct disease entities. Woringer-Kolopp is now considered synonymous with pagetoid reticulosis, while Ketron-Goodman is now thought to be more similar to the deadly CD8+ aggressive epidermotropic T-cell lymphoma (CD8+ AECTCL). Because pagetoid reticulosis and CD8+ AECTCL have such different prognoses and presentations, the terms Woringer-Kolopp and Ketron-Goodman are avoided in order to minimize

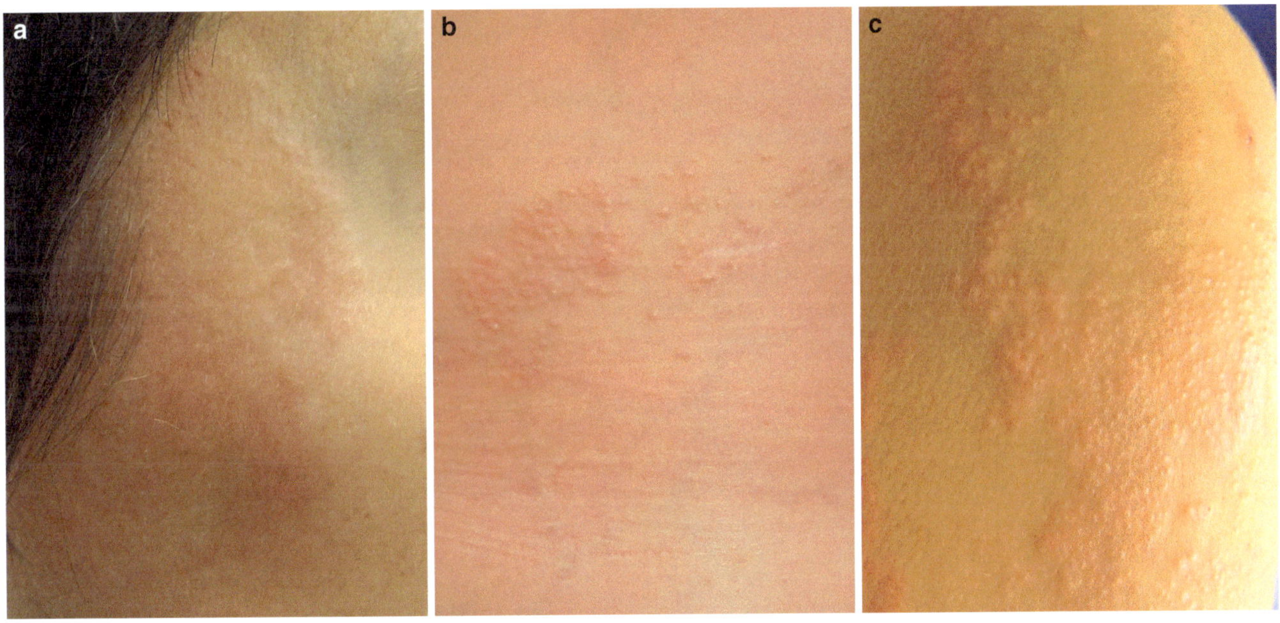

Fig. 5.10 Folliculotropic MF, clinical photographs (*patient featured in clinical case* 5.3). (**a**) An indurated, lightly erythematous, well-demarcated, pruritic plaque on the temple of a 32-year-old woman with folliculotropic MF. (**b**) Grouped follicular erythematous papules on the right flank. (**c**) Innumerable follicularly based papules on an edematous, erythematous plaque on the patient's shoulder and lateral arm

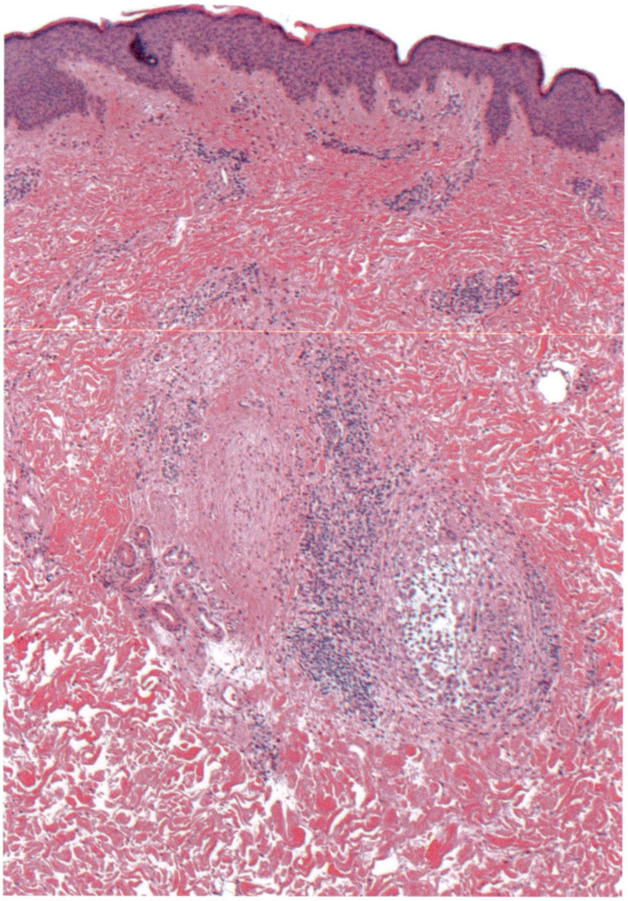

Fig. 5.11 Folliculotropic MF (*patient featured in clinical case* 5.3). Although there is extensive infiltration of the hair follicle by neoplastic T cells, the epidermis and surrounding dermis are largely spared

confusion [1] and are included here only because of their historical significance.

5.3.3 Granulomatous Slack Skin

Granulomatous slack skin (GSS) is an extremely rare but indolent variant of MF [1]. Fewer than 50 cases have been reported in the literature [32]. GSS typically presents with the slow growth of distinctive bulky skin folds in intertriginous areas (Fig. 5.14) [1, 17, 32]. These tend to be particularly prominent in the axillae and groin and may be accompanied by poikilodermatous patches or plaques. Patients often have a longstanding history of the patch and plaque stage of MF [32].

The infiltrate of GSS is composed of a diffuse or band-like dense granulomatous infiltrate of small-to-medium cerebriform T cells, numerous histiocytes, and multinucleate giant cells [1, 17, 32]. The T cells are clonal, express CD3 and CD4, and lack CD8 [1, 32]. The multinucleate giant cells may have as many as 20–30 nuclei and may contain phagocytosed lymphocytes and/or degenerated elastic fibers [17]. Epidermotropism may be subtle or absent. All affected areas will demonstrate loss of elastin, but elastophagocytosis may be subtle [32]. The elastic lamina of large cutaneous vessels is occasionally involved [33].

Of note, although GSS is characterized by a granulomatous infiltrate, it is distinct from granulomatous variants of MF. These two entities cannot be distinguished on the basis of histopathology alone and clinical correlation is necessary (see Sect. 5.3.7) [32].

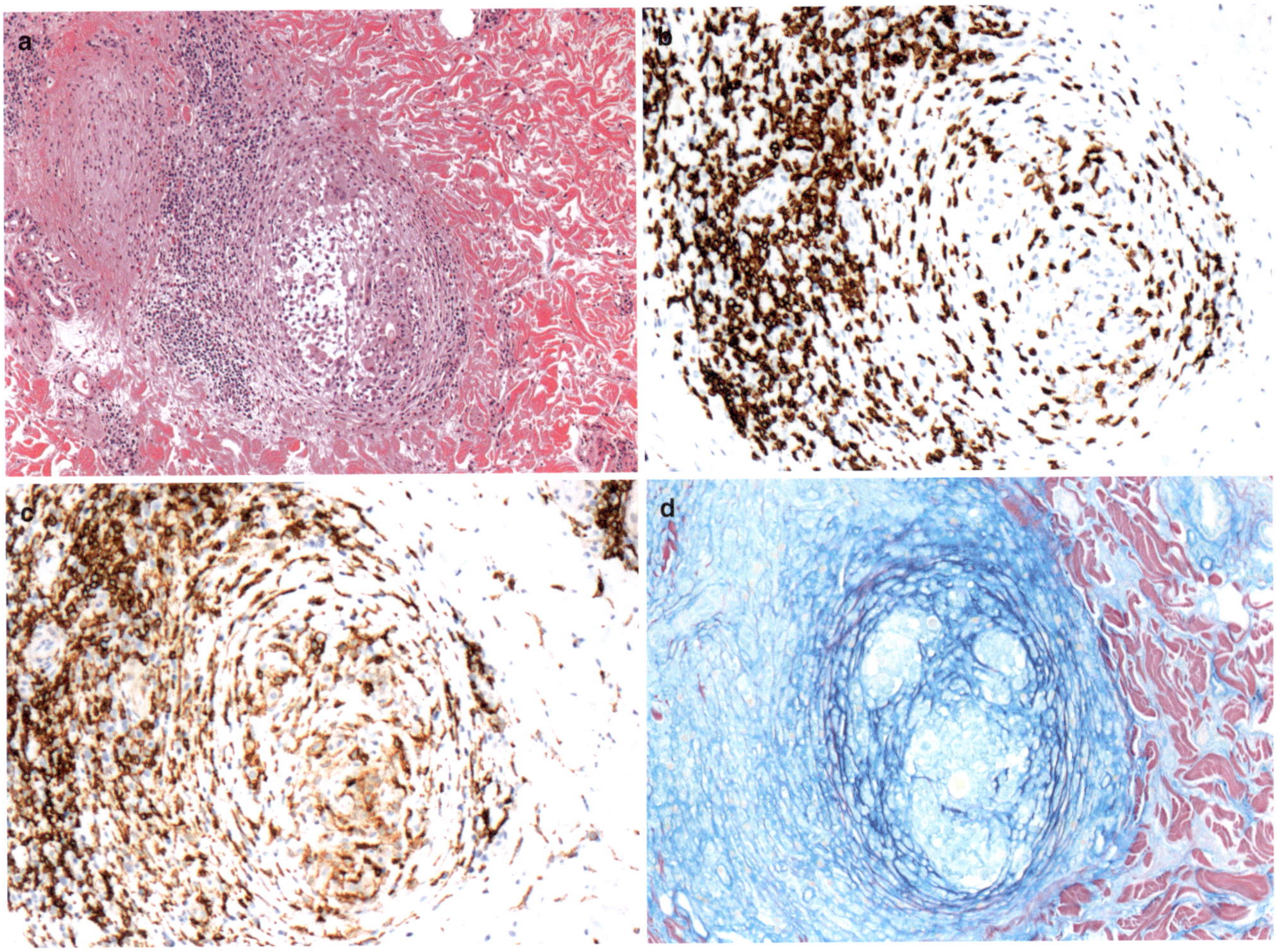

Fig. 5.12 Folliculotropic MF (*patient featured in clinical case* 5.3). (**a**) Dense, perifollicular neoplastic infiltrate of lymphocytes with destruction of the hair follicle (H&E, 10×). (**b**) The invading atypical lymphocytes are CD3+ T cells (CD3, 10×). (**c**) The neoplastic T cells express CD4 (CD4, 10×). (**d**) Colloidal iron stain reveals large amounts of mucin in the hair follicle epithelium with destruction of the hair follicle (colloidal iron, 10×)

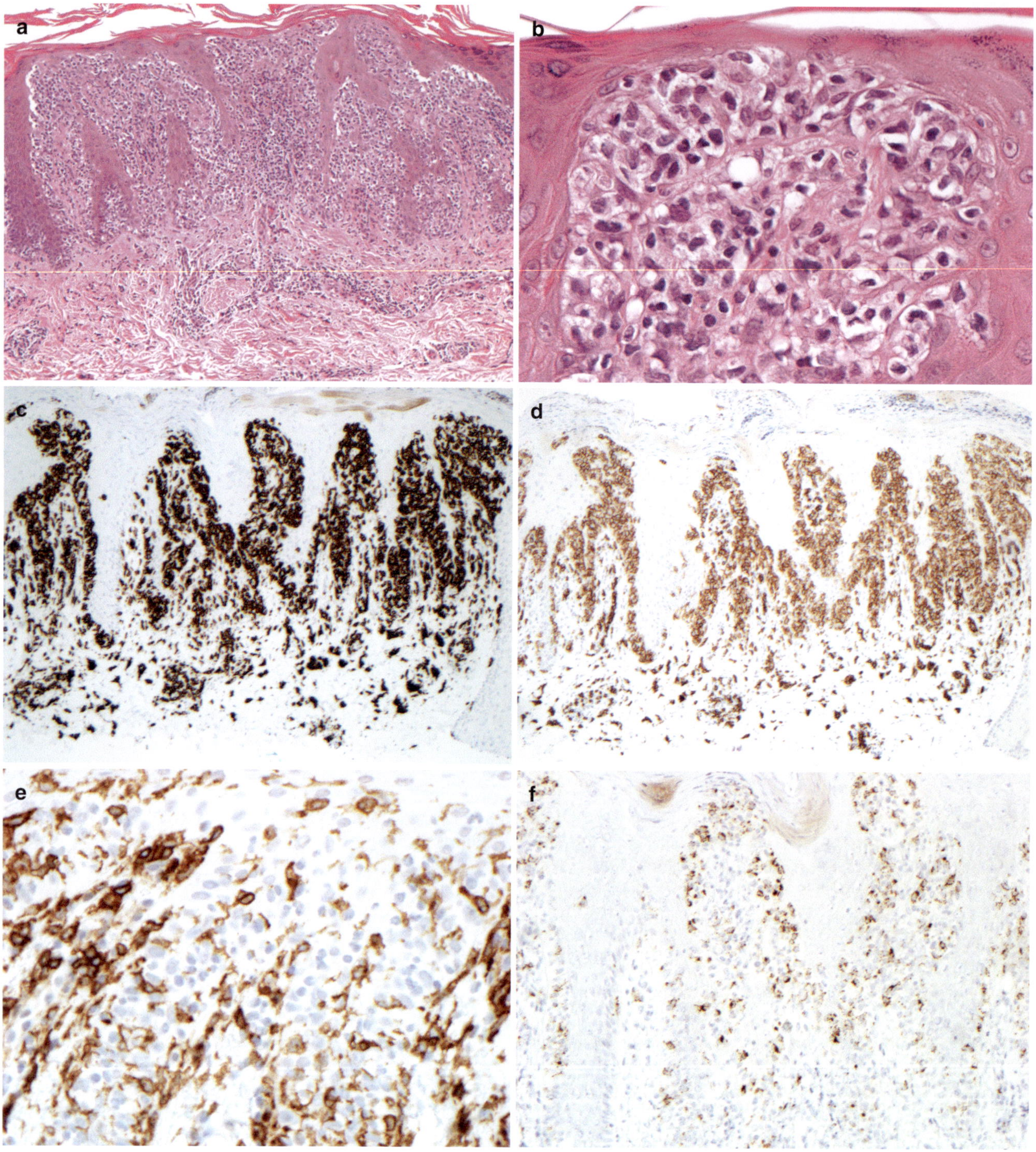

Fig. 5.13 Pagetoid reticulosis (PR). (**a**) Dense lymphoid infiltrate occupies the superficial dermis, directly abutting the epidermis without intervening Grenz zone (H&E 10×). (**b**) The lymphoid cells show minimal cytological atypia (H&E, 40×). (**c**) The infiltrate is composed of CD3+ T cells (CD3, 10×). (**d**) The majority of the lymphoid cells of the infiltrate stain strongly for CD8, indicating a cytotoxic phenotype (CD8, 10×). (**e**) Although some lymphoid cells stain positively for CD4, the majority of the CD4+ cells are histiocytes (CD4, 20×). (**f**) Consistent with a cytotoxic phenotype, many of the lymphoid cells in the infiltrate express granzyme B (Granzyme B, 20×)

5.3.4 Hypopigmented MF

Hypopigmented MF is rare and accounts for just 3 % of patients with MF [10]. Patients typically present with hypopigmented, asymptomatic, slightly pruritic, scaly patches with irregular borders (Fig. 5.15) [17]. Some patients may also have classic patches, plaques, and tumors of MF [34]. Hypopigmented MF has the same indolent nature and excellent prognosis as classic MF [17].

Patients with hypopigmented MF typically have darker skin, but this form of MF has been observed in lighter pigmented or Caucasian patients. Hypopigmented MF may be underreported in Caucasian patients because the loss of pigmentation may be less obvious. Of note, patients with less pigmented skin are more likely to have coincident classic MF lesions [17, 34]. In contrast to other forms of MF, hypopigmented MF often impacts children; nearly 20 % of reported cases are in children [34].

Although the histopathology of the infiltrate is the same as that of classic MF, the T cells of hypopigmented MF are often CD8+ [34]. Hypopigmentation is likely secondary to changes in melanin production rather than to loss of melanocytes. With treatment, perifollicular repigmentation may occur [17, 34].

Of note, there are reports of cases of *hyper*pigmented MF composed of hyperpigmented patches and plaques and also characterized by a CD8+ phenotype [35].

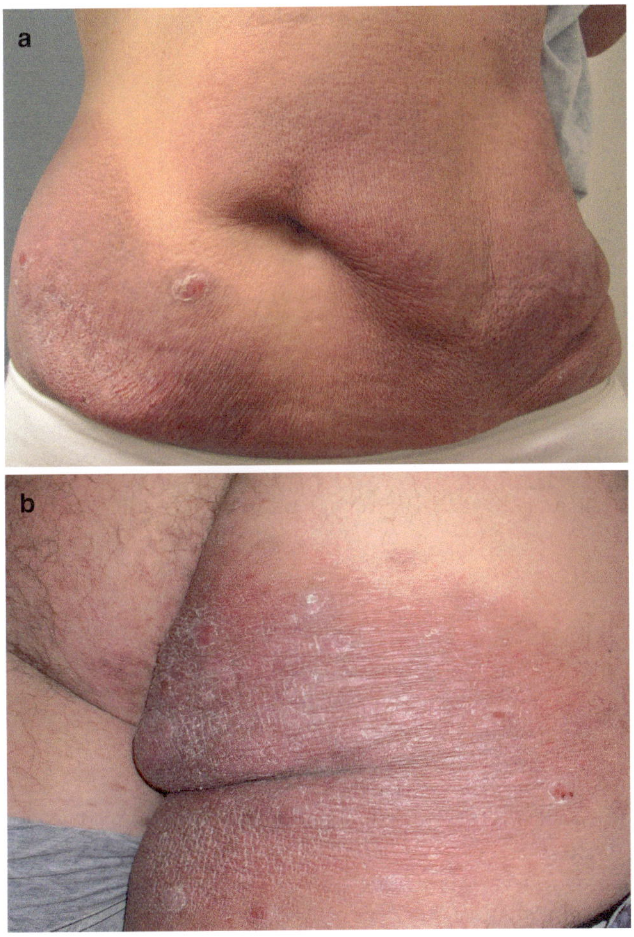

Fig. 5.14 Granulomatous slack skin (GSS). (**a**) Thickened, erythematous-to-violaceous, pendulous plaques of skin with areas of scale and erosion on the abdomen of a young woman. (**b**) Lichenified thickened plaque with erythema, scale, and erosions on the buttock of an 18-year-old man (*patient featured in clinical case* 5.4)

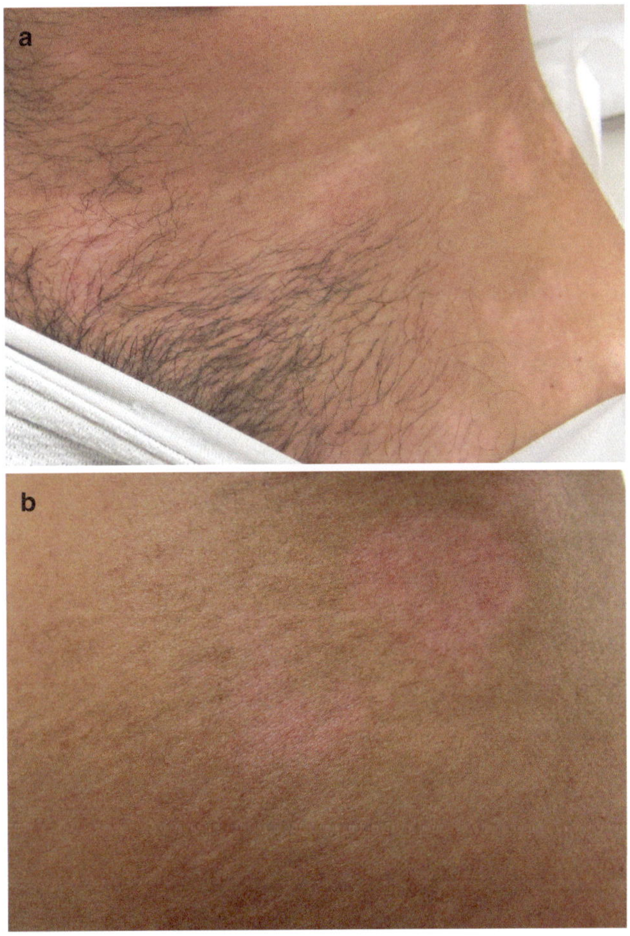

Fig. 5.15 Hypopigmented MF (*patient featured in clinical case* 5.5). (**a**) Numerous, irregularly shaped, hypopigmented-to-erythematous patches on the suprapubic region and upper thigh of a young man. Some patches are atrophic. Areas of hypopigmentation stop abruptly above the waistband, consistent with the classic "bathing suit" distribution of MF. (**b**) Three and 5 cm, pink, hypopigmented patches on the patient's buttock

5.3.5 Syringotropic MF

Syringotropic MF is a rare form of adnexotropic MF, formerly known as "syringotropic MF with alopecia" or "syringotropic cutaneous T-cell lymphoma." It is characterized by red-brown patches, slightly infiltrated scaly plaques, or small skin-colored to erythematous papules (Fig. 5.16) [17, 36]. Alopecia and anhidrosis are common, occurring in up to 70 and 30 % of cases, respectively. There is no location predilection. Patients are almost exclusively male, and many patients carry a previous diagnosis of conventional or classic MF [17, 36]. Nearly 50 % of cases present with solitary or localized lesions [36].

Histopathologically, syringotropic MF is characterized by a dense perieccrine infiltrate of small cerebriform cells with hyperplasia of the secretory portions of the eccrine apparatus (Figs. 5.17 and 5.18) [17, 29]. Conventional histopathologic characteristics of MF, including epidermotropism, are seen in the majority of patients with syringotropic MF (Fig. 5.17a) [36]. Hair follicles may be involved, but unlike in follicular MF, follicular mucinosis is absent [17].

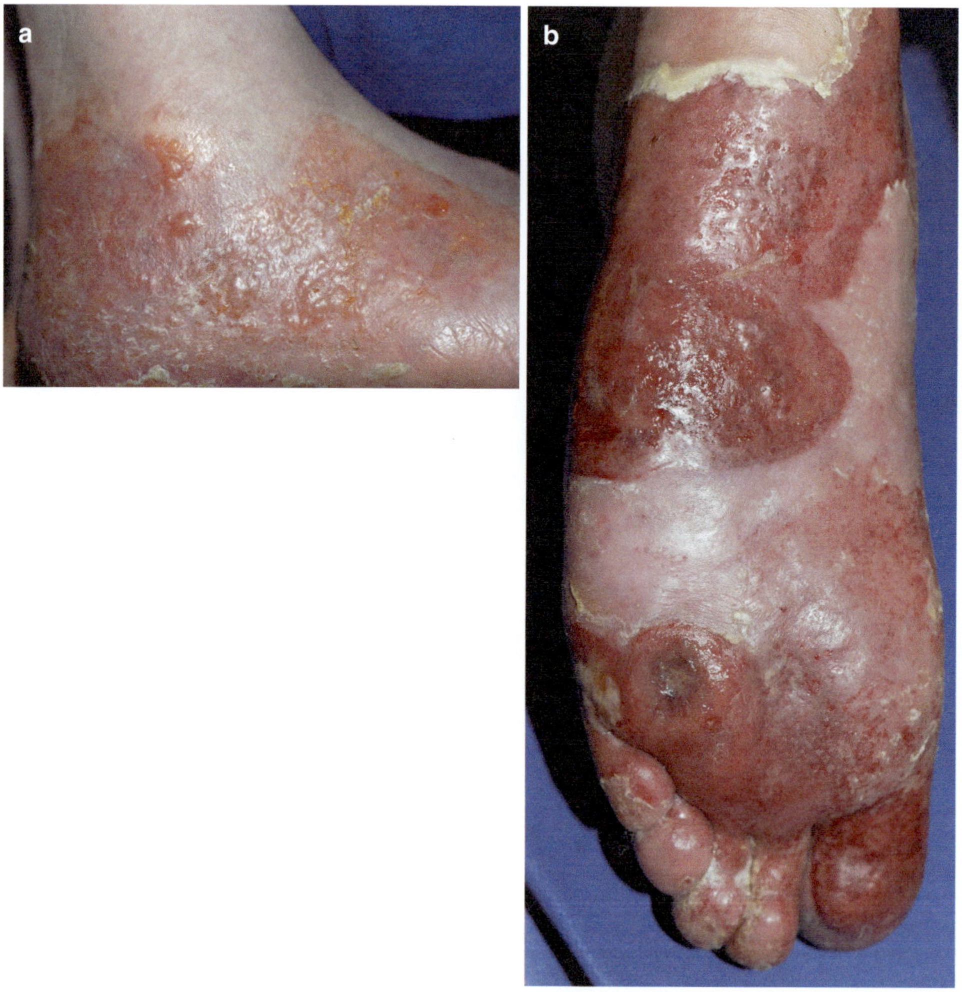

Fig. 5.16 Syringotropic MF (*patient featured in clinical case* 5.6). (**a**) On the lateral aspect of the foot of a 68-year-old man is a pink plaque studded with innumerable flaccid orange vesicles, some with erosion. (**b**) The patient's plantar foot with striking eroded plaques and erythema (Courtesy of Dr. Richard A. Johnson, Massachusetts General Hospital, Boston, MA)

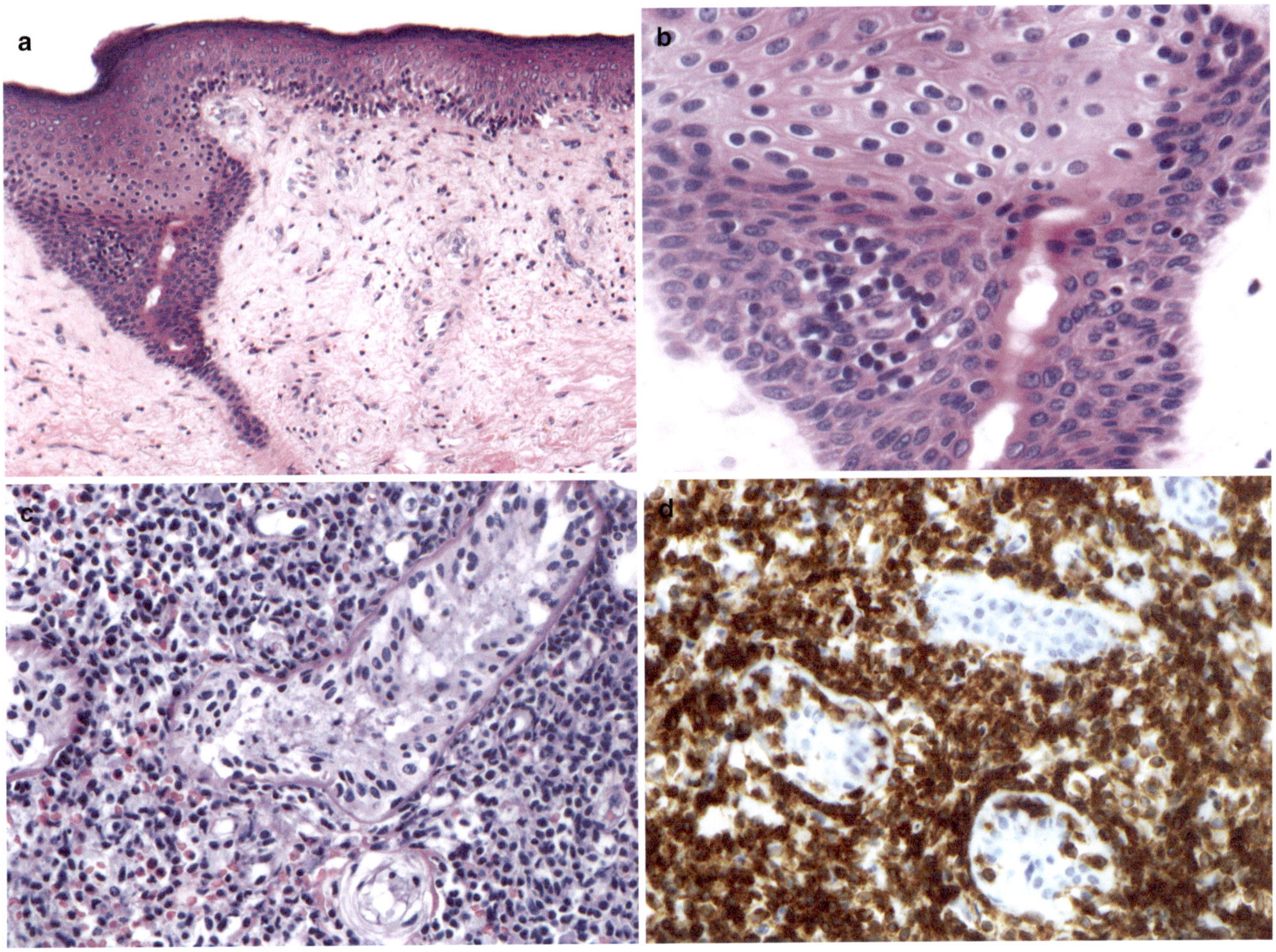

Fig. 5.17 Syringotropic MF (*patient featured in clinical case* 5.6). (**a**) Atypical lymphocytes tag the dermal-epidermal junction and invade the epithelium of the eccrine pore and duct. Eccrine duct hyperplasia is present (H&E, 20×). (**b**) The atypical lymphocytes have irregularly shaped heterochromatic nuclei (H&E, 60×). (**c**) Deeper in the dermis there is a dense perieccrine lymphocytic infiltrate (H&E, 40×). (**d**) Neoplastic CD3+ T cells are present in the eccrine gland apparatus (CD3, 40×)

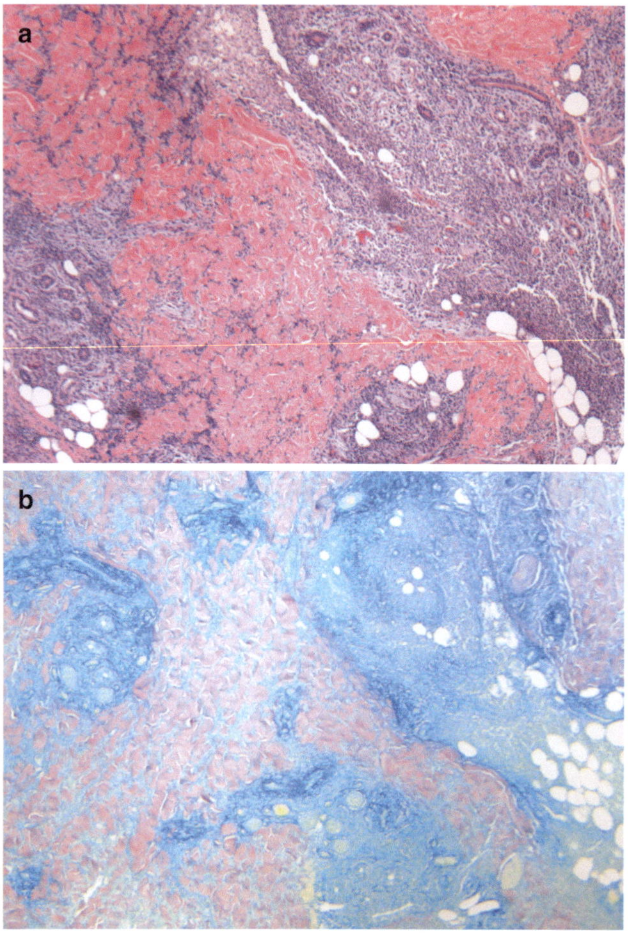

Fig. 5.18 Syringotropic MF (*patient featured in clinical case* 5.6). (**a**) Atypical lymphocytes overrun the eccrine apparatus (H&E, 4×). (**b**) Mucin is present in the dermis and eccrine apparatus (colloidal iron, 4×)

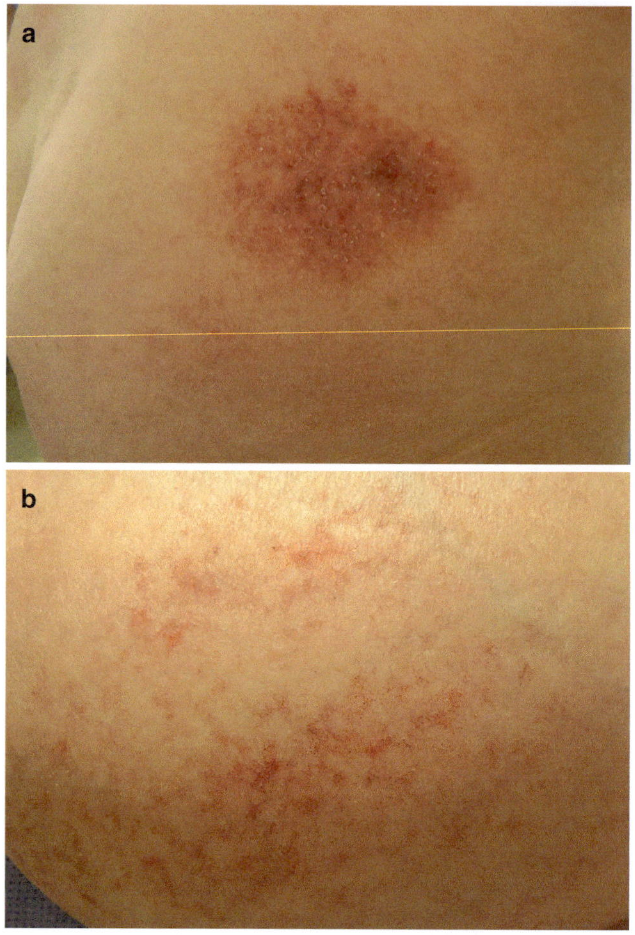

Fig. 5.19 Poikilodermatous (MF). (**a**) A 5 cm poikilodermatous patch with hyperpigmentation, hypopigmentation, and telangiectasias on the buttock of a 75-year-old woman. (**b**) Patches of delicate reticulate erythema are present on the lateral aspect of the same patient's breast

5.3.6 Poikilodermatous MF

Poikilodermatous MF impacts approximately 11 % of patients with MF and is clinically characterized by lesions with alternating hyperpigmentation, hypopigmentation, atrophy, and telangiectasias (Fig. 5.19) [17]. Areas of poikiloderma often develop slowly at the site of other classic MF patches or in areas of chronic friction. Presentation with isolated poikiloderma is possible [17].

Poikilodermatous MF is histopathologically identical to longstanding plaque or patch stage MF [17]. Additional findings include atrophy of the epidermis with flattening or loss of the rete, moderate vacuolization of the basal layer keratinocytes at the dermoepidermal junction, pigment loss, numerous papillary dermal melanophages, telangiectatic vessels, and superficial dermal scarring [17].

5.3.7 Granulomatous MF

Granulomatous MF (GMF) is a rare variant of MF that is often difficult to differentiate from benign granulomatous dermatitis or GSS. Patients typically present with patches and plaques of classic MF, some with atrophy of the skin.

This form of MF is characterized by a diffuse or nodular perivascular or periadnexal lymphocytic, dermal to subcutaneous infiltrate with extensive granuloma formation, numerous histiocytic giant cells, and minimal epidermotropism. Granulomas are typically present in a sarcoid-like pattern. In one study, 80 % of cases were CD4+ CD8−, with the remainder having a CD8+ phenotype. Clonal TCR is present in nearly all cases. Clinical correlation is needed to differentiate granulomatous MF from GSS; patients with granulomatous MF do not develop the pendulous skin folds characteristic of GSS [32, 37]. Patients with GMF have a worse prognosis than those with classic or folliculotropic MF, with a 5-year survival of 66 % [32].

5.4 Differential Diagnosis

5.4.1 Diagnostic Considerations

The differential diagnosis of MF is extremely broad, particularly given the variety of clinical and histopathologic appearances of its many subtypes (*see* Fig. 5.4). In this section, the differential diagnoses are described separately for distinct subtypes of MF. As in all of clinical medicine, diagnosis necessitates a synthesis of clinical presentation and pathophysiology. Important clinical considerations include the clinical evolution of the disease, lesion morphology, and the distribution of lesions [7]. Histopathology, immunohistochemistry, and molecular studies are invaluable in diagnosing MF [7, 38]. Loss of CD2 and/or CD5 supports a diagnosis of MF.

5.4.2 Differential Diagnosis of Classic (Patch/Plaque/Tumor Stage) MF

The differential diagnosis for classic MF alone is quite broad, given the variation in clinical appearance and histopathology at different stages of the disease.

5.4.2.1 Psoriasis

Psoriasis is the most common clinical mimic of classic MF, given that both present with chronic, recurrent, sharply marginated, erythematous patches and plaques. However, in contrast to the lesions of MF, those of psoriasis classically demonstrate silvery-white scales and are located in a symmetric distribution on extensor surfaces [11, 39]. Erythrodermic psoriasis may also mimic MF. Patients with psoriasis may also develop psoriatic arthritis, which is absent in MF. In contrast to MF, psoriasis manifests with hyperkeratosis and parakeratosis, loss of the epidermal granular cell layer, epidermal acanthosis, elongation of the rete, numerous epidermal keratinocytic mitoses, neutrophilic exocytosis with the intraepidermal spongiform pustule of Kojog beneath the stratum corneum, Munro microabscesses within the stratum corneum, thinning of the suprapapillary epidermis, and vascular dilation [40]. While neutrophils may be present in the epidermis and stratum corneum in psoriasis, usually the mononuclear cells, including lymphocytes, are predominantly located in the dermis [40], and neither tagging of the dermoepidermal junction nor Pautrier microabscesses is present. While exocytosis may be seen, epidermotropism is not [41]. Of note, clonal rearrangements can be present in psoriasis [38]. Psoriasis is also an important consideration in the differential diagnosis for pagetoid reticulosis.

5.4.2.2 Atopic Dermatitis

This chronic inflammatory dermatitis often manifests with lichenified patches and is a common mimicker of patch stage/early MF. Atopic erythroderma may also mimic MF. In contrast to MF, the histopathology of chronic atopic dermatitis is characterized by spongiosis, lymphocytic exocytosis, parakeratosis over areas of spongiosis, and a mixed perivascular infiltrate of lymphocytes, histiocytes, and occasionally neutrophils and eosinophils. There may be considerable overlap with the histology of early MF. However, MF typically lacks spongiosis, and the immune infiltrate is primarily lymphocytic; additionally, the cerebriform cytology of lymphocytes in MF and the appearance of tagging and epidermotropism allow for the diagnosis.

5.4.2.3 Hypersensitivity Reactions to Ingested Antigens Such as Drugs

This reactive process is another common mimicker of early MF. There may be considerable overlap between some drug reactions and MF; indeed, MF-like drug hypersensitivity may be histologically indistinguishable from MF. Findings that favor a diagnosis of a hypersensitivity reaction include intraepidermal Langerhans cell microabscesses, keratinocyte dyskeratosis, and the presence of papillary dermal pigment-laden macrophages and eosinophils. Immunohistochemical staining may also be helpful in this differential diagnosis: in cases with a dominant intraepidermal population of cytologically banal CD8+ lymphocytes and a dermal infiltrate of CD4+ T cells, a diagnosis of hypersensitivity is favored. An intraepidermal and dermal infiltrate of purely CD4+ atypical cells favors a diagnosis of MF but may also be observed in MF-like hypersensitivity reactions. TCR rearrangement studies are not helpful because they may be clonal in both MF and hypersensitivity reactions [42].

5.4.2.4 T-Cell Dyscrasia

It often takes many years before a diagnosis of MF can be definitively established. In the interim, many patients are seen with idiopathic chronic dermatoses that relapse after topical treatment and have no known triggering event. Biopsies of these cutaneous lesions lack overtly malignant cytology, do not show loss of T-cell antigens, and do not show a constellation of histologic features that allow for a definitive diagnosis of MF. In retrospect these changes may histopathologically represent early MF, and a clonal TCR rearrangement may or may not be present. Although some of these lesions may ultimately evolve into cutaneous T-cell lymphoma, they are not predictive of this outcome [43]. Differentiating T-cell dyscrasias from overt malignancy can be exceedingly difficult and may require numerous biopsies over time.

5.4.2.5 Adult T-Cell Leukemia/Lymphoma (ATLL)

The histopathology of this HTLV-1-induced T-cell lymphoma can be nearly indistinguishable from that of MF. Common characteristics include epidermotropism and Pautrier microabscesses [44]. ATLL and MF can be differentiated on the basis of HTLV-1 positivity: ATLL is caused by HTLV-1, and the neoplastic cells (circulating and cutaneous) always demonstrate proviral integration, while MF has no known association with HTLV-1. Of note it is possible for patients with MF to be concomitant carriers of HTLV-1, especially in HTLV-1 endemic areas; direct PCR testing of skin lesions for proviral integration is necessary to correctly diagnose these patients [45, 46]. Immunohistochemistry may also be helpful—the cells of MF rarely express CD25, while those of ATLL are often positive for CD25 [17, 47]. Clinical presentation can also be invaluable in differentiating these lymphomas: while MF is indolent and progresses through classic patch, plaque, and tumor stages, acute ATLL is rapid, systemic, and aggressive. The chronic and smoldering forms of ATLL may be more difficult to distinguish from those of MF [46].

5.4.2.6 Lymphomatoid Papulosis (LyP), Type B

This form of LyP is commonly considered to be histopathologically "MF-like." LyP type B also presents with marked epidermotropism, and lesions of tumor stage MF can be very similar clinically to the larger ulcerated nodules of LyP. The clinical presentation often distinguishes these entities, with MF showing an evolution from patch, plaque, to tumor stage versus the self-resolving papules of LyP. Differentiating LyP and MF can be complicated by the fact that patients with LyP are at increased risk of developing secondary lymphoid malignancies, including MF [48]. Although the papules of LyP regress spontaneously, the tumors of MF are persistent.

5.4.2.7 Sézary Syndrome

Although it is an uncommon occurrence, patients with MF may present with widespread erythroderma, clinically similar to that of Sézary syndrome. However, patients with erythrodermic MF typically have preceding clinical features that are classic for MF (e.g., patch-plaque-tumor progression) and lack of significant circulating atypical lymphocytes, whereas in Sézary syndrome patients have erythroderma, lymphadenopathy, and clonality and one or more of the following (1) loss of one or more pan–T-cell antigens, (2) Sezary cells greater than 1,000 cells/μL, or (3) CD4:CD8 ratio greater than 10:1 [17]. The skin biopsy in erythrodermic MF demonstrates more prominent parakeratosis, acanthosis, papillary dermal fibrosis, telangiectasia, and mitotic figures and has a more prominent atypical dermal infiltrate with more striking epidermotropism than is typically found in Sézary syndrome [17].

5.4.3 Differential Diagnosis of Adnexotropic (Folliculotropic and Syringotropic) MF

Given the unique presentation of the adnexotropic forms of MF, it is not surprising that the differential diagnosis for these malignancies differs significantly from that of classic MF. Folliculotropic MF can mimic an array of follicularly-based inflammatory conditions clinically and histopathologically.

5.4.3.1 Follicular Mucinosis (FM)

This nonspecific reactive epithelial condition can be extraordinarily difficult to distinguish from follicular MF given significant clinical and histopathologic overlap [49]. To further complicate the diagnosis, monoclonal populations of T cells may be present in either follicular MF or FM [1, 49], and FM may precede development of follicular MF [49]. Patients with FM are typically young and have areas of alopecia histologically characterized by abundant mucin in hair follicles, hair follicle epithelial destruction, and marked lymphohistiocytic intrafollicular infiltrate [36, 38]. Follicular mucinosis may occur in a number of skin conditions, ranging from inflammatory to infectious to neoplastic [49]. While FM has a benign course and can go into complete remission, follicular MF has a moderate to poor prognosis. Abundant mucin may or may not be present in the follicular epithelium in follicular MF, and biopsies show a dense perifollicular and intrafollicular infiltrate of neoplastic cerebriform T cells [1, 27].

5.4.3.2 Alopecia Areata (AA)

This common form of nonscarring alopecia is a key element in the clinical differential diagnosis for follicular MF and a common misdiagnosis [38]. AA is a lymphocyte-mediated autoimmune condition that presents with round or oval smooth patches of alopecia with a surrounding rim of "exclamation-mark" hairs. Follicular MF often occurs with destruction of hair follicles and loss of hair in circumscribed areas. These can be differentiated on histology: AA shows a classic peribulbar lymphohistiocytic infiltrate ("swarm of bees"), miniaturization of hair follicles, and pigment incontinence [50] but lacks the follicular mucin and atypical neoplastic T-cell infiltrate of follicular MF.

5.4.4 Differential Diagnosis of Granulomatous Slack Skin (GSS)

Because of the unique clinical appearance of GSS, the differential diagnosis is limited. The primary disease that must be distinguished on histopathology is granulomatous MF (see Sect. 5.3.3).

5.4.5 Differential Diagnosis of Granulomatous MF

The differential diagnosis for granulomatous MF includes entities that present with granuloma formation within the skin, including sarcoidosis, granuloma annulare, and other benign granulomatous dermatitis such as drug rash and bug bites. The presence of an aberrant T-cell immunophenotype with pan–T-cell antigen loss and cutaneous lesions characteristic of MF help to support the diagnosis of granulomatous MF.

5.4.6 Differential Diagnosis of Hypopigmented MF

The primary clinical considerations in the differential diagnosis for hypo- or hyperpigmented MF are conditions that cause local alteration in skin pigmentation, including vitiligo, pityriasis versicolor, pityriasis alba, and leprosy.

5.4.6.1 Vitiligo

This autoimmune skin condition is characterized by depigmented areas secondary to complete destruction and the absence of melanocytes. Although the depigmented areas may look similar to those of hypopigmented MF, clinically vitiligo usually lacks poikiloderma, scaling, or pruritus [7]. Unlike in vitiligo, hypopigmentation in MF is caused by abnormal function of melanocytes; they can still be seen on histologic examination [17, 34]. Additional clinical clues are that vitiligo may demonstrate koebnerization and enhancement of the lesion on Wood's lamp examination, characteristics absent in MF [51]. In vitiligo, immunohistochemical stains reveal an absence of intraepidermal melanocytes and no basal layer keratinocytic pigmentation on Fontana stain.

5.4.6.2 Tinea Versicolor

This benign, chronic, noninflammatory, superficial colonization of the stratum corneum by *Malassezia* spp. yeasts presents with hypo- or hyperpigmented macules and patches on the face, arms, and trunk with fine scaling. Delicate hyphal forms and numerous yeast ("spaghetti and meatballs") are readily identified on potassium hydroxide preparation (KOH) or periodic acid–Schiff (PAS) stain [52].

5.4.6.3 Pityriasis Alba (PA)

This chronic dermatosis of childhood presents with white or pink irregular, scaly, well-demarcated patches that occur on the face in 50 % of cases [53]. While both PA and hypopigmented MF are seen in children [34], these conditions can be differentiated on the basis of clinical presentation and histology. PA and MF have very different distributions. Biopsies of pityriasis alba show irregular pigmentation of the basal layer, follicular plugging, follicular spongiosis, and atrophic sebaceous glands [54]. The atypical lymphoid infiltrate and epidermotropism of MF are not seen in PA.

5.4.7 Differential Diagnosis of Poikilodermatous MF

Poikilodermatous MF has a variegated appearance and must be distinguished from a number of other conditions that clinically manifest as acquired poikiloderma [38, 55]. These include the connective tissue disease and iatrogenic conditions such as overuse of topical steroids and radiation dermatitis.

5.4.7.1 Dermatomyositis

The late phase of this connective tissue disease may present with poikiloderma of sun-exposed skin such as on the neck or central upper back (including the classic shawl sign). Histopathologically there is epidermal atrophy, interface dermatitis, increased dermal mucin (identified on colloidal iron or alcian blue stain), telangiectasia, and a sparse inflammatory infiltrate without the atypical T-cell infiltrate and epidermotropism of MF [55].

5.4.7.2 Overuse of Topical Steroids

Overuse of topical steroids can cause thinning of the skin and telangiectasias, leading to a poikilodermatous appearance. Although clinical history will typically yield the correct diagnosis, this may be complicated by the fact that MF is frequently treated with topical steroids. A skin biopsy will not show the atypical T-cell infiltrate and epidermotropism of MF.

5.4.7.3 Radiation Dermatitis

Although iatrogenic exposure to radiation may result in poikilodermatous changes in the skin, this is usually readily differentiated from MF on the basis of clinical history.

5.4.8 Differential Diagnosis of Pigmented Purpuric Variant of MF

This heterogeneous group of dermatoses manifests with petechiae and bronze discoloration of the skin, most often on the lower legs, and can be difficult to distinguish from the rare pigmented purpuric variant of MF. PPD can be subdivided into a number of conditions, including Schamberg disease, Majocchi purpura, Gougerot-Blum purpura, lichen aureus, and eczematid purpura of Doucas and Kapetanakis. Histopathologically, pigmentary purpura is characterized by the presence of papillary dermal pigment-laden macrophages, erythrocyte extravasation, endothelial cell swelling of small superficial dermal vessels, and a lymphoid infiltrate with variable numbers of histiocytes that may be lichenoid or perivascular. It may also be associated with epidermal changes, including spongiosis and parakeratosis. Differentiation from the pigmented purpuric variant of MF may be difficult given that approximately half of cases of PPD are associated with a clonal rearrangement of the TCR [56]. Cellular atypia may be also be present [56].

5.5 Clinical Cases

Case 5.1 Patch/Plaque MF

A 56-year old man with a history of eczematous dermatitis since childhood, previously managed with topical steroids, presented with pruritic, diffuse, light pink scaly patches covering 30–40 % of his body surface area, including the chest, abdomen, axillae, medial upper arms, upper thighs, and buttocks (see Fig. 5.1a). He reported that these plaques worsened in the winter. In the past the plaques had improved with sun exposure, but recently his symptoms had persisted despite sun exposure. Physical examination revealed numerous scaly pruritic patches and thin plaques in a photoprotected distribution.

A biopsy performed 7 years prior had shown a superficial perivascular and papillary dermal lymphocytic infiltrate with minimal cytologic atypica, consistent with mild chronic eczematous dermatitis or an evolving T-cell dyscrasia.

A new biopsy of one of the plaques was performed and revealed a lichenoid lymphocytic infiltrate with tagging of the dermoepidermal junction, significant epidermotropism, and notable cytologic atypia. The intraepidermal lymphocytes were almost exclusively CD3+ CD4+ T cells with loss of CD2 (*see* Fig. 5.5). A CT scan and a complete blood count were performed and showed no evidence of systemic disease. The patient was diagnosed with stage 1B MF.

Total clearing of truncal MF patches was achieved with narrow band ultraviolet-B (NBUVB) phototherapy and topical triamcinolone.

Comment This case of classic patch/plaque stage MF illustrates several important points about disease progression in MF. First, many patients may carry a diagnosis of eczema or chronic dermatitis for decades before they are diagnosed with MF. Second, initial biopsies may be nonspecific, and patients may require multiple biopsies to finally receive a diagnosis. Third, this disease occurs in a bathing suit distribution (in this case the chest, abdomen, axillae, medial upper arms, upper thighs, and buttocks) and is often ameliorated by sunlight.

Case 5.2 MF with LCT

A 70-year-old man presented with a 1-year history of right eyelid swelling and a 3-week history of a new 3-cm indurated plaque by his right eye. Biopsy of the right eye lesion revealed a dense infiltrate of large lymphoid cells expressing CD3, CD4, CD5, and TCR gamma and lacking CD30; the patient was diagnosed with cutaneous T-cell lymphoma, not otherwise specified (CTCL-NOS) and treated with surgical debulking and radiation.

After treatment, he remained disease-free for 4 years. However, he then developed a new nodule in his right eyebrow (*see* Fig. 5.4a) as well as pink scaly patches and smooth dome-shaped papules on his bilateral thighs; the papules on his left thigh progressively enlarged to become violaceous-to-black nodules coalescing into plaques (*see* Fig. 5.4b). This was accompanied by the rapid development of numerous violaceous nodules on the abdomen and chest (*see* Fig 5.4c). Several biopsies were performed. Biopsy of the eyebrow revealed a dense dermal infiltrate with numerous CD30+ large cells and focal folliculotropism, accompanied by atypical CD3+ T cells with irregular nuclei and moderately abundant cytoplasm. Polymerase chain reaction (PCR) revealed a clonal T-cell receptor (TCR). Biopsy of the thigh lesions showed a diffuse dermal infiltrate with epidermal sparing, composed of medium to large lymphoid cells with moderate pale cytoplasm, oval to irregular nuclei, vesicular chromatin, frequent mitoses, and focal necrosis. The atypical cells expressed CD3, CD4, CD5, and CD7. The neoplastic cells lacked expression of CD8, CD30, ALK1, and CD20, consistent with the characteristics a T-cell lymphoma, particularly MF (*see* Fig. 5.8). In spite of the marked variation in the pattern of lymphoid infiltrate and the immunohistochemical staining patterns of the neoplastic cells between the leg and eyebrow lesions, they both showed the same clonal TCR gene rearrangement, suggesting that both represented the same disease process.

Serial CT scans demonstrated no metastatic disease, while flow cytometry revealed the development of a circulating population of neoplastic cells with the same TCR gene rearrangement as those in the skin. The patient was ultimately diagnosed with MF with CD30+ LCT with a small circulating component.

Despite treatment with radiation, methotrexate, targeted therapies, and chemotherapy, the patient's disease continued to progress. Nine years after initial presentation, he died of complications of his MF with LCT.

Comment This case of MF with CD30+ LCT underscores the aggressiveness and poor prognosis associated with LCT. It also highlights the utility of clonality studies in determining if separate lesions are part of the same disease process.

Case 5.3 Folliculotropic MF

A 31-year-old female with an 8-year history of diffuse plaques and pruritus presented with worsening pruritus and increasing plaque thickness and size. Physical examination showed a well-demarcated light pink thin plaque on the right cheek as well as countless diffuse flesh-colored 1-mm follicular papules coalescing into arcuate plaques with alopecia centrally on her arms, back, abdomen, and buttocks (*see* Fig. 5.10). There was no evidence of tumors, nodules, or patches.

Previous biopsy performed 8 years prior revealed mucinous degeneration of the follicular epithelium with a moderately dense superficial and deep perivascular, periadnexal, and perifollicular lymphohistiocytic infiltrate of CD3+ CD5+ CD2+ T cells. Clonal rearrangement of the TCR and immunoglobulin heavy chains was absent. These findings were thus consistent with follicular mucinosis but insufficient for a diagnosis of MF. A repeat biopsy yielded similar results, again insufficient for a diagnosis of MF.

Because of progressive disease despite use of retinoids and phototherapy, a biopsy of her flank was performed and revealed a perivascular and periadnexal atypical lymphoid infiltrate with hair follicle infiltration (pilotropism), disruption of the follicles, and follicular mucin. Significant epidermotropism and Pautrier microabscesses were noted. Immunohistochemical studies revealed the lymphocytes infiltrating the hair follicle to be CD3+ CD4+ T cells with partial loss of CD7 and intact expression of CD2 and CD5. The patient was diagnosed with follicular MF.

She is currently controlled with combination therapy, including bexarotene, PUVA, methotrexate, and intermittent radiation therapy.

Comment This case of follicular MF highlights the variability clinical and histopathologic presentations of MF; one of the major features of this type of MF, which is absent in other types, is the accumulation of mucin within the hair follicles. As with case 5.1, this case demonstrates that it often takes years and multiple biopsies to finally achieve a diagnosis. This patient's clinical course also exhibits the fact that follicular MF may be preceded by follicular mucinosis. Finally, follicular MF can be more recalcitrant to therapy than patch-plaque stage MF.

Case 5.4 Granulomatous Slack Skin (GSS)

An 18-year-old man presented with an 8-year history of pruritus and eczematous-appearing plaques on the forearms and buttocks. In spite of the administration of topical corticosteroids and tacrolimus, over the last year he had developed tender, draining cystic nodules within the eczematous plaque on his buttock, without evidence of any infectious etiology. Physical examination was notable for a confluent, slightly hyperpigmented, reddish-brownish plaque comprised of multiple raised and slightly boggy papules with some overlying scale on the lateral arm. On the lateral aspect of the right buttock a slightly atrophic, shiny red plaque with overlying fine scale was seen. On the medial aspect of the buttock there was a dense infiltrative, violaceous, confluent plaque and an outpouching of pendulous, infiltrated skin with underlying induration (*see* Fig. 5.14b).

A skin biopsy of the right buttock revealed a dense superficial and deep dermal granulomatous infiltrate of atypical lymphoid cells with focal epidermotropism, prominent folliculotropism, and perivascular and periadnexal extension. The infiltrate was composed of small-to-medium sized cells with ovoid to irregular nuclei, variably condensed chromatin, distinct nucleoli, and moderate pale eosinophilic cytoplasm. These cells stained positively for CD3, CD4, and CD5, with some loss of CD7 and focal CD25 positivity. Elastophagocytosis was not seen. A clonal TCR rearrangement was present. Flow cytometry, CBC, and LDH were all within normal limits, and a CT scan of his chest, abdomen, and pelvis revealed no evidence of internal disease. In combination with the clinical presentation, this was consistent with a diagnosis of GSS.

The patient was subsequently treated with PUVA and electron beam therapy in combination with bexarotene and mupirocin, which improved the cutaneous disease.

Comment GSS is a rare variant of MF with an indolent course; this patient had disease for almost a decade without evidence of extracutaneous involvement. As in this patient, the pendulous skin folds tend to occur in the gluteal, inguinal, and axillary regions. As showcased here, diagnosis of GSS necessitates a combination of clinical information and histopathology.

Case 5.5 Hypopigmented MF

A 28-year-old man presented with a 3-year history of progressive, minimally pruritic hypopigmented patches on his hips, trunk, inguinal region, buttocks, inner thighs, and left axilla (*see* Fig. 5.15). He reported a 23-year history of similar hypopigmented macules and patches in a bathing-suit distribution. He noted that he had previously been treated with PUVA for 4 years, with complete resolution of all lesions; however, 4 years after cessation of treatment, asymptomatic truncal lesions with increased erythema began to reappear. Physical examination was notable for scaly, hypopigmented patches and plaques with faint erythema covering 6–8 % of his body surface area.

A punch biopsy of the plaque on his thigh revealed a superficial dermal lymphoid infiltrate composed of small- to medium-sized CD8+ T-cells with epidermotropism and tagging along the dermoepidermal junction. In combination with his clinical presentation, this was consistent with a diagnosis of hypopigmented MF.

Comment Hypopigmented MF is a rare entity usually found in children. In addition, the T cells of hypopigmented MF often have a CD8+ phenotype.

Case 5.6 Syringotropic MF

A 68-year-old man with CLL presented with a 5-year history of painful, debilitating, pruritic bilateral foot dermatitis, previously diagnosed as dyshidrotic eczema or allergic contact dermatitis. He had seen more than ten dermatologists and underwent patch testing four to five times. Despite treatment with topical steroids, lotrisone, griseofulvin, NBUVB, PUVA, and topical tacrolimus, the blistering had become so severe that he was unable to walk. Clinical examination showed large, oozing, painful, malodorous erosions with areas of crusting and innumerable small pustules and vesicles covering the soles of his feet (*see* Fig. 5.16). His nails were dystrophic with anonychia of the left great toe.

An initial biopsy was consistent with dyshidrotic eczema with severe hypersensitivity reaction. However, repeat biopsy showed dense predominantly dermal lymphocytic infiltrate with extension into adipose tissue and skeletal muscle, and focal epidermo- and syringotropism (*see* Fig. 5.17). The atypical neoplastic cells were small to intermediate with irregular nuclei and condensed chromatin. The atypical lymphoid infiltrate is comprised predominantly of T cells showing reactivity for CD3, CD5, and CD4 with loss of CD7; approximately 20 % of cells were positive for CD30, but all were ALK-negative. A PET scan revealed mildly 18-fluoro-deoxyglucose (FDG)-avid left external iliac and inguinal lymph nodes. The patient was diagnosed with syringotrophic MF, worrisome for early LCT.

The patient received two fractions of electron beam therapy to the left foot and had complete resolution of his disease. Two years later he is without recurrence and has been able to resume his normal activities.

Comment This case demonstrates the remarkable efficacy of radiation therapy seen in many cases of localized MF. While other treatments had been ineffective, radiation therapy resolved this patient's disease within two treatments.

References

1. Ralfkiaer E, Cerroni L, Sander CA, Smoller BR, Willemze R. Mycosis fungoides. In: Swerdlow SH, Campo E, Harris NL, Jaffe ES, Pileri SA, Stein H, et al., editors. WHO classification of tumours of haematopoietic and lymphoid tissues. 4th ed. Lyon: International Agency for Research on Cancer; 2008. p. 296–8.
2. Bradford PT, Devesa SS, Anderson WF, Toro JR. Cutaneous lymphoma incidence patterns in the United States: a population-based study of 3884 cases. Blood. 2009;113:5064–73.
3. Willenze R, Jaffees, Burg G, Cerroni L, Berti E, Swerdlow Sh et al. WHO/EORTC classification for Cutaneous Lymphomas. Blood 2005;105:3768–85.
4. Yazganoglu KD, Topkarci Z, Buyukbabani N, Baykal C. Childhood mycosis fungoides: a report of 20 cases from Turkey. J Eur Acad Dermatol Venereol. 2013;27:295–300.
5. Kim YH, Liu HL, Mraz-Gernhard S, Varghese A, Hoppe RT. Long-term outcome of 525 patients with mycosis fungoides and Sezary syndrome: clinical prognostic factors and risk for disease progression. Arch Dermatol. 2003;139:857–66.
6. Marks JG, Miller JJ. In: Marks JG, Miller JJ, editors. Scaling papules, plaques and patches. Lookingbill and Marks' principles of dermatology. 4th ed. Philadelphia: Saunders Elsevier. p. 134–5.
7. Pimpinelli N, Olsen EA, Santucci M, Vonderheid E, Haeffner AC, Stevens S, et al. Defining early mycosis fungoides. J Am Acad Dermatol. 2005;53:1053–63.
8. Ralfkiaer E, Willemze R, Whittaker SJ, et al. Sezary syndrome. In: Swerdlow SH, Campo E, Harris NL, Jaffe ES, Pileri SA, Stein H, editors. WHO classification of tumours of haematopoietic and lymphoid tissues. 4th ed. Lyon: International Agency for Research on Cancer; 2008. p. 299.
9. Vergier B, De Muret A, Beylot-barry M, Vaillant L, Ekouevi D, Chene G, et al. Transformation of mycosis fungoides: clinicopathological and prognostic features of 45 cases. Blood. 2000;95:2212–8.

10. Agar NS, Wedgeworth E, Crichton S, Mitchell TJ, Cox M, Ferreira S, et al. Survival outcomes and prognostic factors in mycosis fungoides/Sézary syndrome: validation of the revised International Society for Cutaneous Lymphomas/European Organisation for Research and Treatment of Cancer staging proposal. J Clin Oncol. 2010;28:4730–9.
11. Hwang S, Janik J, Jaffe E, Wilson W. Mycosis fungoides and Sézary syndrome. Lancet. 2008;371:945–57.
12. Olsen E, Vonderheid E, Pimpinelli N, Willemze R, Kim Y, Knobler R, et al. Revisions to the staging and classification of mycosis fungoides and Sezary syndrome: a proposal of the International Society for Cutaneous Lymphomas (ISCL) and the cutaneous lymphoma task force of the European Organization of Research and Treatment of Ca. Blood. 2007;110:1713–22.
13. Benner MF, Jansen PM, Vermeer MH, Willemze R. Prognostic factors in transformed mycosis fungoides: a retrospective analysis of 100 cases. Blood. 2012;119:1643–9.
14. Molina A, Zain J, Arber DA, Angelopolou M, O'Donnell M, Murata-Collins J, et al. Durable clinical, cytogenetic, and molecular remissions after allogeneic hematopoietic cell transplantation for refractory Sezary syndrome and mycosis fungoides. J Clin Oncol. 2005;23:6163–71.
15. Abbott RA, Whittaker SJ, Morris SL, Russell-Jones R, Hung T, Bashir SJ, et al. Bexarotene therapy for mycosis fungoides and Sézary syndrome. Br J Dermatol. 2009;160:1299–307.
16. Talpur R, Singh L, Daulat S, Liu P, Seyfer S, Trynosky T, et al. Long-term outcomes of 1,263 patients with mycosis fungoides and Sézary syndrome from 1982 to 2009. Clin Cancer Res. 2012;18:5051–60.
17. Kazakov DV, Burg G, Kempf W. Clinicopathological spectrum of mycosis fungoides. J Eur Acad Dermatol Venereol. 2004;18:397–415.
18. Vega F, Luthra R, Medeiros LJ, Dunmire V, Lee S-J, Duvic M, et al. Clonal heterogeneity in mycosis fungoides and its relationship to clinical course. Blood. 2002;100:3369–73.
19. Van Doorn R, van Kester MS, Dijkman R, Vermeer MH, Mulder AA, Szuhai K, et al. Oncogenomic analysis of mycosis fungoides reveals major differences with Sezary syndrome. Blood. 2009;113:127–36.
20. Carbone A, Bernardini L, Valenzano F, Bottillo I, De Simone C, Capizzi R, et al. Array-based comparative genomic hybridization in early-stage mycosis fungoides: recurrent deletion of tumor suppressor genes BCL7A, SMAC/DIABLO, and RHOF. Genes Chromosomes Cancer. 2008;47:1067–75.
21. Fischer TC, Gellrich S, Muche JM, Sherev T, Audring H, Neitzel H, et al. Genomic aberrations and survival in cutaneous T cell lymphomas. J Invest Dermatol. 2004;122:579–86.
22. Gallardo F, Esteller M, Pujol RM, Costa C, Estrach T, Servitje O. Methylation status of the p15, p16 and MGMT promoter genes in primary cutaneous T-cell lymphomas. Haematologica. 2004;89:1401–3.
23. Mao X, Lillington D, Scarisbrick JJ, Mitchell T, Czepulkowski B, Russell-Jones R, et al. Molecular cytogenetic analysis of cutaneous T-cell lymphomas: identification of common genetic alterations in Sézary syndrome and mycosis fungoides. Br J Dermatol. 2002;147:464–75.
24. Navas IC, Ortiz-Romero PL, Villuendas R, Martínez P, García C, Gómez E, et al. p16(INK4a) gene alterations are frequent in lesions of mycosis fungoides. Am J Pathol. 2000;156:1565–72.
25. Prochazkova M, Chevret E, Mainhaguiet G, Sobotka J, Vergier B, Belaud-Rotureau M-A, et al. Common chromosomal abnormalities in mycosis fungoides transformation. Genes Chromosomes Cancer. 2007;46:828–38.
26. Scarisbrick JJ, Mitchell TJ, Calonje E, Orchard G, Russell-Jones R, Whittaker SJ. Microsatellite instability is associated with hypermethylation of the hMLH1 gene and reduced gene expression in mycosis fungoides. J Invest Dermatol. 2003;121:894–901.
27. Van Doorn R, Scheffer E, Willemze R. Follicular mycosis fungoides, a distinct disease entity with or without associated follicular mucinosis. Arch Dermatol. 2002;138:191–8.
28. Lehman J, Cook-Norris RH, Weed BR, Weenig RH, Gibson LE, Weaver AL, et al. Folliculotropic mycosis fungoides: single-center study and systematic review. Arch Dermatol. 2010;146:607–13.
29. Tannous Z, Baldassano MF, Li VW, Kvedar J, Duncan LM. Syringolymphoid hyperplasia and follicular mucinosis in a patient with cutaneous T-cell lymphoma. J Am Acad Dermatol. 1999;41:303–8.
30. Haghighi B, Smoller BR, LeBoit PE, Warnke RA, Sander CA, Kohler S. Pagetoid reticulosis (Woringer-Kolopp disease): an immunophenotypic, molecular, and clinicopathologic study. Mod Pathol. 2000;13:502–10.
31. Steffen C. Ketron-Goodman disease, Woringer-Kolopp disease, and pagetoid reticulosis. Am J Dermatopathol. 2005;27:68–85.
32. Kempf W, Ostheeren-michaelis S, Paulli M, Lucioni M, Wechsler J, Audring H, et al. Granulomatous mycosis fungoides and granulomatous slack skin. Arch Dermatol. 2008;144:1609–17.
33. Kempf W, Kazakov DV, Palmedo G, Fraitag S, Schaerer L, Kutzner H. Pityriasis lichenoides et varioliformis acuta with numerous CD30(+) cells: a variant mimicking lymphomatoid papulosis and other cutaneous lymphomas. A clinicopathologic, immunohistochemical, and molecular biological study of 13 cases. Am J Surg Pathol. 2012;36:1021–9.
34. Ardigó M, Borroni G, Muscardin L, Kerl H, Cerroni L. Hypopigmented mycosis fungoides in Caucasian patients: a clinicopathologic study of 7 cases. J Am Acad Dermatol. 2003;49:264–70.
35. Pavlovsky L, Mimouni D, Amitay-Laish I, Feinmesser M, David M, Hodak E. Hyperpigmented mycosis fungoides: an unusual variant of cutaneous T-cell lymphoma with a frequent CD8+ phenotype. J Am Acad Dermatol. 2012;67:69–75. Elsevier Inc.
36. Pileri A, Facchetti F, Rütten A, Zumiani G, Boi S, Fink-Puches R, et al. Syringotropic mycosis fungoides: a rare variant of the disease with peculiar clinicopathologic features. Am J Surg Pathol. 2011;35:100–9.
37. Scarabello A, Leinweber B. Cutaneous lymphomas with prominent granulomatous reaction: a potential pitfall in the histopathologic diagnosis of cutaneous T-and B-cell lymphomas. Am J Surg Pathol. 2002;26:1259–68.
38. Nashan D, Faulhaber D, Ständer S, Luger TA, Stadler R. Mycosis fungoides: a dermatological masquerader. Br J Dermatol. 2007;156:1–10.
39. Johnson MAN, Armstrong AW. Clinical and histologic diagnostic guidelines for psoriasis: a critical review. Clin Rev Allergy Immunol. 2013;44:166–72.
40. Griffiths C, Barker J. Pathogenesis and clinical features of psoriasis. Lancet. 2007;270:263–71.
41. Fung MA. "Epidermotropism" vs. "exocytosis" of lymphocytes 101: definition of terms. J Cutan Pathol. 2010;37:525–9.
42. Brady SP, Magro CM, Diaz-Cano SJ, Wolfe HJ. Analysis of clonality of atypical cutaneous lymphoid infiltrates associated with drug therapy by PCR/DGGE. Hum Pathol. 1999;30:130–6.
43. Guitart J, Magro C. Cutaneous T-cell lymphoid dyscrasia. Arch Dermatol. 2014;143:921–32.
44. Matutes E. Adult T-cell leukaemia/lymphoma. J Clin Pathol. 2007;60:1373–7.

45. Yamaguchi T, Ohshima K, Karube K, Tutiya T, Kawano R, Suefuji H, et al. Clinicopathological features of cutaneous lesions of adult T-cell leukaemia/lymphoma. Br J Dermatol. 2005;152:76–81.
46. Jaffe E, Cossman J, Blattner W, Robert-Guroff M, Blayney D, Gallo RC, et al. The pathologic spectrum of adult T-cell leukemia/lymphoma in the United States. Am J Surg Pathol. 1984;8:263–75.
47. Tsukasaki K, Hermine O, Bazarbachi A, Ratner L, Ramos JC, Harrington W, et al. Definition, prognostic factors, treatment, and response criteria of adult T-cell leukemia-lymphoma: a proposal from an international consensus meeting. J Clin Oncol. 2009;27:453–9.
48. Kunishige JH, McDonald H, Alvarez G, Johnson M, Prieto V, Duvic M. Lymphomatoid papulosis and associated lymphomas: a retrospective case series of 84 patients. Clin Exp Dermatol. 2009;34:576–81.
49. Cerroni L, Fink-Puches R, Back B, Kerl H. Follicular mucinosis: a critical reappraisal of clinicopathologic features and associated with mycosis fungoides and Sezary syndrome. Arch Dermatol. 2002;138:182–9.
50. Madani S, Shapiro J. Alopecia areata update. J Am Acad Dermatol. 2000;42:549–66.
51. Zhang J-A, Yu J-B. Hypopigmented mycosis fungoides in a Chinese woman. Indian J Dermatol. 2013;58:161.
52. Mendez-Tovar LJ. Pathogenesis of dermatophytosis and tinea versicolor. Clin Dermatol. 2010;28:185–9.
53. Blessmann Weber M, Sponchiado de Avila LG, Albaneze R, Magalhães de Oliveira OL, Sudhaus BD, Cestari TF. Pityriasis alba: a study of pathogenic factors. J Eur Acad Dermatol Venereol. 2002;16:463–8.
54. Vargas-Ocampo F. Pityriasis alba: a histologic study. Int J Dermatol. 1993;32:870–3.
55. Nofal A, Salah E. Acquired poikiloderma: proposed classification and diagnostic approach. J Am Acad Dermatol. 2013;69:e129–40.
56. Magro CM, Schaefer JT, Crowson AN, Li J, Morrison C. Pigmented purpuric dermatosis: classification by phenotypic and molecular profiles. Am J Clin Pathol. 2007;128:218–29.

6 Sézary Syndrome

Amrita Goyal, Joi B. Carter, Aliyah R. Sohani, Jeffrey A. Barnes, Mai P. Hoang, and Lyn McDivitt Duncan

Sézary syndrome is a rare leukemia with a median survival of 3 years. Sézary syndrome patients comprise less than 5 % of all patients with cutaneous T-cell malignancies. Patients present with a triad of symptoms: erythroderma, generalized lymphadenopathy, and a clonal neoplastic proliferation of T cells with cerebriform nuclei in the peripheral blood. They commonly experience intense pruritus and significant derangements of cellular and humoral immunity. Diagnosis is based on clinical presentation, flow cytometric analysis, and histopathology. This chapter discusses the clinical presentation, prognosis, treatment, histopathology, immunophenotype, and differential diagnosis of Sézary syndrome. It closes with two clinical cases, including clinical images, histopathology, and flow cytometry.

A. Goyal, M.D.
Harvard-MIT Division of Health Sciences and Technology, Harvard Medical School, Boston, MA, USA

J.B. Carter, M.D.
Department of Dermatology, Massachusetts General Hospital, Harvard Medical School, Boston, MA, USA

A.R. Sohani, M.D.
Hematopathology Service, Department of Pathology, Massachusetts General Hospital, Harvard Medical School, Boston, MA, USA

J.A. Barnes, M.D., Ph.D.
Comprehensive Cutaneous Lymphoma Program, Department of Medicine, Massachusetts General Hospital Cancer Center, Boston, MA, USA

M.P. Hoang, M.D. • L.M. Duncan, MD (✉)
Dermatopathology Service, Department of Pathology, Massachusetts General Hospital, Harvard Medical School, Boston, MA, USA
e-mail: duncan@helix.mgh.harvard.edu

6.1 Clinical

6.1.1 Clinical Presentation

Sézary syndrome, a rare T-cell leukemia, presents with the triad of erythroderma (erythema of >80 % of body surface area; Figs. 6.1 and 6.2), generalized lymphadenopathy, and a clonal proliferation of neoplastic T cells with cerebriform nuclei (Sézary cells) (Fig. 6.3) [1, 2]. This disease makes up 1–5 % of all cutaneous T-cell malignancies and primarily impacts people over the age of 60; men are affected twice as often as women [3]. Sézary syndrome has a very poor prognosis [1, 2].

A significant proportion of patients experience disabling, intractable pruritus that is refractory to medication. The negative impact on quality of life of this symptom cannot be overstated [2, 4]. Other possible symptoms include alopecia (*see* Fig. 6.1a), onychodystrophy (*see* Fig. 6.2b), palmar and plantar hyperkeratosis, and ocular symptoms, including ectropion and blepharoconjunctivitis [1, 5, 6]. Sézary syndrome is a leukemia and thus a generalized disease. The skin and/or any visceral organ can be involved, but the bone marrow is typically spared. Peripheral blood eosinophilia is common.

Patients with Sézary syndrome may demonstrate significant immune suppression; many ultimately succumb to opportunistic infection [1, 7]. The immune dysfunction seen in patients is multifactorial. Patients show decreased T-cell repertoire diversity, a consequence of clonal expansion of malignant T cells and concomitant reduction in normal T-cell numbers, yielding impairment of adaptive immunity [8]. Patients also have significant dysregulation of innate immu-

J.B. Carter et al. (eds.), *Atlas of Cutaneous Lymphomas: Classification and Differential Diagnosis*,
DOI 10.1007/978-3-319-17217-0_6

nity owing to cytokines secreted by the Sézary cells, which may induce abnormalities in natural killer cells, neutrophils, and dendritic cell function [2, 5, 9]. These defects in adaptive and innate immunity result in dangerous immune suppression [10]. Decreased immune surveillance also results in increased risk of secondary malignancy [1, 7].

Of note, Sézary syndrome is frequently incorrectly called a "leukemic variant of mycosis fungoides." Although this misconception continues to be propagated in the literature, there is nearly indisputable evidence that Sézary syndrome and mycosis fungoides (MF) are biologically and clinically distinct entities. While the leukemic cells of Sézary syndrome are derived from circulating central memory T (T_{CM}) cells and possess a T_H2 phenotype, those of MF are derived from skin resident effector T cells with a T_H1 phenotype [11–13]. Unfortunately, much of the literature on cutaneous T-cell lymphoma groups MF and Sézary syndrome, confounding our understanding of the progression and prognosis of the syndrome.

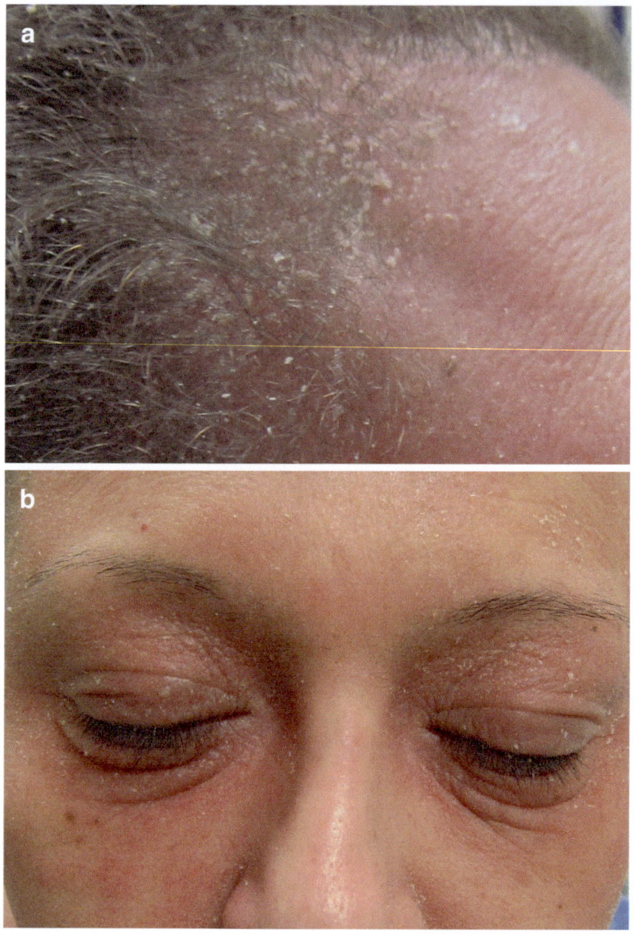

Fig. 6.1 Sézary syndrome, clinical photos from Case 6.1. (**a**) The patient's right temple shows erythema (a representative sample of her diffuse erythroderma), extensive desquamation and scale, and loss of hair. (**b**) Periorbital edema with diffuse erythema and fine scale. There is loss of hair in the right eyebrow

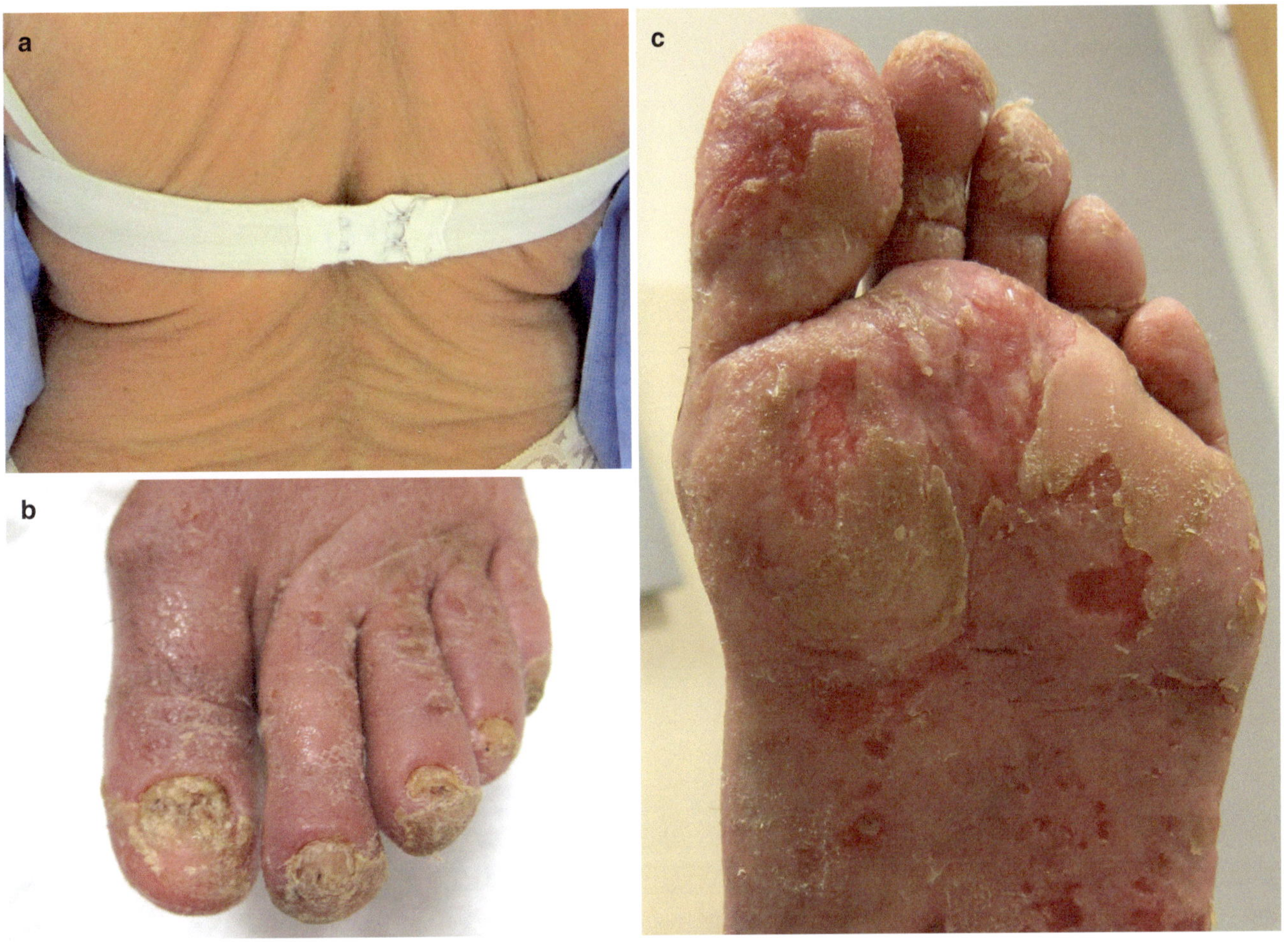

Fig. 6.2 Sézary syndrome, clinical photos from Case 6.2. On clinical examination this patient's skin was diffusely erythematous and thickened with prominent skin markings. (**a**) The patient's lower back shows folds of heavy, redundant skin. There was no involvement of the axillae or groin (not pictured). (**b**) The patient had marked onychodystrophy of all toenails and all fingernails. (**c**) Severe fissuring and desquamation of the skin was present on the hands and feet bilaterally

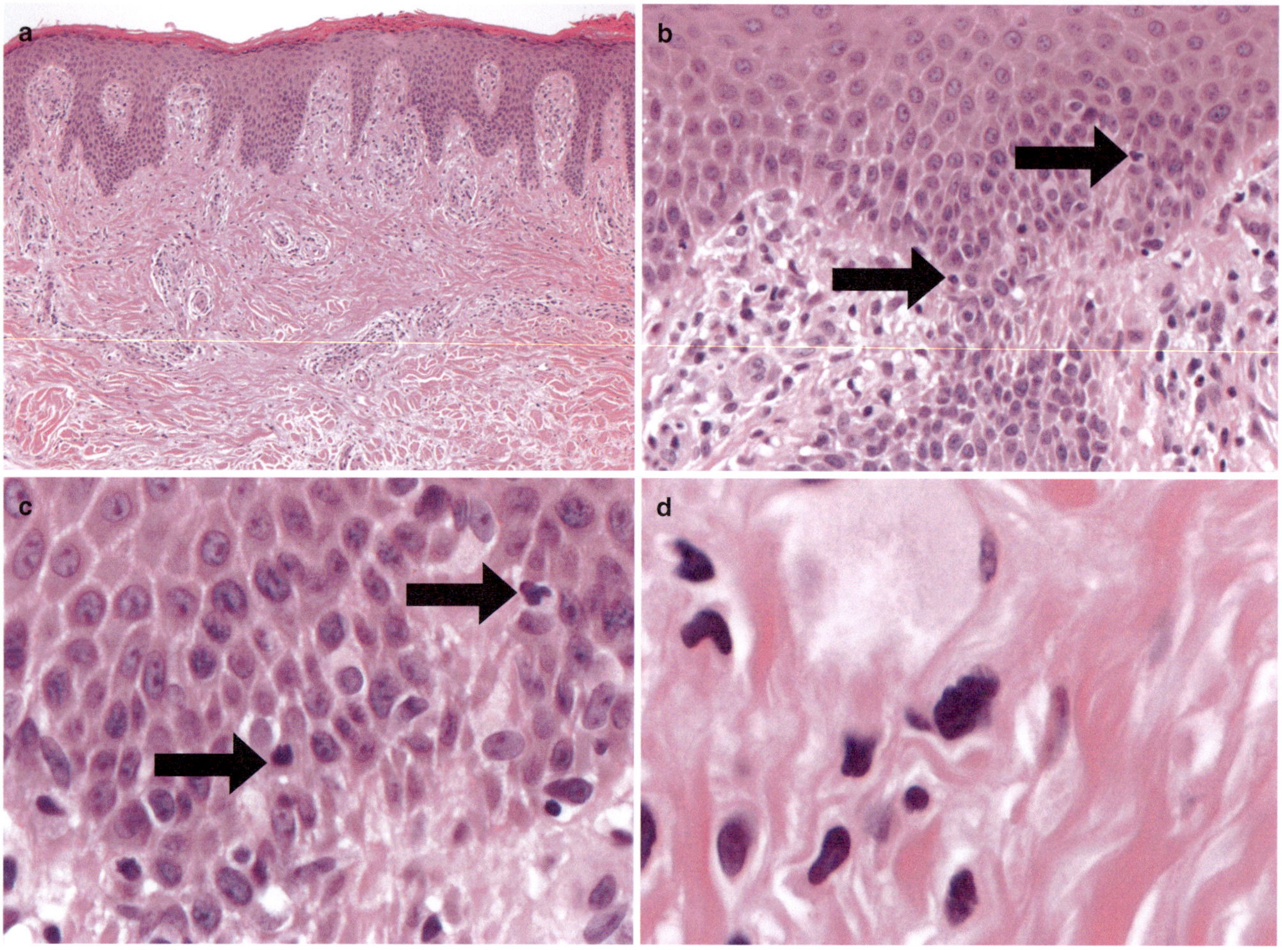

Fig. 6.3 Sézary syndrome, cutaneous biopsy from Case 6.2. (**a**) There is a sparse perivascular infiltrate of atypical lymphocytes (H&E, 10×). (**b**) Some epidermotropism is present, with occasional atypical T cells "tagging" the dermal-epidermal junction (*black arrows*) (H&E, 40×). (**c**) At higher power, the lymphocytes along the dermal-epidermal junction have with irregular nuclear contours (*black arrows*) (H&E, 40×). (**d**) The atypical T cells in the dermal infiltrate have markedly cerebriform nuclei (H&E, 63×)

6.1.2 Prognosis and Treatment

Even with treatment, Sézary syndrome has a dismal prognosis: patients have a median survival of 3 years [14] and a 5-year disease-specific survival of 10–33 % [1, 15].

Although research into the treatment of Sézary syndrome is a rapidly evolving, highly active field, few long-term effective treatments exist. Patients often have short-lived responses to therapy followed by rapid relapse, disease progression, and death. The majority of patients die from opportunistic infections secondary to dysfunction of the immune system induced by neoplastic cells [1, 2, 5]. This disease is rarely curable, and treatment is largely considered palliative [5, 7, 16]. Moreover, many treatments may not resolve the debilitating pruritus experienced by a large proportion of patients [2].

Treatment may incorporate skin-directed therapies [17], immunomodulators [18–21], biologics [22–25], antifolate agents [26, 27], or combinations thereof. Single-agent or multiagent chemotherapy with cyclophosphamide, doxorubicin, vincristine, and prednisone (CHOP) or CHOP-like regimens have also been used [2]. Hematopoietic stem cell transplant (HSCT) holds significant promise as definitive therapy for Sézary syndrome. One large multicenter retrospective analysis found a 3-year survival of 58 % with HSCT, a dramatic improvement over untreated disease [28]; allogeneic transplants are superior to autologous transplants, given the resultant graft-versus-lymphoma effect [7, 16, 28].

6.2 Pathology

6.2.1 Histopathology

The skin biopsy findings in Sézary syndrome may be similar to those of MF but are typically nondiagnostic [29]. Biopsies may show a dermal infiltrate of atypical T cells with convoluted or cerebriform nuclei (Fig. 6.3) [1]. Epidermotropism may be present but is less frequent than in early MF [2, 30]. Biopsies may be nonspecific [1].

On peripheral blood smear review the Sézary cells are heterochromatic with enlarged and markedly irregular indented or folded nuclei (*see* Fig. 6.4) [31]. Peripheral blood flow cytometry reveals an abnormal T-cell population (Fig. 6.5).

6.2.2 Immunophenotype and Molecular Findings

The neoplastic T cells of Sézary syndrome are nearly always CD4+, although rare cases of CD8+ Sézary syndrome have been reported [1]. The neoplastic cells typically express CD2, CD3, TCR-beta, CD5, PD-1, CD27, cutaneous lymphocyte antigen (CLA), and CCR4 [1]. Loss of CD26 and CD7 on CD4+ cells in the blood is a major identifying characteristic on flow cytometry (*see* Fig. 6.5) [2, 32–34].

A clonal T-cell receptor (TCR) gene rearrangement is present [1, 35–38]. Although there are no known recurrent genetic abnormalities, genomic instability likely plays a substantial role in the pathogenesis and progression of this disease. There is a high rate of unbalanced translocations, deletions, and downregulation of chromosomes 1p, 6q, 10q, 17p, and 19 [39].

There is a substantial body of work evaluating the role of micro-RNA expression levels in prognosis and mechanisms of pathogenesis, but these results are not yet ready for clinical applications [40–42].

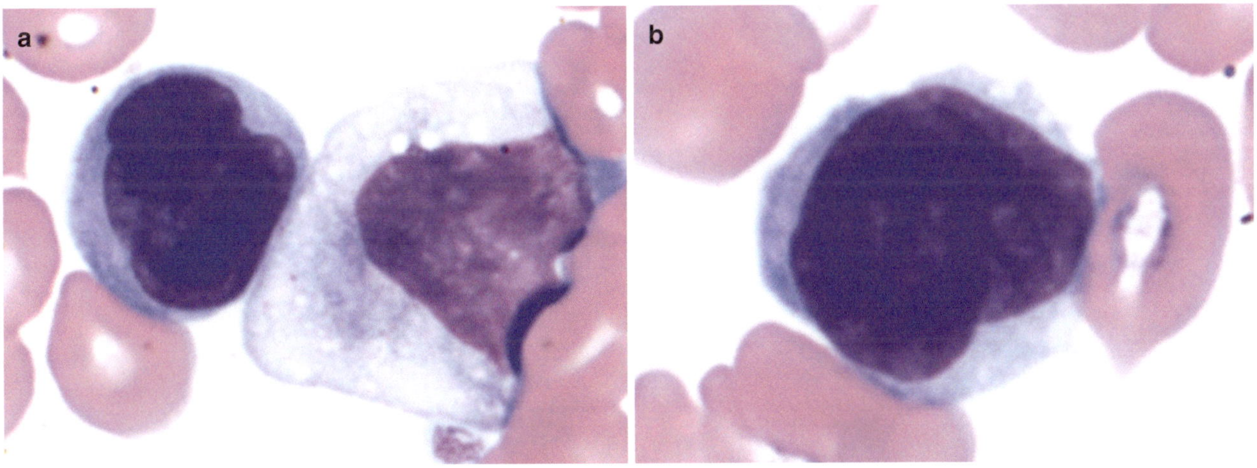

Fig. 6.4 Sézary syndrome, peripheral smear from Case 6.2. (**a**, **b**) Atypical circulating lymphoid cells with cerebriform nuclei containing markedly irregular, folded, and indented nuclear contours and increased nuclear-to-cytoplasmic ratios, consistent with Sézary cells. The cerebriform shape of the nucleus results in a heterochromatic appearance (Wright-Giemsa, 100×)

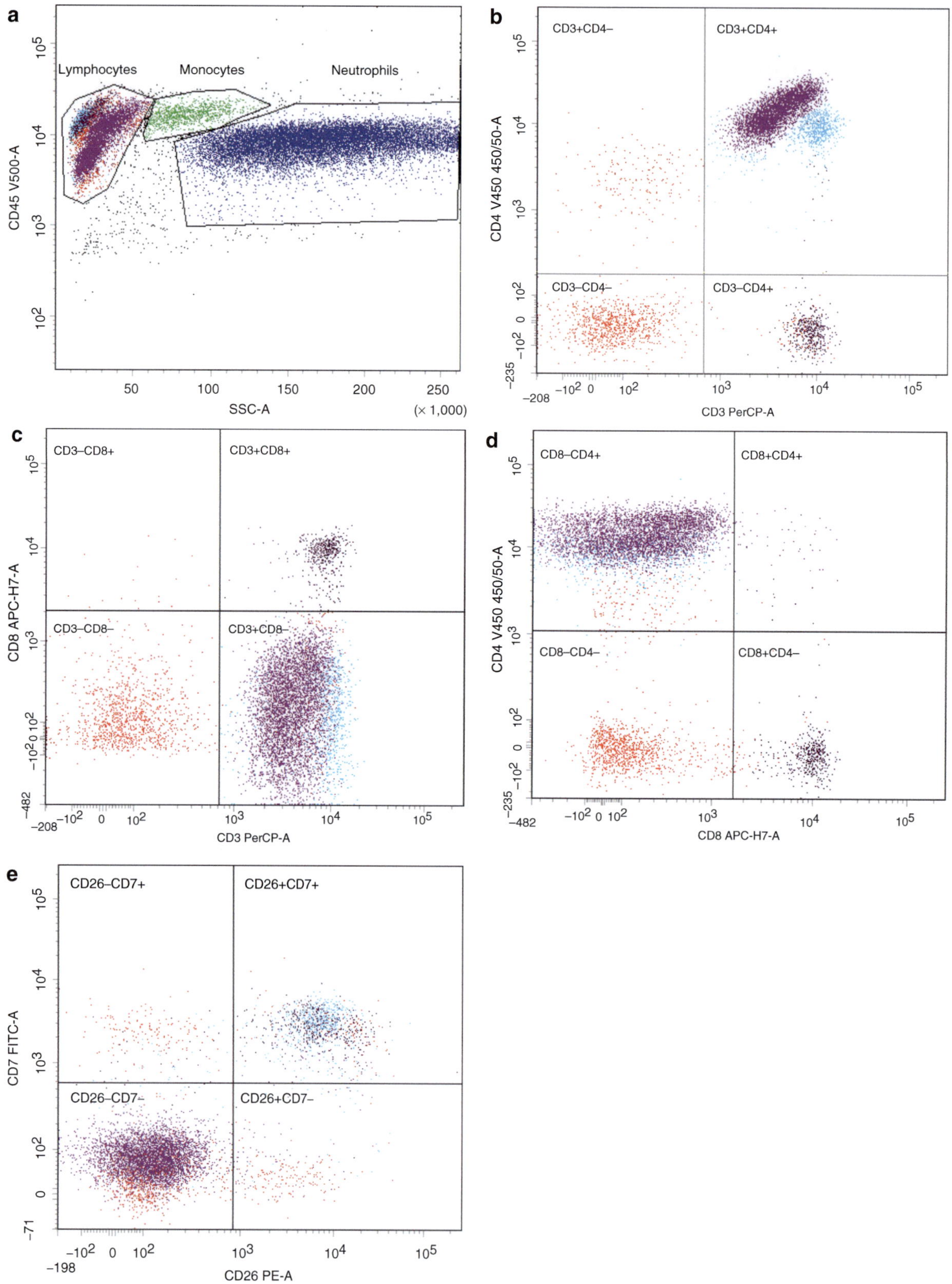

Fig. 6.5 Peripheral blood flow cytometry from Case 6.2. (**a**) CD45 (leukocyte common antigen) stains all leukocytes. Gating CD45+ cells, based on granularity (measured by side scatter [*SSC*]), permits differentiation of lymphocytes, monocytes, and neutrophils. Panels (**b**) through (**e**) include only the cells in the lymphocyte gate. (**b**) CD3+ CD4+ T cells make up nearly 75 % of all lymphocytes. There are two distinct populations of CD3+ CD4+ cells; the T cells of interest have slightly diminished expression of CD3 and are highlighted in purple. (**c, d**) CD3+ CD8+ T cells make up less than 8 % of the total population of lymphocytes, yielding a markedly elevated CD4:CD8 ratio. (**e**) The vast majority of CD3+ CD4+ cells (*purple*) demonstrate loss of CD7 and CD26. *APC* allophycocyanin, *FITC* fluorescein isothiocyanate, *PE* phycoerythrin, *PerCP* peridinin chlorophyll

6.3 Differential Diagnosis

6.3.1 Diagnostic Considerations

In addition to the triad of erythroderma, lymphadenopathy, and clonal neoplastic T cells in the blood, skin, and/or lymph nodes, the following diagnostic criteria must be met [43]:

1. Erythroderma (erythema ≥80 % of the body surface area).
2. Clonal TCR rearrangement in the blood identified by polymerase chain reaction (PCR) or Southern blot analysis.
3. An absolute Sézary cell count of at least 1,000 cells/μL **or** Increased CD4+ or CD3+ cells in the blood with a CD4:CD8 ratio equal to or greater than 10, **or** Increased CD4+ cells in the blood with an abnormal phenotype, including equal to or greater than 40 % of CD4+ CD7− cells or equal to or greater than 30 % of CD4+ CD26− cells.

Many institutions no longer perform Sézary cell counts from the buffy coat of centrifuged blood, given the degree of interobserver variability. Most now rely upon the more consistent technique of peripheral blood flow cytometry, which analyzes expression of CD4, CD8, CD7, and CD26, among other markers. It is possible to have expanded populations of atypical T cells in the blood with loss of CD7 and CD26 in reactive conditions [2]. The differential diagnosis of Sézary syndrome includes a variety of conditions that may present with erythroderma and systemic symptoms. This includes MF with large-cell transformation or erythroderma, adult T-cell leukemia/lymphoma (ATLL), erythrodermic psoriasis, and other lymphoid leukemias.

6.3.2 Differential Diagnosis

6.3.2.1 Mycosis Fungoides (MF)

It is possible for MF to present with marked erythroderma, making it difficult to distinguish from Sézary syndrome clinically. Nevertheless, the two diseases follow very different time courses. Sézary syndrome patients typically develop systemic signs and symptoms, including erythroderma, pruritus, and lymphadenopathy over two years on average and lack the preceding patch-plaque-tumor stages of MF, which evolve over the course of years [1, 5]. Blood involvement with MF may occur in the setting of large-cell transformation (LCT, defined as >25 % of large cells on skin biopsy) [44]. Circulating tumor cells of transformed MF may be indistinguishable from Sézary cells. The histopathology of skin biopsies of Sézary syndrome and late-stage MF are remarkably similar, with the presence of large atypical cerebriform T cells with variable epidermotropism [1, 45]. However, patients with Sézary syndrome have a much more substantial burden of neoplastic cells in the blood than patients with MF [5]. The immunophenotype of the tumor cells may also be helpful in this differential diagnosis. Sézary cells usually express PD-1 and CD27, with loss of CD26 and pan–T cell antigens, including CD2, CD3, and CD5.

6.3.2.2 Erythrodermic Psoriasis

Psoriasis may have a variety of clinical presentations. Although uncommon, it is possible for psoriasis to manifest with marked erythroderma, which may be accompanied by pruritus, hair loss, nail changes, and exfoliative changes. Erythrodermic psoriasis typically occurs rapidly in patients with existing psoriasis. It may be triggered by drug reactions or infections. Patients with a history of psoriasis, rapid disease onset, and/or precipitating factors are much more likely to have erythrodermic psoriasis than Sézary syndrome. Erythrodermic psoriasis accounts for 25 % of cases of erythroderma [46]. Histologically, the presence of intraepidermal neutrophils, psoriasiform epidermal hyperplasia, and the absence of a significant atypical lymphocytic infiltrate favor the diagnosis of psoriasis. Additionally, other than CD7 loss, pan–T cell antigen loss is not a finding in psoriasis.

6.3.2.3 Adult T-Cell Leukemia/Lymphoma (ATLL)

ATLL is a T-cell leukemia/lymphoma characterized by atypical cerebriform cells in the blood. However, ATLL is caused by HTLV-1, while Sézary syndrome has no viral association. ATLL also has a very strong geographic predilection for areas of the world where HTLV-1 is endemic, including the Caribbean, Southeast Asia, and sub-Saharan Africa [47]. While the presence of a positive HTLV-1 titer is supportive of a diagnosis of ATLL, integration of proviral DNA is diagnostic and allows for differentiation from Sézary syndrome. A diagnosis of ATLL cannot be made without HTLV-1 positivity [47].

6.3.2.4 T-Cell Prolymphocytic Leukemia (T-PLL)

As with ATLL and Sézary syndrome, T-PLL is a mature T-cell leukemia derived from post-thymic alpha/beta T cells [48]. T-PLL, a disease of the elderly, is the most common mature T-cell leukemia [48]. T-PLL typically presents with marked leukocytosis and hepatosplenomegaly [48]. Skin involvement is common, occurring in 26 % of patients and may include maculopapular lesions, bruising, or focal erythroderma that becomes generalized over a period of months. However, in contrast to Sézary syndrome, generalized erythroderma is rare in T-PLL [48, 49]. These diseases also have very different time courses. Whereas patients with T-PLL experience a short prodrome of systemic symptoms lasting a median of 2 months prior to diagnosis, the prodrome of Sézary syndrome lasts 24 months on average [49]. The circulating leukemic cells of T-PLL may present with cerebriform morphology indistinguishable from that of Sézary syndrome [49]. These diseases can often be differentiated on peripheral blood flow cytometry. The cells of Sézary syndrome are typically CD7− CD26−, whereas those of T-PLL are usually CD7+ CD26+ [48, 49] (Table 6.1). Chromosomal rearrangement of TCL-1 occurs in T-PLL and may help to differentative from Sézary syndrome [50].

6.3.2.5 Hypereosinophilic Syndromes and Malignancies

Peripheral blood eosinophilia is common in Sézary syndrome, which raises concern for a number of malignant and nonmalignant conditions associated with hypereosinophilia. Relevant malignancies include chronic eosinophilic leukemia, acute myelogenous leukemia, B-cell acute lymphoblastic leukemia, Hodgkin lymphoma, and systemic mastocytosis. Hypereosinophilia can also be seen in parasitic infections, allergic/atopic diseases, and drug hypersensitivity. Primary immunodeficiencies including hyper–IgE syndrome may be considered. Rheumatologic conditions include Churg-Strauss and eosinophilia-myalgia syndromes. Important diagnostic clues include the duration of the eosinophilia, drug exposure, environmental exposure, and concurrent illnesses or systemic symptoms. One key differentiator is that few of these illnesses present with the erythroderma characteristic of Sézary syndrome [51].

Table 6.1 Immunohistochemical features of Sézary syndrome (SS), adult T-cell leukemia/lymphoma (ATLL), and T-cell prolymphocytic leukemia (T-PLL)

Marker	SS	T-PLL	ATLL
CD3	+ Weak/–	+	+
CD2	+/–	+	+
CD4	+	+ Usually	+
CD5	+/–	+	+
CD7	– Usually	+	–
CD8	–	–[a]	–
CD25	Variable	Variable	+
CD26	–	+	–
CD45	+	+	+
CD56	–	–	–
TCR beta	+	+	+

Data from Foucar [48] and Herling et al. [49]

[a]One third of cases of T-PLL may show CD4/CD8 co-expression, and 15 % of cases are CD4–/CD8+

6.4 Clinical Case

Case 6.1

A 32-year-old woman presented with a 3-year history of diffuse erythema and pruritus. She first noticed the development of a rough patch on her inner thigh during her first pregnancy, which over 4–5 months evolved into erythroderma with intractable pruritus. On examination she had diffuse erythroderma, exfoliation, hair loss (*see* Fig. 6.1), onychodystrophy, and palpable inguinal lymphadenopathy. She had received partial treatment at another institution.

Flow cytometry of peripheral blood revealed the presence of 555/μL atypical T cells and a CD4:CD8 ratio of 6.9:1. The peripheral smear showed numerous small to medium-sized lymphoid cells with scant cytoplasm with convoluted, indented nuclei and coarse chromatin. She was diagnosed with partially treated Sézary syndrome. A lymph node biopsy showed dermatopathic changes.

She underwent a course of single-agent targeted therapy and total skin electron beam treatment for residual skin plaques prior to an allogeneic matched hematopoietic stem cell transplant, complicated by mild graft-versus-host disease.

Commentary This patient presented with the classic triad of erythema, lymphadenopathy, and atypical cells in the blood. She also demonstrated other common findings, including hair loss and onychodystrophy. Because she had previously been partially treated, her flow cytometry did not formally meet criteria for a diagnosis of Sézary syndrome, with a CD4:CD8 ratio of only 6.9:1 and just 555/μL atypical cells. As a result of refractory disease despite multiple systemic treatments, she ultimately underwent a hematopoietic stem-cell transplant, the only definitive therapy available for this disease.

Case 6.2

A 62-year-old woman presented with a 2-year history of diffuse pruritus refractory to treatment and a new peripheral eosinophilia. The itch had been intensifying over the last year and was accompanied by erythematous patches on her skin and the development of thickened, loose skin over her joints, back, abdomen, and thighs (*see* Fig. 6.2a). Her axillae and groin were uninvolved, and she had no nail changes. She reported intermittent chills and fever for the last year.

A peripheral blood smear revealed the presence of numerous lymphoid cells with cerebriform nuclei (*see* Fig. 6.4). A skin biopsy demonstrated a perivascular infiltrate of atypical CD4+ lymphoid cells (*see* Fig. 6.3) and a normal tissue elastin stain. Peripheral blood flow cytometry revealed a large population of atypical CD3+ cells, a CD4:CD8 ratio of 15:1, and loss of CD7 and CD26 on 85 % of T cells (*see* Fig. 6.5). The patient was diagnosed with Sézary syndrome.

Although she underwent treatment with extracorporeal photophoresis, her condition continued to deteriorate. She developed severe onychodystrophy (*see* Fig. 6.2b) and thickening and fissuring of the skin complicated by secondary infection (*see* Fig. 6.2c).

Commentary This patient presented with the classic triad of Sézary syndrome: erythroderma, lymphadenopathy, and atypical cells in the blood (a CD4:8 ratio of 15:1 and loss of CD7 and CD26 on 85 % of cells). Her complete blood count also demonstrated a marked eosinophilia, a not uncommon finding in patients with Sézary syndrome. She was treated with extracorporeal photopheresis, a therapy that has shown significant success in treating (but not curing) Sézary syndrome. This case also highlights the point that patients with Sézary syndrome are at risk for frequent skin infections because of their immune-compromised state and damage to the skin, which in some cases can lead to sepsis and even death.

References

1. Ralfkiaer E, Willemze R, Whittaker SJ. Sezary sydrome. In: Swerdlow SH, Campo E, Harris NL, Jaffe ES, Pileri SA, Stein H, et al., editors. WHO classification of tumours of haematopoietic and lymphoid tissues. 4th ed. Lyon: International Agency for Research on Cancer; 2008. p. 299.
2. Olsen EA, Rook AH, Zic J, Kim Y, Porcu P, Querfeld C, et al. Sézary syndrome: immunopathogenesis, literature review of therapeutic options, and recommendations for therapy by the United States Cutaneous Lymphoma Consortium (USCLC). J Am Acad Dermatol. 2011;64:352–404.
3. Bradford PT, Devesa SS, Anderson WF, Toro JR. Cutaneous lymphoma incidence patterns in the United States: a population-based study of 3884 cases. Blood. 2009;113:5064–73.
4. Vij A, Duvic M. Prevalence and severity of pruritus in cutaneous T cell lymphoma. Int J Dermatol. 2012;51:930–4.
5. Hwang S, Janik J, Jaffe E, Wilson W. Mycosis fungoides and Sézary syndrome. Lancet. 2008;371:945–57.
6. Molin S, Ruzicka T. Possible benefit of oral alitretinoin in T-lymphoproliferative diseases: a report of two patients with palmoplantar hyperkeratotic-rhagadiform skin changes and mycosis fungoides or Sézary syndrome. Br J Dermatol. 2009;161:1420–2.
7. Duvic M, Donato M, Dabaja B, Richmond H, Singh L, Wei W, et al. Total skin electron beam and non-myeloablative allogeneic hematopoietic stem-cell transplantation in advanced mycosis fungoides and Sezary syndrome. J Clin Oncol. 2010;28:2365–72.
8. Yawalkar N, Ferenczi K, Jones DA, Yamanaka K, Suh K-Y, Sadat S, et al. Profound loss of T-cell receptor repertoire complexity in cutaneous T-cell lymphoma. Blood. 2003;102:4059–66.
9. Abbas AK, Lichtman AH, Pillai S. Cellular and molecular immunology. 7th ed. Philadelphia: Saunders Elsevier; 2007.
10. Abbas AK, Lichtman AH, Pillai S, editors. Cellular and molecular immunology. 6th ed. Philadelphia: Saunders; 2007.
11. Saed G, Fivenson D. Mycosis fungoides exhibits a Th1-type cell-mediated cytokine profile whereas Sézary syndrome expresses a Th2-type profile. J Invest Dermatol. 1994;103:29–33.
12. Campbell JJ, Clark RA, Watanabe R, Kupper TS. Sezary syndrome and mycosis fungoides arise from distinct T-cell subsets: a biologic rationale for their distinct clinical behaviors. Blood. 2010;116:767–71.
13. Van Doorn R, van Kester MS, Dijkman R, Vermeer MH, Mulder AA, Szuhai K, et al. Oncogenomic analysis of mycosis fungoides reveals major differences with Sezary syndrome. Blood. 2009;113:127–36.
14. Kim YH, Liu HL, Mraz-Gernhard S, Varghese A, Hoppe RT. Long-term outcome of 525 patients with mycosis fungoides and Sezary syndrome: clinical prognostic factors and risk for disease progression. Arch Dermatol. 2003;139:857–66.

15. Agar NS, Wedgeworth E, Crichton S, Mitchell TJ, Cox M, Ferreira S, et al. Survival outcomes and prognostic factors in mycosis fungoides/Sézary syndrome: validation of the revised International Society for Cutaneous Lymphomas/European Organisation for Research and Treatment of Cancer Staging Proposal. J Clin Oncol. 2010;28:4730–9.
16. Molina A, Zain J, Arber DA, Angelopolou M, O'Donnell M, Murata-Collins J, et al. Durable clinical, cytogenetic, and molecular remissions after allogeneic hematopoietic cell transplantation for refractory Sezary syndrome and mycosis fungoides. J Clin Oncol. 2005;23:6163–71.
17. Klein RS, Dunlop JD, Samimi SS, Morrissey KA, Evans KG, Gardner JM, et al. Improvement in peripheral blood disease burden in patients with Sézary syndrome and leukemic mycosis fungoides after total skin electron beam therapy. J Am Acad Dermatol. 2013;68:972–7.
18. Kohn EC, Steis RG, Sausville EA, Veach SR, Stocker JL, Phelps R, et al. Phase II trial of intermittent high-dose recombinant interferon alfa-2a in mycosis fungoides and the Sézary syndrome. J Clin Oncol. 1990;8:155–60.
19. Kaplan EH, Rosen ST, Norris DB, Roenigk HH, Saks SR, Bunn PA. Phase II study of recombinant human interferon gamma for treatment of cutaneous T-cell lymphoma. J Natl Cancer Inst. 1990;82:208–12.
20. Quéreux G, Saint-Jean M, Peuvrel L, Brocard A, Knol A-C, Dréno B. Bexarotene in cutaneous T-cell lymphoma: third retrospective study of long-term cohort and review of the literature. Expert Opin Pharmacother. 2013;14:1711–21.
21. Arulogun S, Prince HM, Gambell P, Lade S, Ryan G, Eaton E, et al. Extracorporeal photopheresis for the treatment of Sézary syndrome using a novel treatment protocol. J Am Acad Dermatol. 2008;59:589–95.
22. Olsen EA, Kim YH, Kuzel TM, Pacheco TR, Foss FM, Parker S, et al. Phase IIb multicenter trial of vorinostat in patients with persistent, progressive, or treatment refractory cutaneous T-cell lymphoma. J Clin Oncol. 2007;25:3109–15.
23. Duvic M, Olsen EA, Breneman D, Pacheco TR, Parker S, Vonderheid EC, et al. Evaluation of the long-term tolerability and clinical benefit of vorinostat in patients with advanced cutaneous T-cell lymphoma. Clin Lymphoma Myeloma. 2009;9:412–6.
24. Whittaker SJ, Demierre M-F, Kim EJ, Rook AH, Lerner A, Duvic M, et al. Final results from a multicenter, international, pivotal study of romidepsin in refractory cutaneous T-cell lymphoma. J Clin Oncol. 2010;28:4485–91.
25. De Masson A, Guitera P, Brice P, Moulonguet I, Mouly F, Bouaziz J-D, et al. Long-term efficacy and safety of alemtuzumab in advanced primary cutaneous T-cell lymphomas. Br J Dermatol. 2014;170:720–4.
26. Zackheim HS, Epstein EH. Low-dose methotrexate for the Sézary syndrome. J Am Acad Dermatol. 1989;21:757–62.
27. Horwitz SM, Kim YH, Foss F, Zain JM, Myskowski PL, Lechowicz MJ, et al. Identification of an active, well-tolerated dose of pralatrexate in patients with relapsed or refractory cutaneous T-cell lymphoma. Blood. 2012;119:4115–22.
28. Duarte RF, Canals C, Onida F, Gabriel IH, Arranz R, Arcese W, et al. Allogeneic hematopoietic cell transplantation for patients with mycosis fungoides and Sézary syndrome: a retrospective analysis of the Lymphoma Working Party of the European Group for Blood and Marrow Transplantation. J Clin Oncol. 2010;28:4492–9.
29. Trotter MJ, Whittaker SJ, Orchard GE, Smith NP. Cutaneous histopathology of Sézary syndrome: a study of 41 cases with a proven circulating T-cell clone. J Cutan Pathol. 1997;24:286–91.
30. Diwan AH, Prieto VG, Herling M, Duvic M, Jone D. Primary Sézary syndrome commonly shows low-grade cytologic atypia and an absence of epidermotropism. Am J Clin Pathol. 2005;123:510–5.
31. Lutzner M, Hobbs JW, Horvath P. Ultrastructure of abnormal cells in Sezary syndrome, mycosis fungoides, and parapsoriasis en plaque. Arch Dermatol. 1971;103:375–86.
32. Bernengo MG, Novelli M, Quaglino P, Lisa F, De Matteis A, Savoia P, et al. The relevance of the CD4+ CD26- subset in the identification of circulating Sézary cells. Br J Dermatol. 2001;144:125–35.
33. Narducci MG, Scala E, Bresin A, Caprini E, Picchio MC, Remotti D, et al. Skin homing of Sézary cells involves SDF-1-CXCR4 signaling and down-regulation of CD26/dipeptidylpeptidase IV. Blood. 2006;107:1108–15.
34. Sokolowska-Wojdylo M, Wenzel J, Gaffal E, Steitz J, Roszkiewicz J, Bieber T, et al. Absence of CD26 expression on skin-homing CLA+ CD4+ T lymphocytes in peripheral blood is a highly sensitive marker for early diagnosis and therapeutic monitoring of patients with Sézary syndrome. Clin Exp Dermatol. 2005;30:702–6.
35. Ponti R, Quaglino P, Novelli M, Fierro MT, Comessatti A, Peroni A, et al. T-cell receptor γ gene rearrangement by multiplex polymerase chain reaction/heteroduplex analysis in patients with cutaneous T-cell lymphoma (mycosis fungoides/Sézary syndrome) and benign inflammatory disease: correlation with clinical, histological and immunophenotypical findings. Br J Dermatol. 2005;153:565–73.
36. Whittaker SJ, Smith NP, Russell Jones R, Luzzatto L. Analysis of β, γ, and δ T-cell receptor genes in mycosis fungoides and Sezary syndrome. Cancer. 1991;68:1572–82.
37. Whittaker SJ, Smith NP. Diagnostic value of T-cell receptor beta gene rearrangement analysis on peripheral blood lymphocytes of patients with erythroderma. J Invest Dermatol. 1992;99:361–2.
38. Bakels V, van Oostveen JW, Gordijn RL, Walboomers JM, Meijer CJ, Willemze R. Diagnostic value of T-cell receptor beta gene rearrangement analysis on peripheral blood lymphocytes of patients with erythroderma. J Invest Dermatol. 1991;97:782–6.
39. Mao X, Lillington DM, Czepulkowski B, Russell-Jones R, Young BD, Whittaker S. Molecular cytogenetic characterization of Sézary syndrome. Genes Chromosomes Cancer. 2003;36:250–60.
40. Ballabio E, Mitchell T, van Kester MS, Taylor S, Dunlop HM, Chi J, et al. MicroRNA expression in Sezary syndrome: identification, function, and diagnostic potential. Blood. 2010;116:1105–13.
41. Narducci MG, Arcelli D, Picchio MC, Lazzeri C, Pagani E, Sampogna F, et al. MicroRNA profiling reveals that miR-21, miR486 and miR-214 are upregulated and involved in cell survival in Sézary syndrome. Cell Death Dis. 2011;2, e151.
42. Van der Fits L, van Kester MS, Qin Y, Out-Luiting JJ, Smit F, Zoutman WH, et al. MicroRNA-21 expression in CD4+ T cells is regulated by STAT3 and is pathologically involved in Sézary syndrome. J Invest Dermatol. 2011;131:762–8.
43. Olsen E, Vonderheid E, Pimpinelli N, Willemze R, Kim Y, Knobler R, et al. Revisions to the staging and classification of mycosis fungoides and Sezary syndrome: a proposal of the International Society for Cutaneous Lymphomas (ISCL) and the cutaneous lymphoma task force of the European Organization of Research and Treatment of Cancer (EORTC). Blood. 2007;110:1713–22.
44. Vergier B, de Muret A, Beylot-Barry M, Vaillant L, Ekouevi D, Chene G, et al. Transformation of mycosis fungoides: clinicopathological and prognostic features of 45 cases. Blood. 2000;95:2212–8.
45. Ralfkiaer E, Cerroni L, Sander CA, Smoller BR, Willemze R. Mycosis fungoides. In: Swerdlow SH, Campo E, Harris NL,

Jaffe ES, Pileri SA, Stein H, et al., editors. WHO classification of tumours of haematopoietic and lymphoid tissues. 4th ed. Lyon: International Agency for Research on Cancer; 2008. p. 296–8.

46. Rosenbach M, Hsu S, Korman NJ, Lebwohl MG, Young M, Bebo BF, et al. Treatment of erythrodermic psoriasis: from the medical board of the National Psoriasis Foundation. J Am Acad Dermatol. 2010;62:655–62.
47. Ohshima K, Jaffe ES, Kikuchi M. Adult T-cell leukaemia/lymphoma. In: Swerdlow SH, Campo E, Harris NL, Jaffe ES, Pileri SA, Stein H, et al., editors. WHO classification of tumours of haematopoietic and lymphoid tissues. 4th ed. Lyon: International Agency for Research on Cancer; 2008. p. 281–4.
48. Foucar K. Mature T-cell leukemias including T-prolymphocytic leukemia, adult T-cell leukemia/lymphoma, and Sézary syndrome. Am J Clin Pathol. 2007;127:496–510.
49. Herling M, Khoury JD, Washington LT, Duvic M, Keating MJ, Jones D. A systematic approach to diagnosis of mature T-cell leukemias reveals heterogeneity among WHO categories. Blood. 2004;104:328–35.
50. Hsi AC, Robivds DH, Luo J, Kreisel FH, Frater JL, Nguyen TT. T-cell pro lymphocytic leukemia frequently shows cutaneous involvement and is associated with gains of MYC, loss of ATM and TCLIA rearrangement. Am J Surg Pathol. 2014;38:1468–86.
51. Nutman TB. Evaluation and differential diagnosis of marked, persistent eosinophilia. Immunol Allergy Clin North Am. 2007;27:529–49.

Adult T-Cell Leukemia/Lymphoma

7

Amrita Goyal, Joi B. Carter, and Lyn McDivitt Duncan

Adult T-cell leukemia/lymphoma (ATLL) is an aggressive peripheral T-cell lymphoma caused by long-term infection with human T-lymphotropic virus 1 (HTLV-1). Patients with ATLL have an extremely poor prognosis, their disease complicated by multidrug resistance of malignant cells, infection due to impaired T-cell mediated immunity, hypercalcemia, and multiple organ failure. Half of patients develop cutaneous manifestations. The cutaneous lesions of ATLL are highly varied and include erythroderma, purpuric papules, and plaques. This chapter addresses the clinical presentation, prognosis, treatment, histopathology, immunohistochemistry, and molecular characteristics of this disease. It closes with a differential diagnosis and clinical case.

A. Goyal, M.D.
Harvard-MIT Division of Health Sciences and Technology, Harvard Medical School, Boston, MA, USA

J.B. Carter, M.D.
Department of Dermatology, Massachusetts General Hospital, Harvard Medical School, Boston, MA, USA

L.M. Duncan, M.D. (✉)
Dermatopathology Service, Department of Pathology, Massachusetts General Hospital, Harvard Medical School, Boston, MA, USA
e-mail: duncan@helix.mgh.harvard.edu

J.B. Carter et al. (eds.), *Atlas of Cutaneous Lymphomas: Classification and Differential Diagnosis*,
DOI 10.1007/978-3-319-17217-0_7

7.1 Clinical

7.1.1 Clinical Presentation

Adult T-cell leukemia/lymphoma (ATLL) is a rapidly progressive lymphoma of mature, peripheral, activated T lymphocytes, caused by HTLV-1 [1–3]. This lymphoma was first described in Japan in 1977 by Uchiyama et al. [4]. ATLL occurs in adults at a median age of 55–58 years (range, 20–80 years) [1, 3]. There is a slight female predominance [1].

Both ATLL and its causative virus, HTLV-1, are endemic to southwestern Japan, the Caribbean, central Africa, and parts of South America [1, 2, 5]. Around the world, an estimated 20 million people are infected with the virus [6]. Approximately 2.5 % of those carriers of HTLV-1 will develop ATLL [1, 2]. Risk of transformation may be higher in men than in women [6]. ATLL has a long latency period, and affected patients were likely infected at a very young age via breastfeeding or exposure to blood products, or later, via sexual transmission [1, 2]. HTLV-1 is a deltaretrovirus; infected cells demonstrate integration of proviral DNA into host cell genomes, which is likely responsible for the oncogenic nature of the virus [7].

There are four variants of ATLL: acute, lymphomatous, chronic, and smoldering [1, 8]. Skin lesions develop in 43–72 % of patients with ATLL. Cutaneous manifestations of ATLL include papules or nodules that are erythematous or violaceous and occasionally ulcerated, scaly patches and plagues and rarely, erythroderma (see Figs. 7.1 and 7.2) [4, 9–11]. Discrete cutaneous lesions are most common in the acute and lymphomatous variants; erythroderma is more common in chronic or smoldering ATLL [1].

The acute and lymphomatous forms of ATLL are more aggressive than the chronic or smoldering variants [6]. In 65 % of patients, ATLL presents in the acute stage, characterized by abrupt onset of leukocytosis, lymphadenopathy, hypercalcemia, lytic bone lesions, hepatosplenomegaly, skin lesions, constitutional symptoms, increased lactate dehydrogenase (LDH) level, and T-cell immunodeficiency. Patients typically have a very high white blood cell count with circulating neoplastic lymphocytes, and eosinophilia and/or neutrophilia [1, 2, 9, 12].

Lymphomatous ATLL, occurring in 20 % of patients, is characterized by peripheral blood involvement and prominent lymphadenopathy. Hypercalcemia may be present, and skin lesions (papules, nodules, tumors, and plaques) are common.

Patients with chronic ATLL have stable lymphocytosis, no organomegaly, no hypercalcemia, and a normal LDH [13]. Smoldering ATLL is the mildest variant and occurs in 5 % of patients. These patients have a normal white blood cell count with >5 % atypical circulating lymphocytes, normal calcium, and no lymphadenopathy or hepatosplenomegaly. LDH may be slightly elevated. Twenty five percent of patients with smoldering or chronic ATLL will develop acute disease [1, 13].

Opportunistic infections are the most common cause of death in patients with ATLL. Common lethal opportunistic pathogens include *Pneumocystis jiroveci*, cytomegalovirus, *Candida* spp., and *Strongyloides stercoralis* [1, 7, 9, 14].

7.1.2 Prognosis and Treatment

Acute ATLL has a grave prognosis: patients treated with chemotherapy have a median survival of 12 months (range, 6–13 months) and a mean 4-year survival of 5 % [2, 7, 13, 15]. Chronic and smoldering ATLL patients fare slightly better, with 4-year survival rates of 27 % for chronic ATLL and 62 % for smoldering ATLL [13]. The nature of the cutaneous findings also impact survival: the mean survival rates are 9 months for patients with nodules, 11 months for those with papules, and 32 months for those with erythroderma [11]. This correlates with the finding that discrete lesions are more often seen in acute or lymphomatous disease, while erythroderma is generally found in patients with chronic or smoldering disease.

Negative prognostic indicators include poor baseline performance status, high LDH, age older than 40 years, hypercalcemia, and involvement of three or more sites. Additional markers of poor prognosis include thrombocytopenia, eosinophilia, bone marrow involvement, high circulating levels of interleukin-5, expression of CCR4 on malignant cells, p53 mutations, and p16 deletions [12]. Notably, patients with expression of CCR4 are more likely to develop cutaneous lesions [3].

Testing for proviral integration is recommended to make a diagnosis of ATLL with cutaneous involvement. Cases of ATLL with HTLV-1 infection detected by PCR amplification but without proviral integration in the skin are considered to be cutaneous T-cell lymphoma (CTCL) arising in HTLV-1 carriers; patients without proviral integration have a better prognosis than those with integration, with median survival times of 72 and 14 months, respectively [11]. The density of the cutaneous infiltrate and cytological features correlate with outcome: patients with nodular or diffuse infiltration with medium- to large-sized lymphoma cells have a worse prognosis than those with a perivascular infiltrate of small- to medium-sized cells [11].

Multiagent chemotherapy is first-line therapy for acute ATLL, but prognosis remains poor [2, 7, 14]. The response to chemotherapy of acute or lymphomatous ATLL is at best transient; recent reports attribute the transient response to expression by lymphoma cells of P-glycoprotein and lung resistance-related protein [2, 13]. Combination therapy with zidovudine and interferon alpha is much more promising, with a response rate between 65 and 92 %. Patients receiving this treatment experienced a dramatic improvement in overall survival, with a 4-year mean survival of 55 % for patients who respond to therapy [16]. Allogeneic stem cell transplants have been attempted with some success [12, 15]. The aggressive course and minimal response to therapy underscores the importance of prevention by reducing HTLV-1 transmission [7]. Chronic and smoldering ATLL, on the other hand, are considered indolent and their clinical course is not altered by conventional chemotherapy [16].

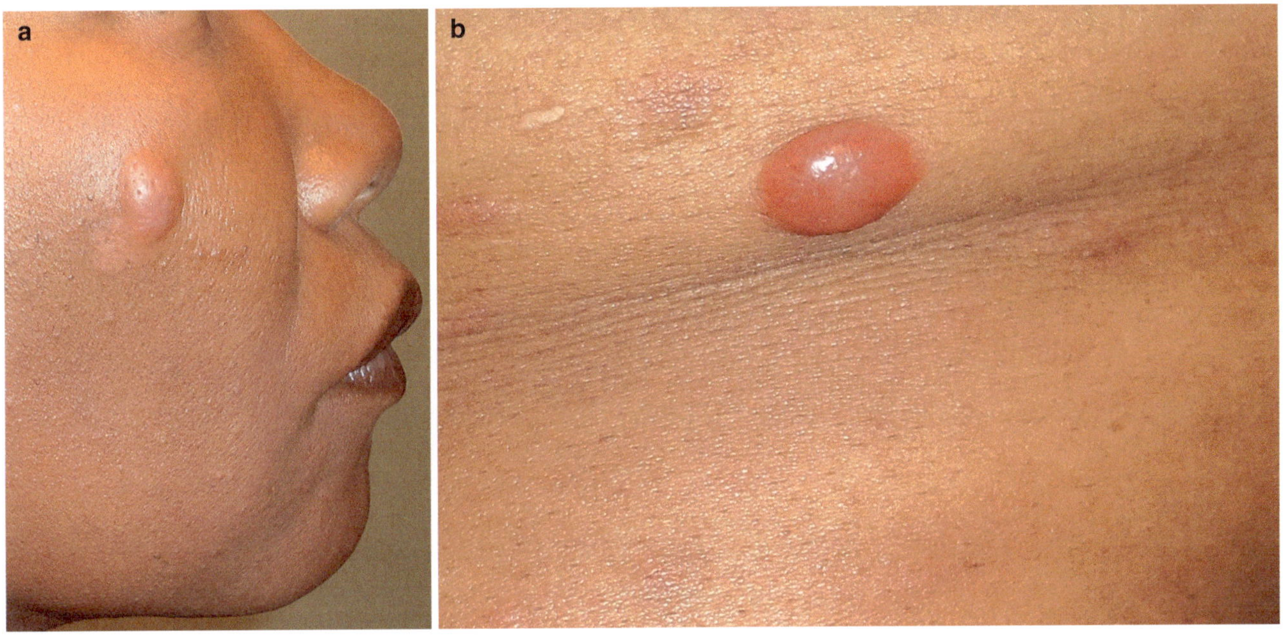

Fig. 7.1 Adult T-cell leukemia/lymphoma (ATLL) tumors from the patient in case 7.1. (**a**) Firm, domed, skin-colored to erythematous 2-cm tumor on the cheek with adjacent hypopigmentation but no surrounding erythema. (**b**) A bright pink, sharply demarcated, domed tumor on the flank. To the left and right of the nodule are flat, pink, scaly macules

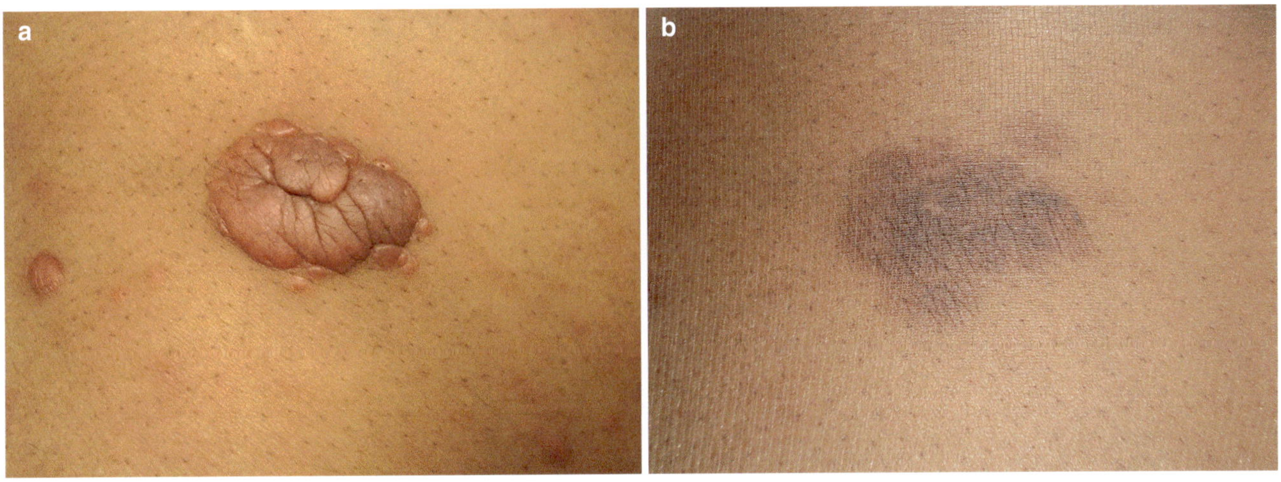

Fig. 7.2 Adult T-cell leukemia/lymphoma (ATLL) tumors from the patient in case 7.1, before and after local radiation therapy. (**a**) Shown prior to radiation treatment is a pink to violaceous, cerebriform tumor measuring 3 cm, located on the patient's right anterior upper thigh, with numerous surrounding smaller violaceous papules and nodules and flat erythematous macules. (**b**) After local radiation therapy, the tumor and nodules resolved with residual hyperpigmentation

7.2 Pathology

7.2.1 Histopathology

ATLL is histopathologically characterized by a diffuse dermal or perivascular infiltrate of pleomorphic neoplastic T cells [9]. Large nodules of neoplastic cells may present in the dermis and subcutaneous fat (see Fig. 7.3) [1]. ATLL may show striking epidermotropism and formation of Pautrier's microabscesses mimicking mycosis fungoides (Fig. 7.3b) [1, 10, 11, 13]. Areas of cutaneous erythema correlate with areas of perivascular or diffuse infiltration by small-to-medium neoplastic cells, whereas papules and nodules often demonstrate nodular or diffuse infiltration of medium-to-large atypical T cells [11].

Of note, the peripheral blood contains atypical lymphocytes with irregular, convoluted nuclei, also known as "flower cells" (see Fig. 7.4) [2, 10].

7.2.2 Immunophenotype and Molecular Findings

The neoplastic T cells of ATLL are typically positive for CD4 and pan-T-cell markers CD2, CD3, and CD5. They also typically express CD25, CD45RO, TCRα/β, and HLA-DR [12]. The vast majority of cells lack CD7 and CD26 [12]. CD3 expression is often diminished [12]. The neoplastic T cells are usually negative for CD8, but cases positive for CD8, both CD4+ CD8+ and CD4− CD8+, have been reported. The tumor cells also express markers found on regulatory T cells, including CCR4 and FoxP3 [1, 17]. Large, transformed lymphocytes may be positive for CD30 but are negative for anaplastic lymphoma kinase (ALK) [1]. The minimum immunophenotypic analysis required for diagnosis includes CD3, CD4, CD7, CD8, and CD25 (Table 7.1) [12].

Both clonal rearrangement of the T-cell receptor and clonal HTLV-1 provirus integration into the ATLL lymphoma cells are nearly always present [1, 2]. Proviral integration most likely plays a key role in the leukemogenic nature of the infection [6]. Transmission requires a live infected cell and occurs via cell-cell contact and formation of a viral synapse. The virus integrates randomly into the host genome, and infected cells then undergo clonal proliferation [7].

Most cases of ATLL demonstrate aneuploidy and clonal abnormalities in chromosome structure. Although no chromosomal abnormalities are recognized as specific to ATLL [1], mutations in p53 and deletions of p16 are associated with a poor prognosis [12].

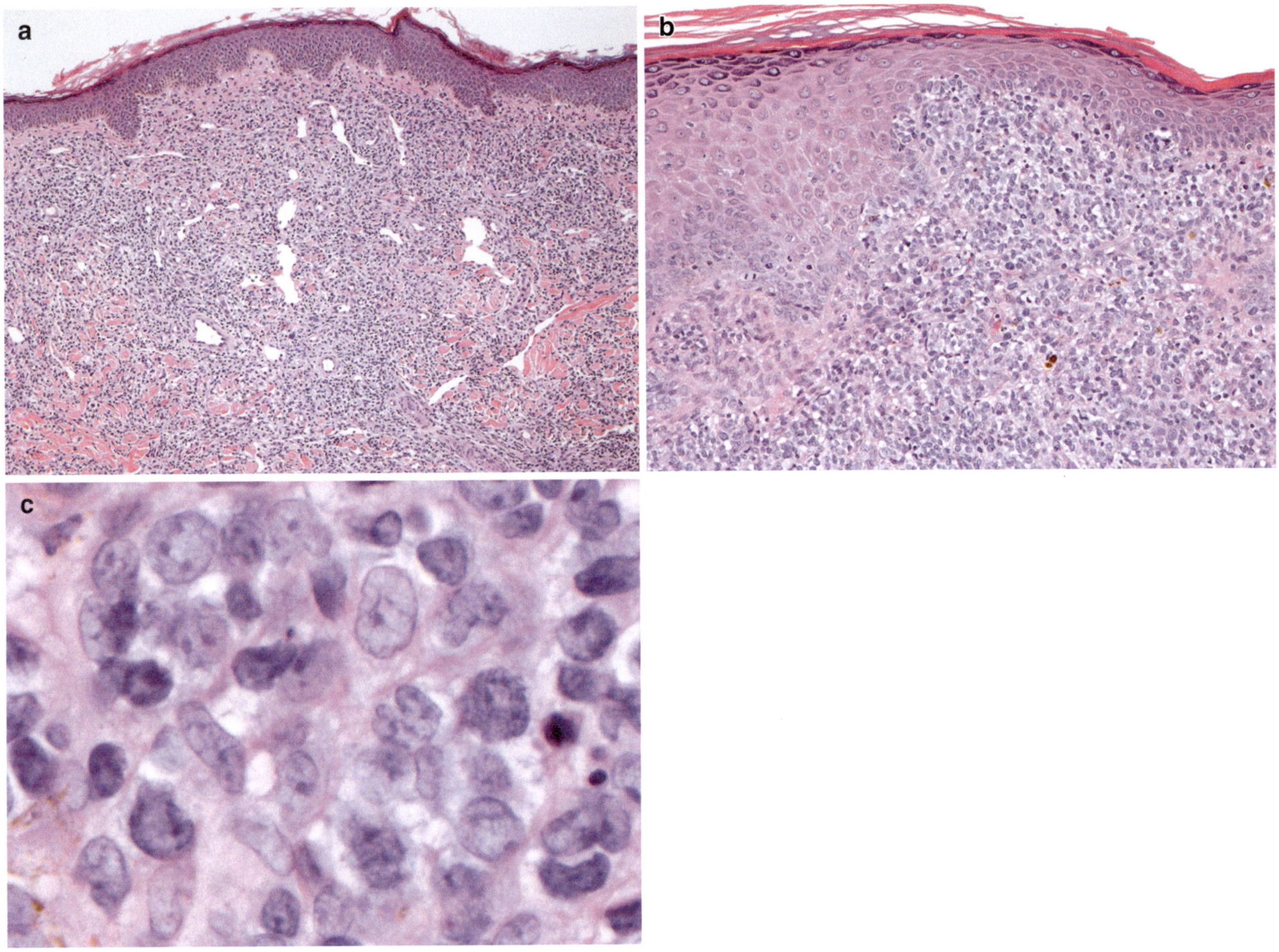

Fig. 7.3 Adult T-cell leukemia/lymphoma, histopathology from the patient in case 7.1. (**a**) Low magnification reveals a dense, dermal lymphoid infiltrate in the superficial and midreticular dermis (H&E, 10×). (**b**) Epidermotropism and Pautrier's microabscesses are present (H&E, 20×). (**c**) The lymphoid infiltrate is composed of medium to large, atypical cells. The atypical cells have irregularly shaped nuclei with dispersed chromatin. Note the cerebriform contours of many of the larger cells (H&E, 40×)

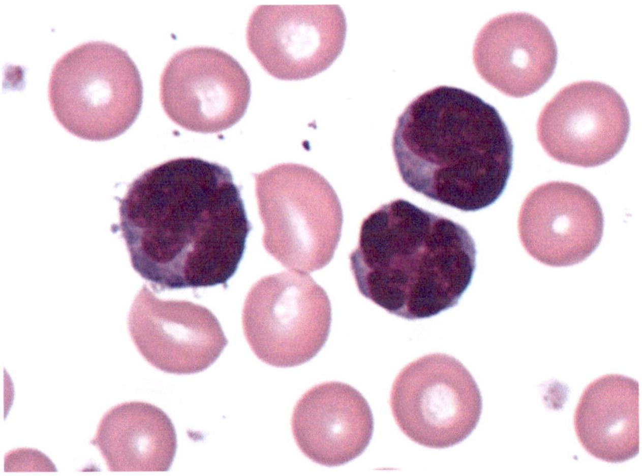

Fig. 7.4 Peripheral smear from the patient in case 7.1 shows numerous large, atypical T lymphocytes with cerebriform, lobulated nuclei, known as flower cells (H&E, 100×)

Table 7.1 Immunohistochemical staining patterns in adult T-cell leukemia/lymphoma

Positive markers
CD2
CD3 (diminished)
CD4 (rare negative cases)
CD5
CD25
CD30 (in some cases of large-cell transformation)
CD45RO
TCR α/β
CCR4
FoxP3
HLA-DR
Negative markers
CD7
CD8 (rare positive cases)
CD26
ALK

ALK anaplastic lymphoma kinase, *CCR* CC chemokine receptor, *TCR* T-cell receptor

7.3 Diagnosis

7.3.1 Diagnostic Considerations

While ATLL is not a primary cutaneous lymphoma, diagnosis is commonly made on skin biopsy. Because of the variable histopathological presentations, the differential diagnosis may include many other cutaneous T-cell lymphomas [14]. Diagnosis often rests on HTLV-1 testing, including detection of anti–HTLV-1 antibodies and clonal proviral integration [13, 15].

7.3.2 Differential Diagnosis

7.3.2.1 Mycosis Fungoides (MF)

This indolent, primary cutaneous T-cell lymphoma, classically progresses through patch, plaque, and tumor stages, in contrast to the rapid, systemic, aggressive onset of acute ATLL [18]. Nevertheless, epidermal involvement in ATLL, including epidermotropism and Pautrier's microabscesses, can be nearly indistinguishable from that seen in MF [13]. The chronic and smoldering forms of ATLL may mimic MF. ATLL can usually be distinguished from MF on the basis of HTLV-1 positivity: ATLL is caused by HTLV-1, and the neoplastic cells nearly always demonstrate proviral integration, whereas MF has no known association with HTLV-1. It is important to note that there are reports of MF in which the patients are infected with HTLV-1, particularly in HTLV-1 endemic areas, but because no HTLV-1 proviral integration is present in the tumor cells, these patients have a diagnosis of MF rather than cutaneous manifestations of ATLL [11, 18]. Finally, ATLL cells typically stain positive for CD25, but the neoplastic cells of MF less commonly express CD25 [12, 19].

7.3.2.2 Sézary Syndrome (SS)

Although SS shows histologic findings similar to those of ATLL and MF, SS is defined by the presence of atypical cerebriform "Sézary cells" in the bloodstream. The most notable differentiating factor between SS and ATLL is HTLV-1 positivity—ATLL cells are necessarily HTLV-1 positive, but SS has no association with HTLV-1 [20].

7.3.2.3 CD30+ Lymphoproliferative Disease (CD30+ LPD)

CD30+ LPD represents a spectrum of CD30+ disorders, including lymphomatoid papulosis (LyP) and anaplastic large-cell lymphoma (ALCL). Owing to the occasional presence of large CD30+ cells in ATLL, CD30+ LPD may be considered in the differential diagnosis for ATLL. However, CD30+ LPD generally remains skin-limited, whereas involvement of peripheral blood is a primary feature of ATLL. CD30+ ALCL may be immunophenotypically similar to ATLL in the skin. The neoplastic cells of ATLL are negative for CD15, ALK, and epithelial membrane antigen (EMA) [13]. Identification of proviral integration of HTLV-1 supports the diagnosis of ATLL.

7.4 Clinical Case

Case 7.1

A 58-year-old Haitian woman presented with a 5-month history of an evolving eruption of more than 100 skin-colored to erythematous nodules on her face, trunk, arms, thighs, and lower legs (see Figs. 7.1 and 7.2a). Her lesions began as pink macules and over the course of weeks developed into pruritic nodules. She had no adenopathy or other systemic symptoms.

A skin biopsy demonstrated a dense dermal lymphoid infiltrate of medium-to-large atypical cells with marked epidermotropism and rare Pautrier's microabscesses (see Fig. 7.3b). Immunohistochemistry revealed the atypical cells to be predominantly CD3+ CD25+ T cells with partial loss of CD2, CD5, and CD7. The CD4:CD8 ratio was approximately 10:1.

HTLV-1 serologies confirmed the presence of anti–HTLV-1 antibodies, and flow cytometry revealed the presence of atypical flower cells in the blood (see Fig. 7.4). The patient underwent a PET-CT scan, which showed no adenopathy or visceral disease, and smoldering ATLL was diagnosed. She underwent antiviral and interferon treatment, but her disease progressed and required combination chemotherapy and radiation treatment. Local radiation therapy to her upper thigh resulted in complete clearance of several nodules (see Fig. 7.2b).

Commentary This patient is from Haiti, a country where HTLV-1 is endemic. ATLL most commonly strikes women in their sixth decade, the same demographic as this patient. ATLL is a systemic disease; the presence of CD25+ atypical cells, seen on this patient's skin biopsies and peripheral blood flow cytometry, is characteristic of ATLL.

Case 7.2

A 65-year-old Haitian man presented with a 3-month history of a pruritic rash and new onset end-stage renal disease secondary to focal segmental glomerulosclerosis (FSGS), on hemodialysis. The pruritic eruption started on right forearm at his dialysis fistula site and then generalized to involve more than 80 % of his body surface area. On examination, skin showed slightly hyperpigmented to erythematous papules and nummular plaques with surrounding collarette and central scale on the trunk and extremities, sparing the bathing suit distribution; there was involvement of the abdomen, back, axillae, arms, legs, palms, and soles (Fig. 7.5).

A skin biopsy was performed and revealed intraepidermal Pautrier microabscesses and a perivascular infiltrate composed of enlarged atypical lymphoid cells. The atypical lymphoid infiltrate was composed of T cells with a CD3+, CD4+, CD8−, CD2^{dim} phenotype and felt to be consistent with a CD4+ cutaneous T-cell lymphoma; diagnostic considerations included mycosis fungoides (MF) and adult T-cell leukemia/lymphoma (ATLL) (Fig. 7.6).

Serologies performed as part of his renal transplant workup revealed the presence of anti-HTLV-1 antibodies. Subsequent polymerase chain reaction on biopsy tissue revealed the presence of HTLV-1 virus and a clonal T-cell receptor (TCR) gene rearrangement in the skin. Blood smear showed rare lymphoid cells with irregular to lobated or clefted nuclei. Given the clinical and histopathologic findings, in conjunction with evidence of HTLV-1 infection, the patient was diagnosed with smoldering ATLL (Fig. 7.7).

The patient was started on topical steroids for pruritus relief and systemic therapy with interferon-alpha and zidovudine (AZT) with significant skin improvement.

Commentary This patient's demographic again highlights the geographic distribution of HTLV-1 virus: it is endemic to Haiti and the Caribbean. Another key point in this case is that cutaneous biopsy from MF and ATLL can be indistinguishable. Evidence of HTLV-1 virus in the blood is supportive of a diagnosis of cutaneous involvement of ATLL. However, given that it is possible for patients with MF to have concomitant ATLL infection, diagnosis of ATLL in the skin can only be rendered by performing tissue PCR for the HTLV-1 virus.

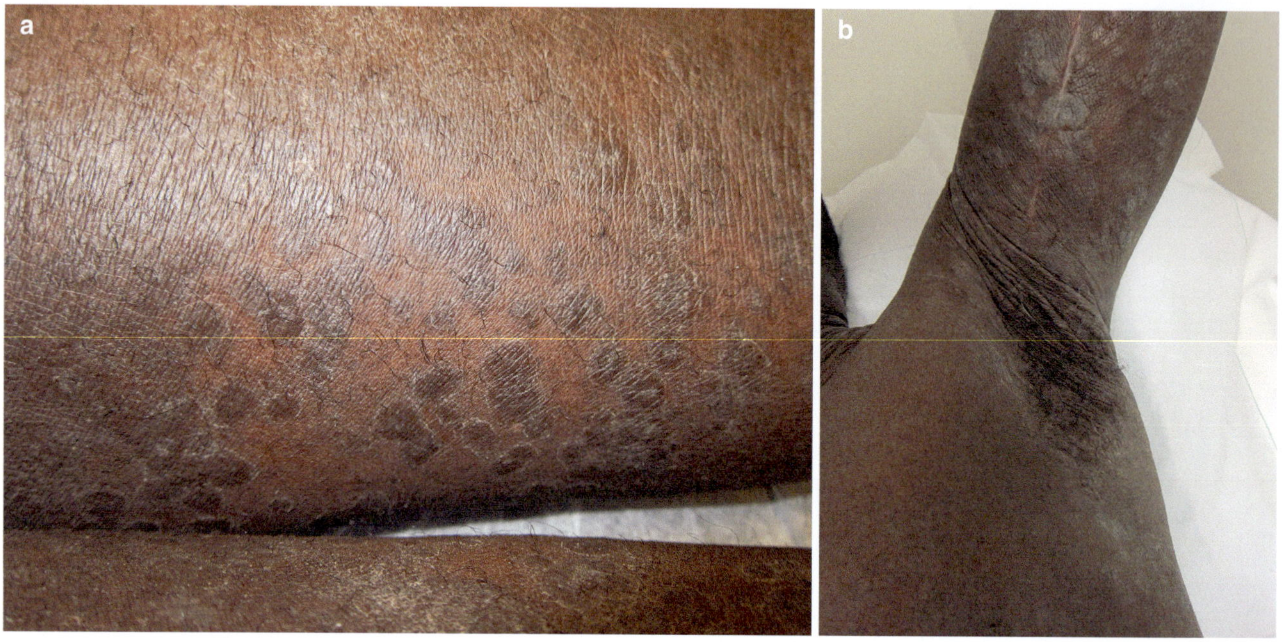

Fig. 7.5 Adult T-cell leukemia/lymphoma (case 7.2) (**a**) On the patient's thighs are innumerable, coin-sized, skin-colored to erythematous to hyperpigmented patches and plaques with fine scale. (**b**) In the axillae, there are nummular skin-colored to erythematous plaques with surrounding collarette and central scale

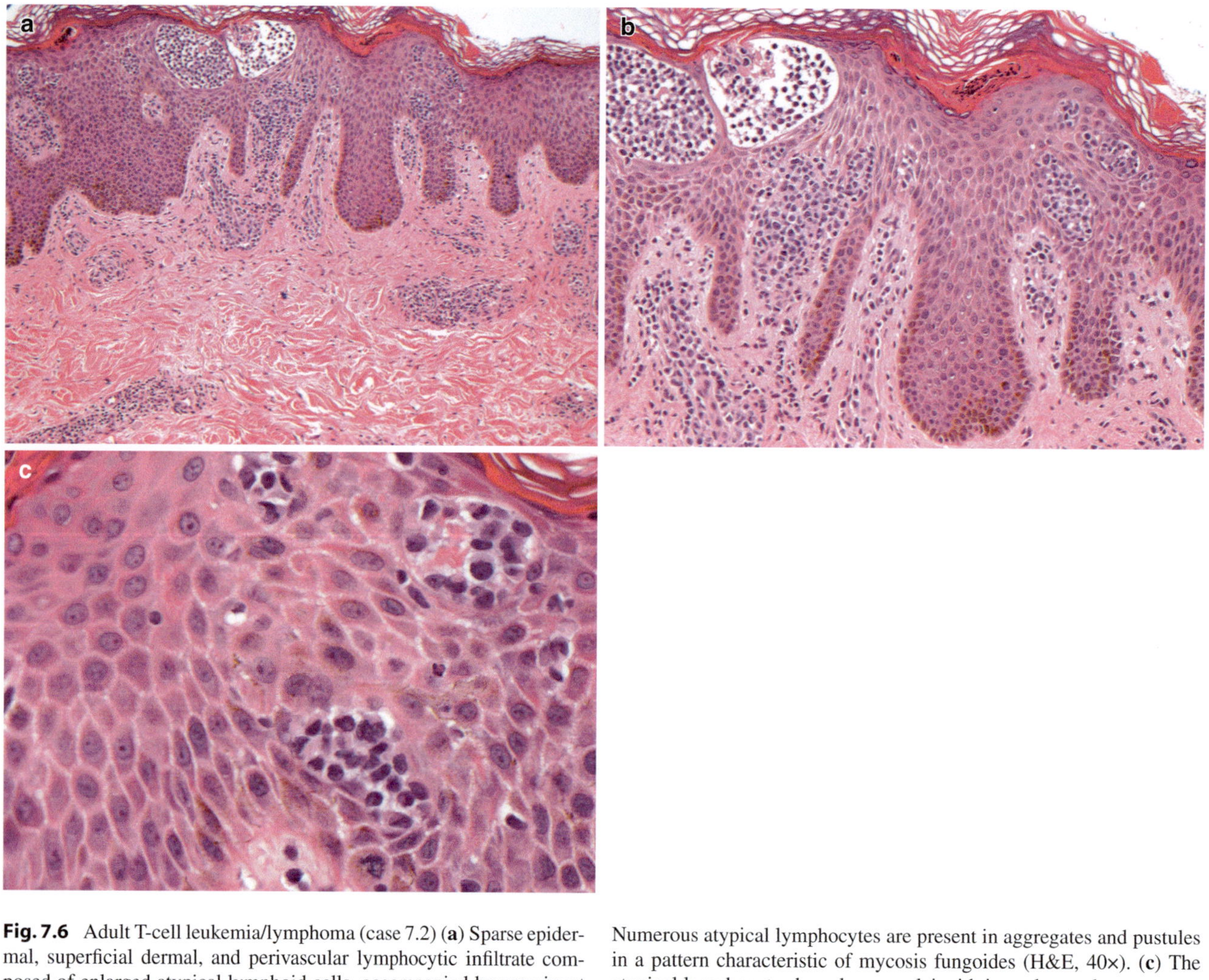

Fig. 7.6 Adult T-cell leukemia/lymphoma (case 7.2) (**a**) Sparse epidermal, superficial dermal, and perivascular lymphocytic infiltrate composed of enlarged atypical lymphoid cells, accompanied by prominent Pautrier microabscesses in the superficial epidermis (H&E, 10×). (**b**) Numerous atypical lymphocytes are present in aggregates and pustules in a pattern characteristic of mycosis fungoides (H&E, 40×). (**c**) The atypical lymphocytes have large nuclei with irregular nuclear contours (H&E, 63×)

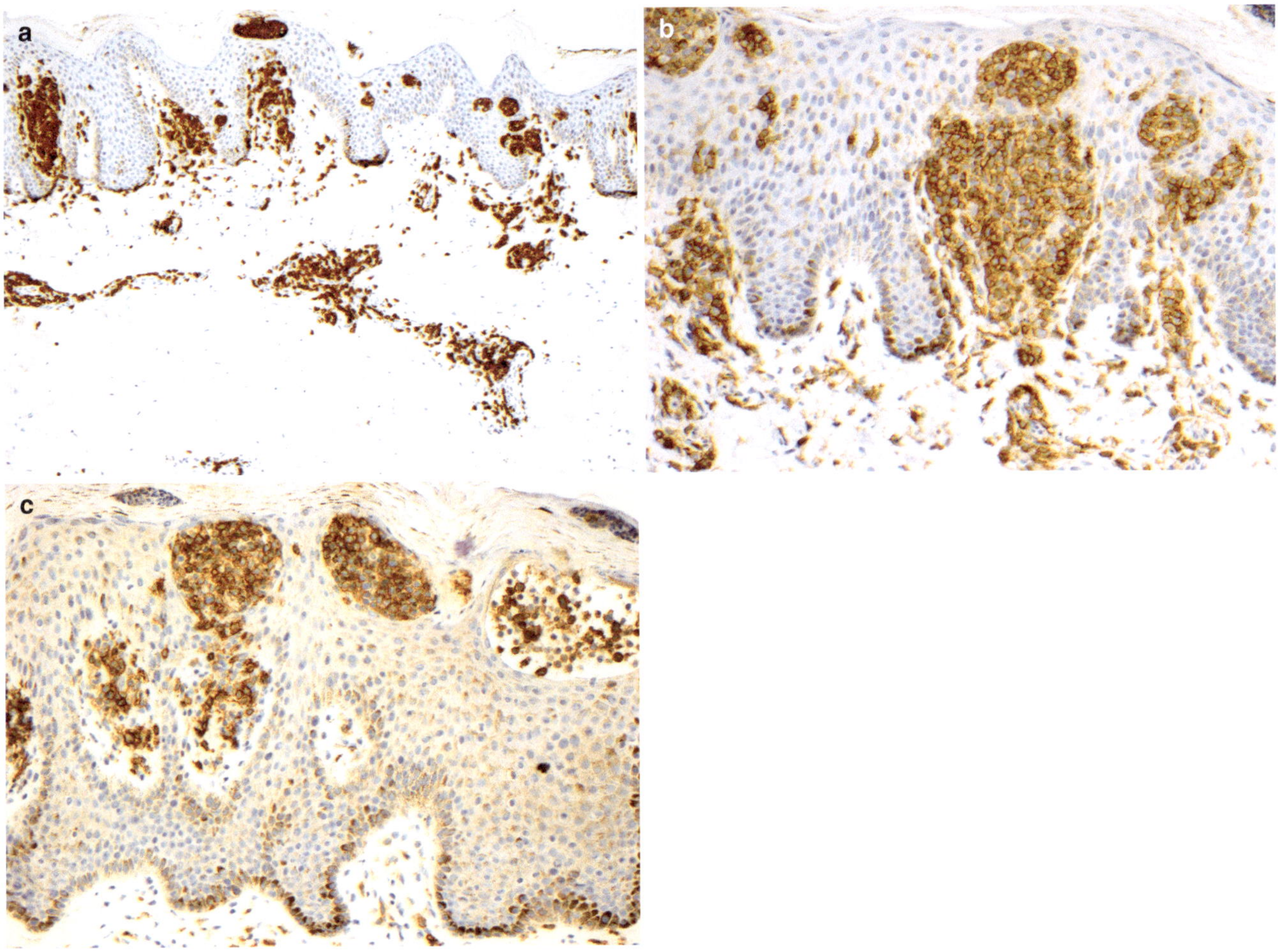

Fig. 7.7 Adult T-cell leukemia/lymphoma (case 7.2) (**a**) The atypical lymphocytes stain positively for CD3 (CD3, 10×). (**b**) The lymphocytes also express CD4 (CD4, 40×). (**c**) The atypical cells also demonstrate expression of CD25 (CD25, 40×)

References

1. Ohshima K, Jaffe ES, Kikuchi M. Adult T-cell leukaemia/lymphoma. In: Swerdlow SH, Campo E, Harris NL, Jaffe ES, Pileri SA, Stein H, et al., editors. WHO classification of tumors of haematopoietic and lymphoid tissues. 4th ed. Lyon: International Agency for Research on Cancer; 2008. p. 281–4.
2. Ishitsuka K, Tamura K. Treatment of adult T-cell leukemia/lymphoma: past, present, and future. Eur J Haematol. 2008;80:185–96.
3. Ishida T, Utsunomiya A, Iida S, Inagaki H, Takatsuka Y, Kusumoto S, et al. Clinical significance of CCR4 expression in adult T-cell leukemia/lymphoma: its close association with skin involvement and unfavorable outcome. Clin Cancer Res. 2003;9:3625–34.
4. Uchiyama T, Yodoi J, Sagawa K, Takatsuki K, Uchino H. Adult T-cell leukemia: clinical and hematologic features of 16 cases. Blood. 1977;50:481–92.
5. Swerdlow SH, Habeshaw JA, Rohatiner AZ, Lister TA, Stansfeld AG. Caribbean T-cell lymphoma/leukemia. Cancer. 1984;54:687–96.
6. Matsuoka M, Jeang K-T. Human T-cell leukaemia virus type 1 (HTLV-1) infectivity and cellular transformation. Nat Rev Cancer. 2007;7:270–80.
7. Taylor GP, Matsuoka M. Natural history of adult T-cell leukemia/lymphoma and approaches to therapy. Oncogene. 2005;24:6047–57.
8. Shimoyama M. Diagnostic criteria and classification of clinical subtypes of adult T-cell leukaemia-lymphoma. Br J Haematol. 1991;79:428–37.
9. Ohshima K. Pathological features of diseases associated with human T-cell leukemia virus type I. Cancer Sci. 2007;98:772–8.
10. Chan HL, Su IJ, Kuo TT, Kuan YZ, Chen MJ, Shih LY, et al. Cutaneous manifestations of adult T cell leukemia/lymphoma. Report of three different forms. J Am Acad Dermatol. 1985;13:213–9.
11. Yamaguchi T, Ohshima K, Karube K, Tutiya T, Kawano R, Suefuji H, et al. Clinicopathological features of cutaneous lesions of adult T-cell leukaemia/lymphoma. Br J Dermatol. 2005;152:76–81.
12. Tsukasaki K, Hermine O, Bazarbachi A, Ratner L, Ramos JC, Harrington W, et al. Definition, prognostic factors, treatment, and response criteria of adult T-cell leukemia-lymphoma: a proposal from an international consensus meeting. J Clin Oncol. 2009;27:453–9.
13. Matutes E. Adult T-cell leukaemia/lymphoma. J Clin Pathol. 2007;60:1373–7.
14. Bunn PA, Schechter GP, Jaffe ES, Blayney D, Young RC, Matthews MJ, et al. Clinical course of retrovirus-associated adult T-cell lymphoma in the United States. N Engl J Med. 1983;309:257–64.
15. Nakase K, Hara M, Kozuka T, Tanimoto K, Nawa Y. Bone marrow transplantation from unrelated donors for patients with adult T-cell leukaemia/lymphoma. Bone Marrow Transplant. 2006;37:41–4.
16. Hermine O, Bouscary D, Gessain A, Turlure P, Leblond V, Franck N, et al. Brief report: treatment of adult T-cell leukemia-lymphoma with zidovudine and interferon alfa. N Engl J Med. 1995;332:1749–51.
17. Karube K, Ohshima K, Tsuchiya T, Yamaguchi T, Kawano R, Suzumiya J, et al. Expression of FoxP3, a key molecule in CD4CD25 regulatory T cells, in adult T-cell leukaemia/lymphoma cells. Br J Haematol. 2004;126:81–4.
18. Jaffe E, Cossman J, Blattner W, Robert-Guroff M, Blayney D, Gallo RC, et al. The pathologic spectrum of adult T-cell leukemia/lymphoma in the United States. Am J Surg Pathol. 1984;8:263–75.
19. Kazakov DV, Burg G, Kempf W. Clinicopathological spectrum of mycosis fungoides. J Eur Acad Dermatol Venereol. 2004;18:397–415.
20. Waldmann TA, Greene WC, Sarin PS, Saxinger C, Blayney DW, Blattner WA, et al. Functional and phenotypic comparison of human T cell leukemia/lymphoma virus positive adult T cell leukemia with human T cell leukemia/lymphoma virus negative Sézary leukemia, and their distinction using anti-Tac. Monoclonal antibody identifying the human receptor for T cell growth factor. J Clin Invest. 1984;73:1711–8.

8 Subcutaneous Panniculitis-Like T-Cell Lymphoma

Amrita Goyal, Joi B. Carter, and Lyn McDivitt Duncan

Subcutaneous panniculitis-like T-cell lymphoma (SPTCL) is a cytotoxic T-cell lymphoma with an excellent prognosis. Patients present with recurrent, generally painless, erythematous subcutaneous tumors on the trunk and extremities, often followed by lipoatrophy. Of note, this diagnosis previously encompassed two different diseases: lymphomas composed of alpha/beta-type T cells and lymphomas of gamma/delta T cells [1]. In the most recent WHO-EORTC guidelines, these have now been separated into SPTCL and primary cutaneous gamma/delta T-cell lymphoma (pcGDTCL), respectively [2]. Older studies, which lumped together both the alpha/beta and gamma/delta lymphomas, may report lower 5-year survival rates and poorer prognosis, reflecting the more aggressive course of pcGDTCL. This chapter discusses the clinical presentation, prognosis, and treatment of SPTCL, as well as its histopathology and immunohistochemistry. The chapter closes with a differential diagnosis and a clinical case.

A. Goyal, M.D.
Harvard-MIT Division of Health Sciences and Technology, Harvard Medical School, Boston, MA, USA

J.B. Carter, M.D.
Department of Dermatology, Massachusetts General Hospital, Harvard Medical School, Boston, MA, USA

L.M. Duncan, M.D. (✉)
Dermatopathology Service, Department of Pathology, Massachusetts General Hospital, Harvard Medical School, Boston, MA, USA
e-mail: duncan@helix.mgh.harvard.edu

J.B. Carter et al. (eds.), *Atlas of Cutaneous Lymphomas: Classification and Differential Diagnosis*, DOI 10.1007/978-3-319-17217-0_8

8.1 Clinical

8.1.1 Clinical Presentation

Subcutaneous panniculitis-like T-cell lymphoma (SPTCL) is a cytotoxic T-cell lymphoma of alpha/beta T cells involving the subcutaneous fat [3–5]. SPTCL represents less than 1 % of all non-Hodgkin's lymphomas. It occurs twice as often in females than in males. SPTCL is primarily a disease of young patients: Patients have a median age of 35 years, and 20 % are under the age of 20 [3].

Patients present with solitary or multiple violaceous to erythematous, deep-seated subcutaneous tumors or plaques on the trunk and extremities, which may mimic panniculitis [3]. The skin lesions are recurrent and self-healing, are often painless, and may or may not ulcerate [6]. Many patients are left with areas of lipoatrophy after regression of nodules (Fig. 8.1) [7].

Systemic symptoms are common and may include fever, malaise, fatigue, myalgias, chills, and weight loss [1]. Although more than half of patients also experience mild cytopenias, metastatic or visceral involvement by the lymphoma is rare. Less than 20 % of SPTCL patients develop hemophagocytic syndrome (HPS), which is associated with poor prognosis [2].

Of note, SPTCL is strongly associated with autoimmune diseases. Up to 20 % of patients have a concurrent autoimmune condition, most commonly lupus [2, 3, 8, 9]; there have also been documented cases with juvenile rheumatoid arthritis, Sjögren's syndrome, type 1 diabetes, idiopathic thrombocytopenia, multiple sclerosis, Raynaud's disease, and Kikuchi syndrome [2, 3].

8.1.2 Prognosis and Treatment

SPTCL has an excellent prognosis, with or without treatment. The 5-year disease-specific survival rate is 85 %. Although it is rare in SPTCL, patients who experience HPS have a markedly poorer prognosis, with a 5-year survival rate of 36 %. When patients with HPS are excluded, the mean 5-year survival rate increases to 91 % [2].

Patients with SPTCL are often treated with prednisone, methotrexate, and (in refractory cases) chemotherapy regimens based on doxorubicin. Therapy-induced remission occurs in 50–65 % of patients [2].

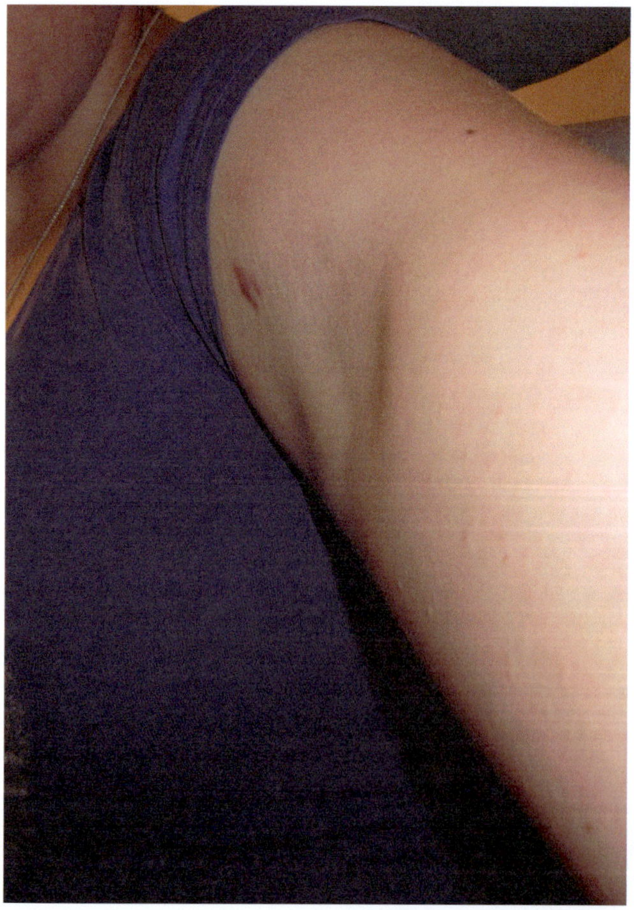

Fig. 8.1 Subcutaneous panniculitis-like T-cell lymphoma (Case 8.1). This clinical image shows a 5-cm area of lipoatrophy at the site of a prior nodule. Superior to that is a well-healed 1-cm biopsy scar

8.2 Pathology

8.2.1 Histopathology

Biopsies of SPTCL demonstrate an atypical subcutaneous lymphoid infiltrate. This infiltrate involves the fat lobules but usually spares the septae, mimicking lobular panniculitis (see Fig. 8.2). There is only occasional infiltration into the reticular dermis, most often involving adnexal structures including eccrine glands, hair follicles, and sebaceous glands. Angioinvasion and angiodestruction are uncommon [2].

The neoplastic cells infiltrate the fat lobules as a diffuse infiltrate of predominantly small to medium-sized lymphocytes with scattered large cells. Circumferential rimming of individual adipocyte spaces by the neoplastic cytotoxic T cells is a characteristic finding (see Fig. 8.3). Fat necrosis and nuclear karyorrhexis are almost always present [2].

The associated inflammatory infiltrate is typically composed of small, reactive, CD4+ T cells and histiocytes. Histiocytes contain lipid and cell debris. Multinucleated giant cells, neutrophils, eosinophils, and plasma cells are rarely present in significant numbers [2].

8.2.2 Immunophenotype and Molecular Findings

SPTCL is composed of CD4–, CD8+, CD56–, betaF1+ T cells [1–3]. They have strong expression of cytotoxic proteins, including granzyme B, TIA-1, and perforin [1, 2, 10]. Loss of CD2 occurs in 10 % of cases, loss of CD5 in 50 %, and loss of CD7 in 44 % (Table 8.1) [2].

Clonal T-cell receptor (TCR) gene rearrangements are typically present [1]. Tumor cells are negative for Epstein-Barr virus (EBV). No specific cytogenetic features have been consistently identified [3].

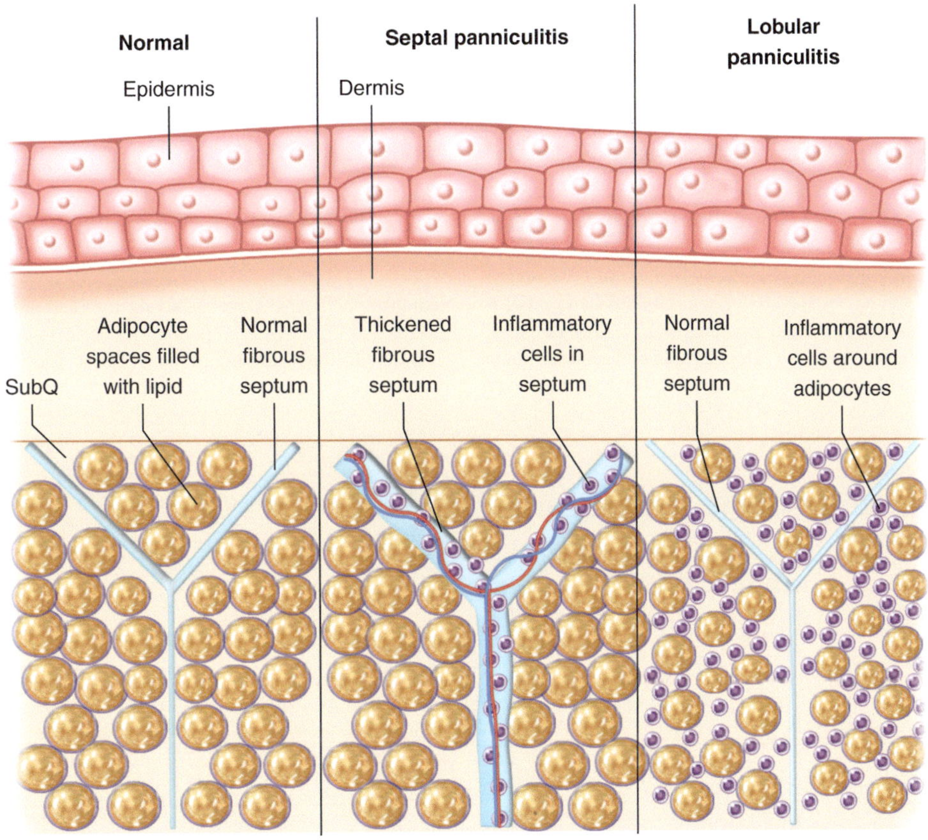

Fig. 8.2 Histopathology of septal versus lobular panniculitis. There are two major histopathologic types of panniculitis—septal and lobular. Many conditions demonstrate characteristics of both (see Table 8.2.) The subcutaneous fat is composed of adipocytes, with their lipid-filled cytoplasm, and fibrous septae containing the vasculature that feeds the fat. The normal subcutaneous fat (*left*) is composed of lobules separated by thin, fibrous septae with vasculature and few inflammatory cells. The adipocyte cytoplasm contains abundant lipid forming a clear space. In septal panniculitis (*center*), the inflammatory cells are primarily found in the fibrous septum, near the vasculature; the fat lobules are minimally affected. In lobular panniculitis (*right*), the fibrous septum is normal, but the fat lobules contain numerous inflammatory cells. SPTCL is a lobular panniculitis, *SubQ* subcutis

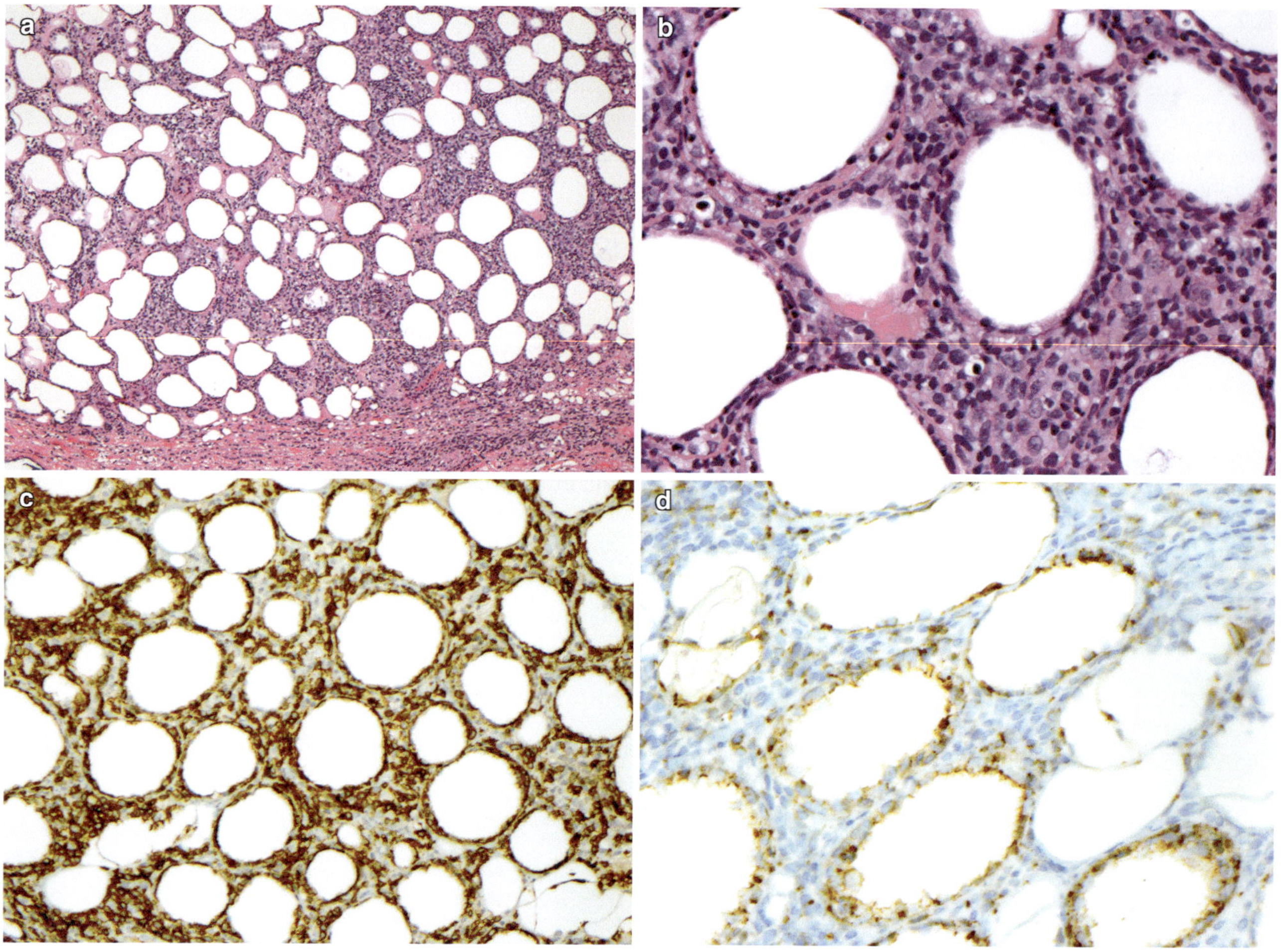

Fig. 8.3 Subcutaneous panniculitis-like T-cell lymphoma, histopathology (Case 8.1). (**a**) The subcutaneous fat is infiltrated with small to medium-sized lymphocytes in a lobular pattern (H&E, 20×). (**b**) Small to medium-sized lymphocytes with irregular hyperchromatic nuclei occupy the fat lobule and rim the fat spaces (H&E, 40×). (**c**) The atypical cells stain positively for the T-cell marker CD8 (CD8, 40×). The neoplastic cells also stain positively for CD3 and CD5 but lack CD4, CD20, and CD56 (*not pictured*). (**d**) Perforin-expressing cytotoxic T cells demonstrate rimming of the fat spaces (perforin, 40×)

Table 8.1 Immunohistochemical phenotype of subcutaneous panniculitis-like T-cell lymphoma

Positive markers	Negative markers
CD8	CD4
BetaF1	CD56
TIA-1	CD5 (lost in 50 %)
Granzyme B	CD7 (lost in 44 %)
Perforin	
CD2 (90 % of cases)	

8.3 Differential Diagnosis

8.3.1 Diagnostic Considerations

Diagnosis is based on a patient's clinical presentation, the time-course of the lesions, and histopathology. Numerous benign and malignant conditions present with deep-seated nodules on physical examination, panniculitis-like morphology on microscopic examination, or both. Differentiating the type of panniculitis (septal *vs* lobular) may be helpful (see Fig. 8.2). Immunohistochemical stains are particularly important to identify the cytotoxic phenotype and to differentiate T cells expressing the alpha/beta TCR from those with the gamma/delta TCR; the cells of SPTCL have a TCR composed of alpha/beta chains [2]. Table 8.2 includes a comparison of histopathologic and immunohistochemical characteristics for several entities included in the differential diagnosis of SPTCL.

8.3.2 Differential Diagnosis

8.3.2.1 Primary Cutaneous Gamma/Delta T-Cell Lymphoma (pcGDTCL)

SPTCL has an excellent prognosis, but pcGDTCL is nearly always fatal, with a median survival of 15 months [11]. As with SPTCL, pcGDTCL can present with a panniculitis-like morphology and is composed of cytotoxic T cells, but the

Table 8.2 Clinical and histopathologic differential diagnosis of Subcutaneous panniculitis-like T-cell lymphoma (SPTCL)

	SPTCL	pcGDTCL[a]	Erythema nodosum	Lupus panniculitis	Benign panniculitis
Type of disease	Neoplasm	Neoplasm	Autoimmune	Autoimmune	Infectious, traumatic, others
Clinical presentation	Generally painless, recurrent, self-resolving subcutaneous nodules; often heal with lipoatrophy	Deep-seated dermal or subcutaneous nodules with ulceration and overlying epidermal necrosis	Painful, recurring, self-resolving subcutaneous nodules	Painful, recurrent dermal or subcutaneous nodules that almost always heal with lipoatrophy	Painful, erythematous subcutaneous nodules
Tissue site	Trunk and extremities	Extremities, thighs, buttocks	Anterior shin	Trunk and proximal extremities	Varied
Associated symptoms	B symptoms, mild cytopenias	B symptoms, hemophagocytic syndrome, pancytopenia	Malaise, fever	Constitutional symptoms	Varied
Median age, *y*	35	42	30	25	Varied
Gender predilection	Female	None	Female	Female	None
Associated conditions	Lupus, juvenile rheumatoid arthritis, Sjögren's syndrome, multiple sclerosis, and other autoimmune	Hemophagocytic syndrome	Autoimmune disease, infection, visceral neoplasia, pregnancy	Systemic lupus erythematosus, discoid lupus	Varied
Prognosis	Excellent	Nearly always fatal	Excellent	Excellent	Excellent
Cellular phenotype	Neoplastic CD4– CD8+ CD56– TIA-1+ BetaF1+ Cytotoxic T cells	Neoplastic CD4– CD8– CD56+ TIA-1+ BetaF1– Cytotoxic T cells	Mixed infiltrate: lymphocytes, histiocytes, giant cells, occasional eosinophils	CD4+ T-cell predominance; occasionally CD8+ predominant; CD123+ plasmacytoid dendritic cells present	T cells with a CD4:CD8 ratio of 2:1
Cellular atypia present?	Yes	Yes	Absent	Usually absent	Absent
Distribution of lymphoid infiltrate	Lobular subcutaneous	Lobular and focal septal subcutaneous, occasionally with dermal involvement	Interlobular septal inflammation with spilling into the fat lobule in a lacelike pattern	Lobular and focal septal subcutaneous, occasionally with dermal involvement	Lobular subcutaneous and dermal
Distinctive feature	Rimming of adipocyte spaces by atypical cytotoxic T cells	Gamma delta phenotype	Polymorphous infiltrate with spilling into fat lobule	Increased dermal mucin, lymphoid follicles and eosinophilic hyalinization of the fat lobule	Infectious processes may have neutrophilic debris or granulomas
TCR clonality	Monoclonal (alpha/beta)	Monoclonal (gamma/delta)	Polyclonal	Polyclonal, may be monoclonal	Polyclonal

[a]*pcGDTCL* primary cutaneous gamma delta T-cell lymphoma, *TCR* T-cell receptor

phenotypes differ. SPTCL cells have a CD4−, CD8+, CD56− phenotype, whereas the more aggressive pcGDTCL tumor cells usually have a CD4−, CD8−, CD56+ phenotype [3, 11]. SPTCL by definition is a tumor of alpha/beta T cells and is thus betaF1 positive (except for rare betaF1 silent cases), whereas pcGDTCL is always betaF1 negative. Expression of the cytotoxic enzyme granzyme M favors a diagnosis of pcGDTCL over SPTCL [12].

8.3.2.2 Infectious Panniculitis

Inflammation of the subcutaneous fat secondary to infection may present with deep-seated subcutaneous tumors or nodules, but the nodules of benign panniculitis are often painful, whereas the nodules of SPTCL are generally painless. Histologically, benign panniculitis is characterized by a polymorphous infiltrate of CD20+ B cells and CD3+ T cells. CD4+ and CD8+ cells are present in roughly a 2:1 ratio and are usually TIA-1 negative. The inflammatory infiltrate usually extends into the dermis, and epidermal hyperplasia is common. In SPTCL, on the other hand, there is a preponderance of CD8+ cells rimming the fat spaces, and the cytologically atypical cells nearly always express TIA-1 [4]. Finally, infectious panniculitis typically lacks the clonal TCR gene rearrangements and cytological atypia characteristic of SPTCL.

8.3.2.3 Erythema Nodosum (EN)

The clinical presentation of EN resembles SPTCL, with deep-seated papules and nodules that are self-resolving and recurrent. Though the lesions of SPTCL are painless, however, those of EN are almost always painful. As with SPTCL, systemic symptoms such as malaise and fever are common, and both conditions are most common in young women [13]. SPTCL and EN can be differentiated on biopsy by the pattern of the inflammation: SPTCL is characterized by a lobular lymphocytic infiltrate, whereas EN shows a septal infiltrate composed of lymphocytes, histiocytes, giant cells, and occasional eosinophils, which may appear to spill into the fat lobule in a lacelike pattern [14].

8.3.2.4 Lupus Erythematosus Panniculitis (LEP)

Also known as *lupus profundus*, LEP poses the most common diagnostic dilemma in the differential diagnosis of SPTCL. Both disorders present as firm nodules, but SPTCL nodules are usually painless and are based entirely in the subcutaneous layer, whereas the nodules of LEP are often painful and can be present in mid-dermis, deep dermis, or subcutaneous fat. Diagnosis can be complicated by the fact that more than 20 % of patients with SPTCL have coexisting autoimmune disorders [3, 15]; 30 % of patients with LEP have concomitant discoid lupus and 10 % have systemic lupus erythematosus [16, 17]. Histologically, LEP does not usually show complete circumferential rimming of fat cells with CD8+ T cells, and it typically demonstrates a preponderance of CD4+ cells rather than the CD8+ cells typical of SPTCL. Germinal center formation and the presence of CD123+ plasma cells are common in LEP but rare in SPTCL. LEP may show mucin deposition in the reticular dermis, which is absent in SPTCL [8]. Other histological findings often seen in LEP and rarely observed in SPTCL include reactive lymphoid follicles and eosinophilic hyalinization of the fat lobule with a honeycomb-like pattern. As with SPTCL, LEP may demonstrate clonality of the TCR [8].

8.3.2.5 Extranodal NK/T-Cell Lymphoma, Nasal Type (eNK/TCL)

Both eNK/TCL and SPTCL may present with deep-seated masses, but they have some important histological and immunophenotypic differences. Unlike SPTCL, eNK/TCL typically shows angiocentricity and angiodestruction, and it usually prominently involves the dermis [7]. As the name implies, the cells of eNK/TCL have an NK/T-cell phenotype (CD56+, CD4−, CD8−) and are EBV+, whereas those of SPTCL have a cytotoxic T-cell phenotype (CD56−, CD4−, CD8+, TIA-1$^+$, grauzyme B$^+$, perforin$^+$) without EBV association [7].

8.3.2.6 Mycosis Fungoides (MF)

Tumor-stage mycosis fungoides may be clinically difficult to differentiate from the nodular skin lesions and deep-seated plaques of SPTCL. The clinical course can be extremely helpful, as MF typically progresses through patch, plaque, and tumor stages but SPTCL does not. There are also important histopathological distinctions: SPTCL is based in the subcutaneous fat, with minimal involvement of the dermis and epidermis. When tumor-stage MF involves the fat, the CD4+ cells usually do not demonstrate the rimming characteristic of SPTCL.

8.3.2.7 Blastic Plasmacytoid Dendritic Cell Neoplasm (BPDCN)

This primary cutaneous lymphoma also presents with cutaneous nodules or tumors, but BPDCN is derived from plasmacytoid dendritic cells, and its cells express CD4, CD56, and CD123 [18]. The cells of SPTCL, on the other hand, are derived from cytotoxic T cells and have a CD4-, CD8+, TIA-1$^+$, grauzyme B$^+$, perforin$^+$ phenotype.

8.3.2.8 Lymphomatoid Granulomatosis (LyG)

This EBV-related B-cell lymphoproliferative disease may present with subcutaneous panniculitis. In contrast to the monomorphic, cytologically atypical cytotoxic T-cell infiltrate of SPTCL, however, LyG is characterized by occasional large, atypical B cells with a background polymorphous infiltrate. Biopsies of LyG show scant CD8+ T cells and the absence of rimming of fat spaces by cytotoxic cells. Unlike LyG, SPTCL is negative for EBV [19].

8.4 Clinical Case

Case 8.1

A 16-year-old girl presented with a 4-month history of extraordinarily painful subcutaneous nodules on the bilateral arms and chest. Over the course of weeks, the nodules were observed to enlarge, form smaller nodules at the periphery, and subsequently resolve, leaving a large area of lipoatrophy (see Fig. 8.1). The tumors were associated with a 10-lb weight loss over the past several months but no other constitutional symptoms. The patient has a family history of rheumatoid arthritis but no personal history of autoimmune disease.

A skin biopsy revealed subcutaneous lobular inflammation composed of atypical CD8+ cytotoxic T cells expressing the beta chains of the T-cell receptor (see Fig. 8.2). A monoclonal TCR rearrangement was present. A PET-CT scan revealed multifocal cutaneous disease but no visceral involvement. A diagnosis of subcutaneous panniculitis-like T-cell lymphoma was made.

Commentary Although this patient's nodules were painful, atypical for SPTCL, the remainder of her clinical and histopathologic presentation is consistent with SPTCL. She is in the typical age group and experienced the weight loss commonly seen in this lymphoma; however, she did lack accompanying constitutional symptoms. Other elements consistent with SPTCL included the resolution skin nodules spontaneously with resultant areas of marked lipoatrophy, the lack of extra-cutaneous involvement, and expression of the alpha-beta TCR by the lymphoma cells.

References

1. Salhany K, Macon W. Subcutaneous panniculitis-like T-cell lymphoma: clinicopathologic, immunophenotypic, and genotypic analysis of alpha/beta and gamma/delta subtypes. Am J Surg Pathol. 1998;22:881–93.
2. Willemze R, Jansen PM, Cerroni L, Berti E, Santucci M, Assaf C, et al. Subcutaneous panniculitis-like T-cell lymphoma: definition, classification, and prognostic factors: an EORTC Cutaneous Lymphoma Group Study of 83 cases. Blood. 2008;111:838–45.
3. Jaffe ES, Gaulard P, Ralfkiaer E, Cerroni L, Meijer CJLM. Subcutaneous panniculitis-like T-cell lymphoma. In: Swerdlow SH, Campo E, Harris NL, Jaffe ES, Pileri SA, Stein H, et al., editors. WHO classification of tumors of haematopoietic and lymphoid tissues. Lyon: International Agency for Research on Cancer; 2008. p. 294–5.
4. Kumar S, Krenacs L, Medeiros J, Elenitoba-Johnson KS, Greiner TC, Sorbara L, et al. Subcutaneous panniculitic T-cell lymphoma is a tumor of cytotoxic T lymphocytes. Hum Pathol. 1998;29:397–403.
5. Gonzalez CL, Medeiros LJ, Braziel RM, Jaffe ES. T-cell lymphoma involving subcutaneous tissue. A clinicopathologic entity commonly associated with hemophagocytic syndrome. Am J Surg Pathol. 1991;15:17–27.
6. Wang HH, Myers T, Lach LJ, Hsieh CC, Kadin ME. Increased risk of lymphoid and nonlymphoid malignancies in patients with lymphomatoid papulosis. Cancer. 1999;86:1240–5.
7. Parveen Z, Thompson K. Subcutaneous panniculitis-like T-cell lymphoma: redefinition of diagnostic criteria in the recent World Health Organization-European Organization for Research and Treatment of Cancer classification for cutaneous lymphomas. Arch Pathol Lab Med. 2009;133:303–8.
8. Magro CM, Crowson A, Kovatich A, Burns F. Lupus profundus, indeterminate lymphocytic lobular panniculitis and subcutaneous T-cell lymphoma: a spectrum of subcuticular T-cell lymphoid dyscrasia. J Cutan Pathol. 2001;28:235–47.
9. Von den Driesch P, Staib G, Simon M, Sterry W. Subcutaneous T-cell lymphoma. J Am Acad Dermatol. 1997;36:285–9.
10. Santucci M, Pimpinelli N, Massi D, Kadin ME, Meijer CJLM, Müller-Hermelink HK, et al. Cytotoxic/natural killer cell cutaneous lymphomas. Report of EORTC Cutaneous Lymphoma Task Force Workshop. Cancer. 2003;97:610–27.
11. Gaulard P, Berti E, Willemze R, Jaffe ES. Primary cutaneous peripheral T-cell lymphomas, rare subtypes. In: Swerdlow SH, Campo E, Harris NL, Jaffe ES, Pileri SA, Stein H, et al., editors. WHO classification of tumors of haematopoietic and lymphoid tissues. Lyon: International Agency for Research on Cancer; 2008. p. 302–5.
12. Krenacs L, Smyth MJ, Bagdi E, Krenacs T, Kopper L, Rudiger T, et al. The serine protease granzyme M is preferentially expressed in NK-cell, gamma delta T-cell, and intestinal T-cell lymphomas: evidence of origin from lymphocytes involved in innate immunity. Blood. 2003;101:3590–3.
13. Cribier B, Caille A, Heid E, Grosshans E. Erythema nodosum and associated diseases. A study of 129 cases. Int J Dermatol. 1998;37:667–72.
14. Thurber S, Kohler S. Histopathologic spectrum of erythema nodosum. J Cutan Pathol. 2006;33:18–26.
15. Pincus LB, LeBoit PE, McCalmont TH, Ricci R, Buzio C, Fox LP, et al. Subcutaneous panniculitis-like T-cell lymphoma with overlapping clinicopathologic features of lupus erythematosus: coexistence of 2 entities? Am J Dermatopathol. 2009;31:520–6.
16. Watanabe T, Tsuchida T. Lupus erythematosus profundus: a cutaneous marker for a distinct clinical subset? Br J Dermatol. 1996;134:123–5.
17. Martens P, Moder K, Ahmed I. Lupus panniculitis: clinical perspectives from a case series. J Rheumatol. 1999;26:68–72.
18. Facchetti F, Jones D, Petrella T. Blastic plasmacytoid dendritic cell neoplasm. In: Swerdlow SH, Campo E, Harris NL, Jaffe ES, Pileri SA, Stein H, et al., editors. WHO classification of tumors of haematopoietic and lymphoid tissues. Lyon: International Agency for Research on Cancer; 2008. p. 145–7.
19. Beaty MW, Toro J, Sorbara L, Stern JB, Pittaluga S, Raffeld M, et al. Cutaneous lymphomatoid granulomatosis: correlation of clinical and biologic features. Am J Surg Pathol. 2001;25:1111–20.

Extranodal NK/T-Cell Lymphoma, Nasal-Type

9

Amrita Goyal, Joi B. Carter, Jeffrey A. Barnes, Aliyah R. Sohani, and Lyn McDivitt Duncan

Extranodal NK/T-cell lymphoma (eNK/TCL) is an aggressive Epstein-Barr virus (EBV)–associated lymphoma with a very poor prognosis. It commonly presents in the midline face or skin with large ulcerative nodules, may disseminate rapidly to the viscera and lymph nodes, and is complicated by hemophagocytic syndrome and disseminated intravascular coagulation (DIC). Alternative terms in the literature include angiocentric T-cell lymphoma, malignant midline reticulosis, lethal midline granuloma, polymorphic reticulosis, and angiocentric immunoproliferative lesion [1, 2]. One extremely important point to note is that this is not a lymphoma of natural killer T cells (NKT cells), but rather a neoplasm of NK cells or cells with a cytotoxic T-cell phenotype. Hence they are termed NK/T-cell lymphomas [1]. Some differentiate eNK/TCLs that occur in the aerodigestive tract (nasal eNK/TCL) from those that occur elsewhere (nasal-type), but regardless of the primary site, the histology is identical [1]. This chapter discusses the clinical presentation, prognosis, treatment, histopathology, immunohistochemistry, molecular characteristics, and differential diagnosis of eNK/TCL. The chapter closes with a clinical case featuring a patient with eNK/TCL arising in the nose with subsequent cutaneous involvement.

A. Goyal, M.D.
Harvard-MIT Division of Health Sciences and Technology, Harvard Medical School, Boston, MA, USA

J.B. Carter, M.D.
Department of Dermatology, Massachusetts General Hospital, Department of Medicine, Harvard Medical School, Boston, MA, USA

J.A. Barnes, M.D., Ph.D.
Comprehensive Cutaneous Lymphoma Program, Department of Medicine, Massachusetts General Hospital Cancer Center, Boston, MA, USA

A.R. Sohani, M.D.
Hematopathology Service, Department of Pathology, Massachusetts General Hospital, Harvard Medical School, Boston, MA, USA

L.M. Duncan, M.D. (✉)
Dermatopathology Service, Department of Pathology, Massachusetts General Hospital, Harvard Medical School, Boston, MA, USA
e-mail: duncan@helix.mgh.harvard.edu

J.B. Carter et al. (eds.), *Atlas of Cutaneous Lymphomas: Classification and Differential Diagnosis*, DOI 10.1007/978-3-319-17217-0_9

9.1 Clinical

9.1.1 Clinical Presentation

Extranodal NK/T-cell lymphomas, nasal type (eNK/TCL) are aggressive, angioinvasive, angiodestructive, necrotizing lymphomas that can cause extensive tissue destruction and have an extremely poor prognosis [1, 2]. eNK/TCL is far more common in East Asians [3] and in patients of Native American descent East Mexico and Central and South America (particularly from Peru) [4, 5]. eNK/TCL accounts for 1.5 % of all lymphomas in the United States and 3.3–8 % of lymphomas in East Asia [6]. This form of lymphoma is more common in adults and is two to three times more common in men than in women [1, 7]. The mean age of onset is 44 years [8].

eNK/TCL is strongly associated with the Epstein-Barr virus (EBV) [1, 7, 9]. Although the role of EBV in eNK/TCL pathogenesis is poorly understood, it is thought that East Asians are more likely to develop this lymphoma because of the higher prevalence of EBV in East Asian populations [7, 8, 10].

Nasal eNK/TCL arises in the mucosa of the aerodigestive tract, and typically presents as ulcerative nodules in the midline of the face; these lesions can result in dramatic facial destruction. Other associated findings may include nasal obstruction, epistaxis, nasal discharge, purulent rhinorrhea, proptosis, extraocular muscle restriction, oronasal fistulas, and facial edema [1, 2, 7, 9]. eNK/TCL occurring at extranasal sites (nasal-type eNK/TCL) has identical histopathology, phenotype, and genotype [2]. Approximately 10 % of cases of nasal-type eNK/TCL arise primarily in the skin; these tend to be disseminated at presentation [2, 6]. Cutaneous manifestations typically include numerous, painful, generalized, ulcerated nodules on the trunk and extremities [1, 11] (Fig. 9.1). Patients generally present with localized disease (76 %) at diagnosis and tend to have good performance status, normal lactate dehydrogenase (LDH) (63 %), and lack B symptoms (35 %) [12]. Other common primary sites of eNK/TCL include the testis and gastrointestinal tract [2, 6].

Lymph node involvement can occur secondarily in eNK/TCL, but bone marrow involvement is rare [13]. Patients with eNK/TCL can experience rapid spread to the gastrointestinal tract, testes, cervical lymph nodes, lungs, liver, brain, and rarely the eye or orbit [1, 7, 8, 13–15]. Once the lymphoma spreads beyond the skin, patients often develop fever, hemophagocytic syndrome, and disseminated intravascular coagulation (DIC) [1, 6, 15].

9.1.2 Prognosis and Treatment

Patients with eNK/TCL have an estimated survival of 6–30 months. The mean 5-year survival rate for eNK/TCL patients ranges from 30 to 50 %, even with treatment [1, 6–8, 16]. Poor prognostic indicators include advanced stage (III or IV), invasion of bone or skin, high levels of EBV DNA in the blood, and detection of EBV in the bone marrow [1]. Specific prognostic models for eNK/TCL have been proposed; adverse risk factors included in a model presented by Lee et al. [12] include advanced stage, the presence of B symptoms, lymph node involvement, and elevated LDH. In this model, the 5-year overall survival rate was 81 % for patients with none of these risk factors, 64 % with one risk factor, 34 % with two risk factors, and 7 % with three or more [12]. Extranasal eNK/TCLs (nasal-type) tend to be even more aggressive than nasal eNK/TCL and are minimally responsive to therapy [1]. Circulating EBV DNA released by dead tumor cells can help predict tumor burden and prognosis, and can assist with diagnosis and monitoring [1, 6].

The standard of care for limited-stage disease is multiagent chemotherapy in combination with localized radiation therapy [6, 7]. eNK/TCL is likely to be highly resistant to chemotherapy because of high levels of expression of the multidrug resistance protein (MRP), which pumps some chemotherapeutic agents out of neoplastic cells [6, 17]. Although allogeneic stem cell transplantation has been effective in a handful of patients, patients who relapse after transplant have a markedly poor outcome [7]. Studies have reported excellent responses to high-dose radiation therapy [18], and several promising chemotherapy regimens are under investigation [19–22].

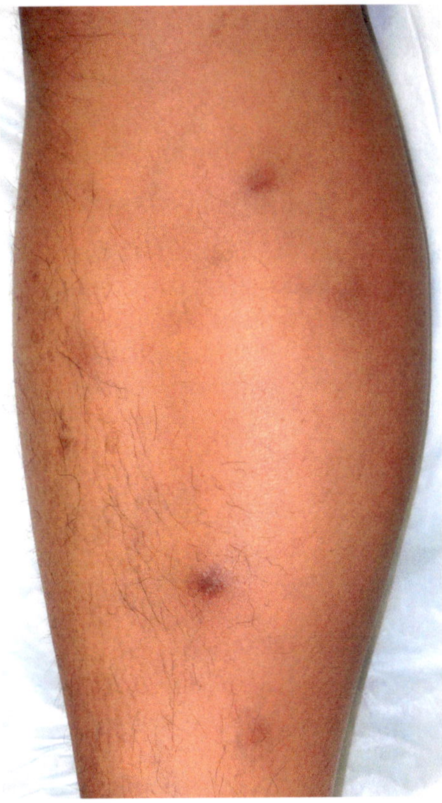

Fig. 9.1 Nasal extranodal NK/T-cell lymphoma (eNK/TCL) (case 9.1). This clinical photograph shows numerous tender, 1- to 2-cm, violaceous, deep-seated subcutaneous nodules on the posterior calf of the patient in case 9.1. One nodule has a punctum of ulceration and a small amount of overlying hemorrhagic crust. Biopsy showed these lesions to be cutaneous involvement by the patient's known nasal eNK/TCL

9.2 Pathology

9.2.1 Histopathology

Although eNK/TCLs may be differentiated based on primary site (nasal *vs* nasal-type) the histopathology is identical [1].

Skin biopsy shows a diffuse dermal infiltrate of neoplastic NK/T cells [1, 7–10]. The overlying epidermis or mucosa typically shows extensive ulceration and loss of mucosal glands. Alternatively, marked pseudoepitheliomatous hyperplasia of the above epithelium can occur [1].

Prominent angiocentricity and angiodestruction is the hallmark of this lymphoma [1, 7–10] (Figs. 9.2 and 9.3). Necrosis and apoptosis may occur secondary to vascular occlusion and the release of cytokines or chemokines by neoplastic cells [1] (Fig. 9.4). Because these tumors are often associated with marked necrosis, a large biopsy sample is often needed to ensure that viable tumor is present and that key findings such as angiocentricity are not missed [6, 7, 23].

The neoplastic NK/T-cell infiltrate is typically composed of medium-sized cells or a mixture of small and large cells, which are occasionally anaplastic. The tumor cells have a moderate amount of pale-to-clear cytoplasm and characteristic irregularly folded and elongated nuclei; they have thus been deemed "cucumber cells." The tumor cells may demonstrate small, inconspicuous nucleoli and granular or vesicular chromatin; cytoplasmic azurophilic granules are visible on Giemsa stain [1, 6]. A dense, inflammatory infiltrate of small lymphocytes, plasma cells, histiocytes, and eosinophils may also be present [1].

9.2.2 Immunophenotype and Molecular Findings

The neoplastic NK cells are positive for CD56, CD2, cytoplasmic CD3epsilon, CD45RO, HLA-DR, CD25, FAS/CD95, and FAS ligand [1, 9, 10] (Table 9.1). The cells frequently express cytotoxic molecules including granzyme B, TIA-1, and perforin [1, 10]. The tumor cells are generally negative for surface CD3, CD4, CD5, CD8, TCR delta, betaF1, and CD57, and only occasionally express CD7 or CD30 [1]. Rare cases derived purely from cytotoxic T cells show a similar immunophenotype, but may express CD8 and surface CD3 (Fig. 9.5).

T-cell receptor and immunoglobulin genes are in the germline configuration. Loss of 6p, 11q, 13p, or 17p is common [1, 9]. Some cases demonstrate partial deletions of *FAS*, *TP53*, beta-catenin, *KRAS*, or *KIT*, although these mutations are of uncertain significance in disease pathogenesis or progression. The presence of a *p53* mutation may hold some prognostic value [1, 24].

eNK/TCL are almost always positive for EBV by in situ hybridization (ISH) for EBV-encoded small RNAs (EBER) [9, 10] (see Fig. 9.3). If cells are EBV negative, a diagnosis of eNK/TCL is highly unlikely [1]. Importantly, because only one third to one half of cases demonstrate expression of the EBV protein LMP-1, this test not an appropriate surrogate for EBV detection [10].

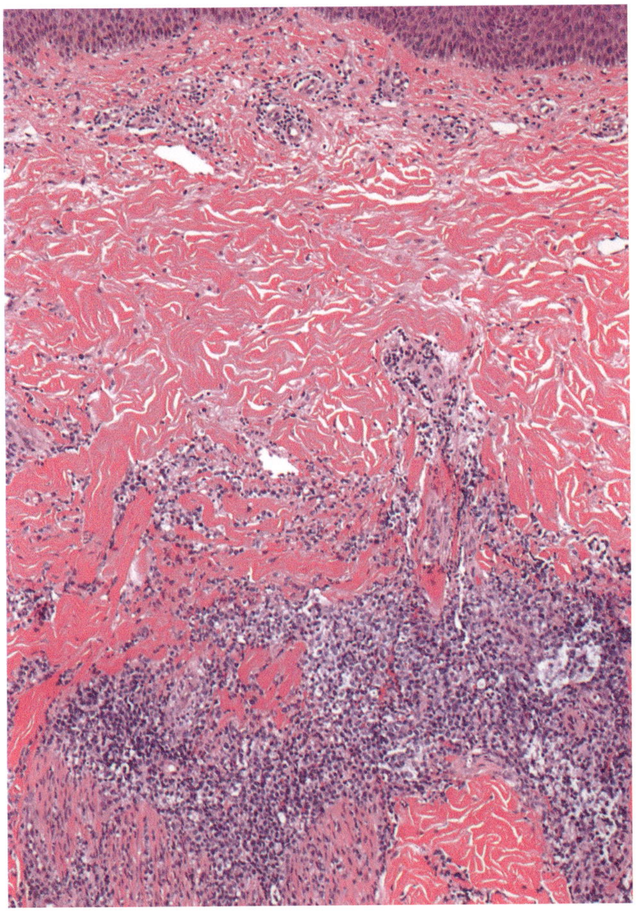

Fig. 9.2 Extranodal NK/T-cell lymphoma (eNK/TCL). Cutaneous biopsy from the patient in case 9.1 demonstrates the hallmark histopathologic characteristics of angiotropism, angioinvasion, and angiodestruction, with marked involvement of the superficial and deep vascular plexuses. The deep vessels are surrounded and invaded by large numbers of neoplastic NK/T cells (H&E, 10×)

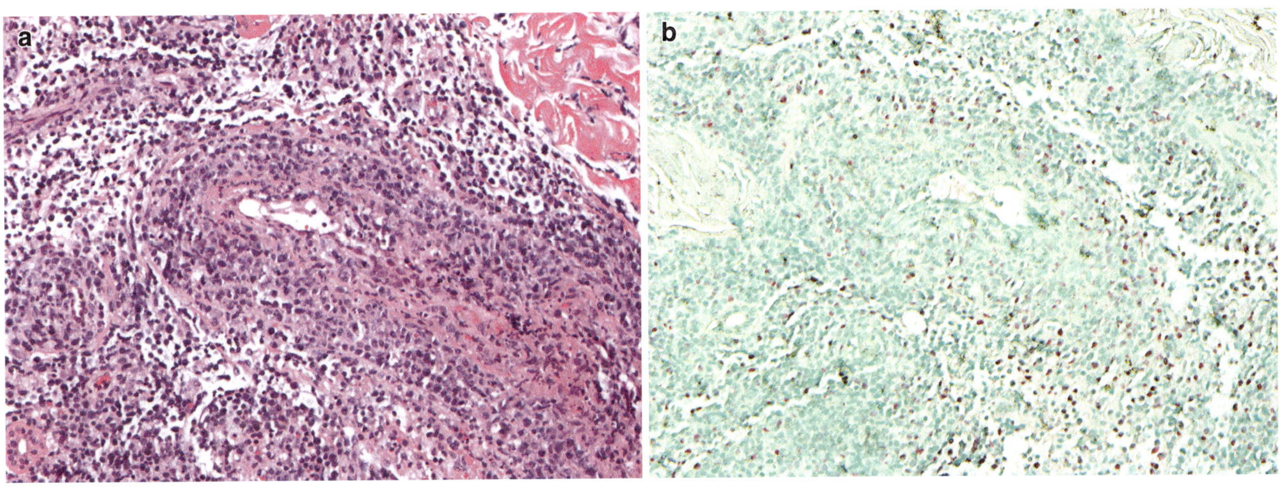

Fig. 9.3 Histopathology and in situ hybridization for Epstein-Barr virus (EBV)–encoded small RNAs (EBER) from the patient in case 9.1. (**a**) The biopsy specimen is characterized by marked angioinvasion and angiocentricity. In the deep dermis, invasion and destruction of a large vessel by neoplastic NK/T cells is seen (H&E, 20×). (**b**) In situ hybridization reveals that many of the neoplastic cells destroying the vessel in **a** express EBER and are thus infected with EBV shown as red staining (*in situ* hybridization for EBER, 20×)

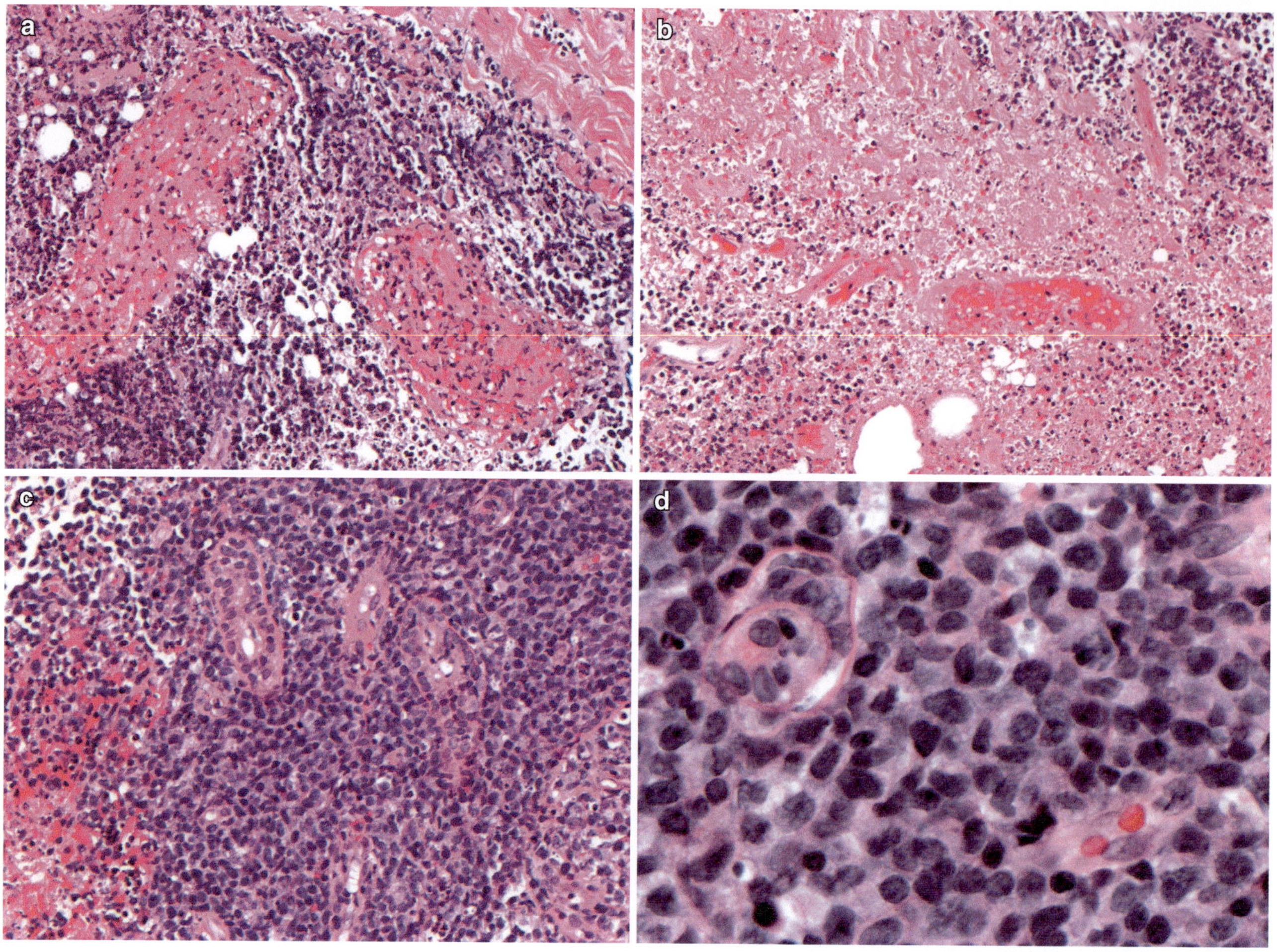

Fig. 9.4 Extranodal NK/T-cell lymphoma (eNK/TCL), histopathology from the patient in case 9.1. (**a**) Large necrotic vessels in the dermis are surrounded and invaded by neoplastic cells (H&E, 20×). (**b**) Destruction of vasculature by the NK/T cells results in widespread tissue necrosis (H&E, 20×). (**c**) Sheets of tumor cells surround eccrine duct, with hemorrhage on the left (H&E, 20×). (**d**) This angiocentric tumor surrounds and invades the walls of two dermal vessels. The tumor cells have round to oval or elongated nuclei with inconspicuous nucleoli and a moderate amount of pale cytoplasm (H&E, 63×)

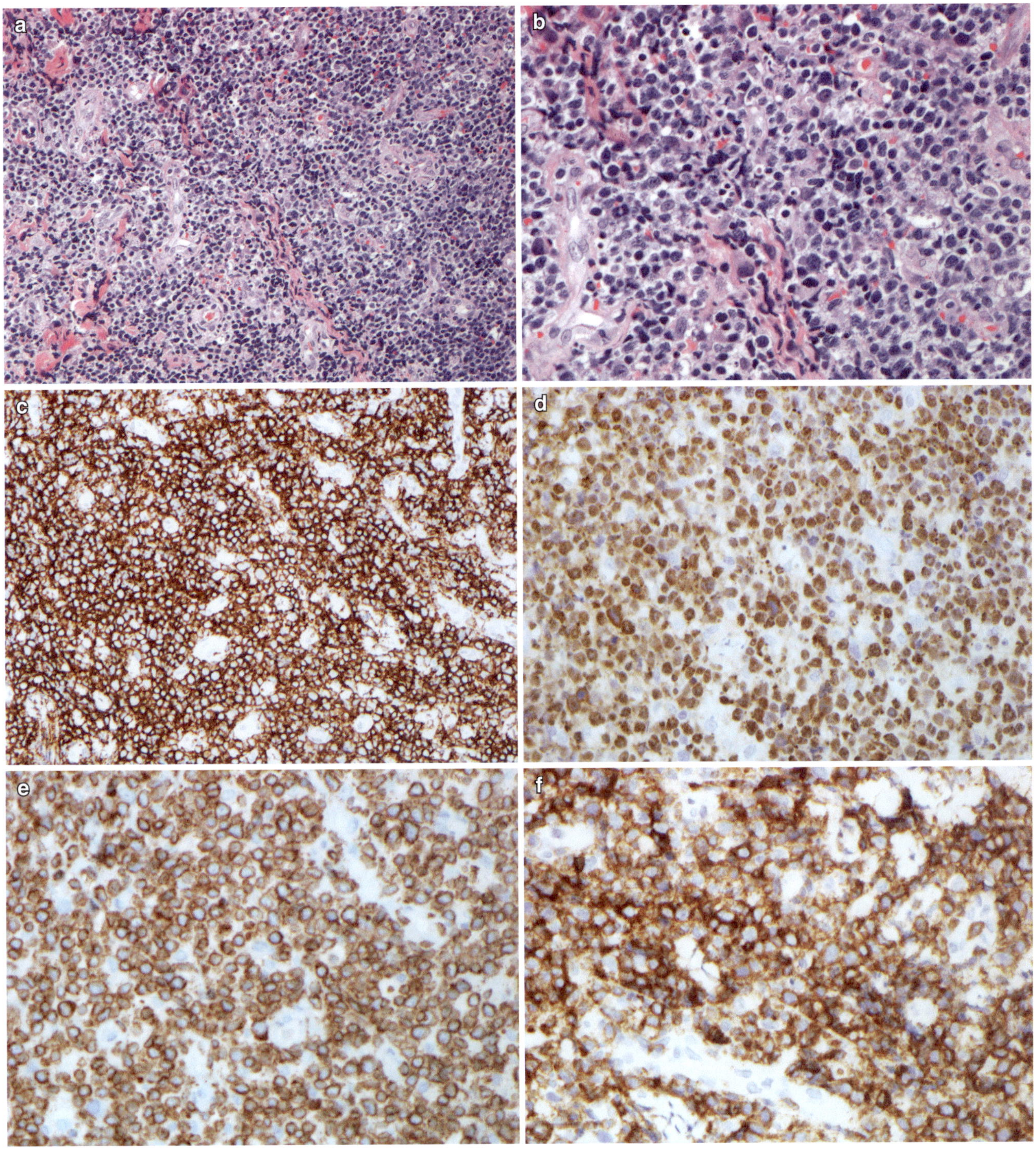

Fig. 9.5 Extranodal NK/T-cell lymphoma (eNK/TCL), histopathology and immunohistochemistry from a case with a cytotoxic T-cell phenotype. (**a**) The dermis is infiltrated by neoplastic cells with angioinvasion and angiodestruction (H&E, 20×). (**b**) The tumor cells have a moderate amount of cytoplasm and irregularly shaped, hyperchromatic nuclei and inconspicuous nuclei (H&E, 40×). (**c**) The neoplastic cells express CD56 (CD56, 20×). (**d**) Tumor cells are positive for EBER on *in situ* hybridization, supporting a diagnosis of eNK/TCL (EBER, 40×). (**e**) Unlike cases of eNK/TCL with a predominantly NK-cell phenotype, these cells express large amounts of surface CD3 (sCD3), consistent with a primarily T-cell phenotype (CD3, 40×). (**f**) Also consistent with the T-cell phenotype is the expression of CD8 by neoplastic cells (CD8, 40×)

Table 9.1 Common immunohistochemical staining patterns in extranodal NK/T-cell lymphoma (eNK/TCL)

Positive	Negative
CD2	Surface CD3[a]
Cytoplasmic CD3epsilon	CD4
CD25	CD7 (occasionally +)
CD56	CD5
CD45RO	CD8[a]
HLA-DR	CD30 (occasionally +)
Granzyme B (frequent)	CD57
TIA-1 (frequent)	TCR delta
Perforin (frequent)	BetaF1
FAS/CD95	
FAS ligand	

TCR T-cell receptor
[a]Rarely positive in cases with a primarily cytotoxic T-cell phenotype

9.3 Differential Diagnosis

9.3.1 Diagnostic Considerations

Diagnosis requires an integration of clinical, immunologic, and genetic data. Midline location can be a key diagnostic feature for eNK/TCLs on the face. Immunohistochemical stains characteristically demonstrate at least one NK-cell marker (CD56, CD16, or CD57) without surface CD3 expression. B-cell markers (CD19 and CD20) or myeloperoxidase (MPO) should not be expressed. These tumors are EBV positive. Unlike many other lymphomas, the T-cell receptor and immunoglobulin genes are typically in their germ-line configuration [1, 2, 9], with the exception of rare cases of cytotoxic T-cell lineage, which may demonstrate clonal T-cell receptor rearrangements (see Fig. 9.5).

9.3.2 Differential Diagnosis

9.3.2.1 Hydroa Vacciniforme-Like Lymphoma (HVLL)

HVLL is a rare, EBV-positive, aggressive cutaneous T-cell lymphoma characterized by angioinvasion and angiodestruction. It generally occurs in children from Latin America or Asia. It can present as ulcerated nodules with scarring, a vesicopapular skin eruption resembling hydroa vacciniforme, and/or edema of the lips and periorbital region [25]. Immunophenotyping helps in achieving the correct diagnosis: HVLL typically lacks CD56 expression, whereas eNK/TCL is CD56+ [11].

9.3.2.2 Lymphomatoid Granulomatosis (LyG)

LyG is an angiocentric, angiodestructive, EBV-associated B-cell lymphoma that nearly always involves the lungs. Cutaneous involvement occurs in approximately half of patients, with a variable presentation that ranges from ulcerated subcutaneous and dermal nodules to violaceous, maculopapular eruptions [26]. One of the key differentiating features is that LyG is a B-cell lymphoproliferative disease; eNK/TCL is not. Although eNK/TCL is much more common in East Asian populations, LyG shows no such ethnic predilection but often occurs in the setting of immunosuppression [2].

9.3.2.3 CD8+ Aggressive Epidermotropic Cutaneous T-Cell Lymphoma (AECTCL)

In the setting of angioinvasion/angiodestruction and rapid onset of ulcerative nodules, CD8+ AECTCL is a diagnostic consideration. Immunohistochemical stains are usually helpful in this differential diagnosis: CD8+ AECTCL manifests as an epidermotropic infiltrate of CD8+ T cells, but the tumor cells in eNK/TCL are usually negative for CD8. eNK/TCL is associated with EBV; CD8+ AECTCL is not [1, 27].

9.3.2.4 Blastic Plasmacytoid Dendritic Cell Neoplasm (BPDCN)

Given the CD56 positivity of the atypical cells and the presence of TCR in the germline configuration, BPDCN may be considered in the differential diagnosis of eNK/TCL [9]. This tumor is derived from blastic plasmacytoid dendritic cells rather than from mature NK cells, as is eNK/TCL. The neoplastic blastic plasmacytoid dendritic cells of BPDCN are EBV negative, lack cytoplasmic granules, and are strongly positive for CD4 and CD123, which are not expressed in eNK/TCL [9]. BPDCN also lacks the angiocentricity and angiodestruction characteristic of eNK/TCL [28].

9.3.2.5 Pyoderma Gangrenosum (PG)

When eNK/TCL occurs at sites other than the face, the clinical differential diagnosis may include PG. Characterized by large, ulcerated lesions, PG may clinically resemble eNK/TCL, but PG is a neutrophilic dermatosis featuring prominent edema and a dense neutrophilic infiltrate, in contrast to the NK/T-cell infiltrate of eNK/TCLs. The EBV positivity, angiocentricity, and angiodestruction characteristic of eNK/TCL are absent in PG [29].

9.4 Clinical Case

Case 9.1

A 39-year-old immigrant from Southeast Asia with a history of EBV-positive nasal extranodal NK/T cell lymphoma presented with a 1-month history of approximately 15 new, painful, rapidly enlarging, violaceous subcutaneous nodules on his calf, measuring 1–3 cm (see Fig. 9.1). His nasal NK/T-cell lymphoma was diagnosed 4 years ago, after 2 years of facial pain, drainage, eyelid ptosis, and nasal obstruction. At that time, he had no evidence of hemophagocytic syndrome or systemic involvement. Treatment with high-dose radiation therapy initially led to clearance of the lesions and complete remission for nearly 2 years. His radiation therapy was complicated by severe radiation dermatitis, mucositis, esophagitis, and thrush. His recovery was further complicated by repeated necrotizing pneumonias.

Cutaneous biopsy of one of the new painful subcutaneous nodules revealed angiotropism, angioinvasion, and angiodestruction with marked involvement of the superficial and deep vascular plexuses (see Figs. 9.2, 9.3, and 9.4). ISH revealed EBER expression by the neoplastic cells (see Fig. 9.3). Although he had no sinonasal symptoms, a nasal biopsy was performed and revealed similar pathology. He was diagnosed with sinonasal recurrence of his eNK/TCL with new cutaneous involvement.

Commentary This patient comes from a region where EBV is endemic. Of note, his eNK/TCL was of nasal origin and secondarily cutaneous, with histology identical to that of primary cutaneous eNK/TCL. The angiotropism, angioinvasion, and angiodestruction seen in this case are classic for eNK/TCL. In addition, this case illustrates how aggressive this lymphoma can be: in spite of multiagent chemotherapy and high-dose radiation to treat his nasal disease, the patient experienced recurrence of disease and cutaneous dissemination.

References

1. Chan J, Quintanilla-Martinez L, Ferry J, Peh S-C. Extranodal NK/T-cell lymphoma, nasal type. In: Swerdlow SH, Campo E, Harris NL, Jaffe ES, Pileri SA, Stein H, et al., editors. WHO classification of tumors of haematopoietic and lymphoid tissues. 4th ed. Lyon: International Agency for Research on Cancer; 2008. p. 285–8.
2. Jaffe E, Chan J, Su I. Report of the workshop on nasal and related extranodal angiocentric T/natural killer cell lymphomas: definitions, differential diagnosis, and epidemiology. Am J Surg Pathol. 1996;20:2–11.
3. Vose J, Armitage J, Weisenburger D. International peripheral T-cell and natural killer/T-cell lymphoma study: pathology findings and clinical outcomes. J Clin Oncol. 2008;26:4124–30.
4. Arber DA, Weiss LM, Albújar PF, Chen YY, Jaffe ES. Nasal lymphomas in Peru. High incidence of T-cell immunophenotype and Epstein-Barr virus infection. Am J Surg Pathol. 1993;17:392–9.
5. Elenitoba-Johnson KS, Zarate-Osorno A, Meneses A, Krenacs L, Kingma DW, Raffeld M, et al. Cytotoxic granular protein expression, Epstein-Barr virus strain type, and latent membrane protein-1 oncogene deletions in nasal T-lymphocyte/natural killer cell lymphomas from Mexico. Mod Pathol. 1998;11:754–61.
6. Suzuki R, Takeuchi K. Extranodal NK/T-cell lymphoma: diagnosis and treatment cues. Hematol Oncol. 2008;26:66–72.
7. Metgud RS, Doshi JJ, Gaurkhede S, Dongre R, Karle R. Extranodal NK/T-cell lymphoma, nasal type (angiocentric T-cell lymphoma): a review about the terminology. J Oral Maxillofac Pathol. 2011;15:96–100.
8. Ng SB, Lai KW, Murugaya S, Lee KM, Loong SLE, Fook-Chong S, et al. Nasal-type extranodal natural killer/T-cell lymphomas: a clinicopathologic and genotypic study of 42 cases in Singapore. Mod Pathol. 2004;17:1097–107.
9. Liang X, Graham DK. Natural killer cell neoplasms. Cancer. 2008;112:1425–36.
10. Gaal K, Sun NC, Hernandez AM, Arber DA. Sinonasal NK/T-cell lymphomas in the United States. Am J Surg Pathol. 2000;24:1511–7.
11. Wang M, Wang S, Yang Q-P, Liu Y-M, Gao L-M, Sun H, et al. Hydroa vacciniforme-like lymphoma of an adult: a case report with review of the literature. Diagn Pathol. 2013;8:72.
12. Lee J, Suh C, Park YH, Ko YH, Bang SM, Lee JH, et al. Extranodal natural killer T-cell lymphoma, nasal-type: a prognostic model from a retrospective multicenter study. J Clin Oncol. 2006;24: 612–8.
13. Wong KF, Chan JK, Cheung MM, So JC. Bone marrow involvement by nasal NK cell lymphoma at diagnosis is uncommon. Am J Clin Pathol. 2001;115:266–70.
14. Kuwabara H, Tsuji M, Yoshii Y, Kakuno Y, Akioka T, Kotani T, et al. Nasal-type NK/T cell lymphoma of the orbit with distant metastases. Hum Pathol. 2003;34:290–2.
15. Cuadra-Garcia I, Proulx G. Sinonasal lymphoma: a clinicopathologic analysis of 58 cases from the Massachusetts General Hospital. Am J Surg Pathol. 1999;23(11):1–16.
16. Kim K, Chie EK, Kim CW, Kim IH, Park CI. Treatment outcome of angiocentric T-cell and NK/T-cell lymphoma, nasal type: radiotherapy versus chemoradiotherapy. Jpn J Clin Oncol. 2005;35:1–5.
17. Natkunam Y, Smoller BR, Zehnder JL, Dorfman RF, Warnke RA. Aggressive cutaneous NK and NK-like T-cell lymphomas: clinicopathologic, immunohistochemical, and molecular analyses of 12 cases. Am J Surg Pathol. 1999;23:571–81.
18. Li Y-X, Yao B, Jin J, Wang W-H, Liu Y-P, Song Y-W, et al. Radiotherapy as primary treatment for stage IE and IIE nasal natural killer/T-cell lymphoma. J Clin Oncol. 2006;24:181–9.
19. Yamaguchi M, Tobinai K, Oguchi M, Ishizuka N, Kobayashi Y, Isobe Y, et al. Concurrent chemoradiotherapy for localized nasal natural killer/T-cell lymphoma: an updated analysis of the Japan clinical oncology group study JCOG0211. J Clin Oncol. 2012;30:4044–6.
20. Kim SJ, Kim K, Kim BS, Kim CY, Suh C, Huh J, et al. Phase II trial of concurrent radiation and weekly cisplatin followed by VIPD chemotherapy in newly diagnosed, stage IE to IIE, nasal, extranodal

NK/T-cell lymphoma: Consortium for Improving Survival of Lymphoma study. J Clin Oncol. 2009;27:6027–32.
21. Yamaguchi M, Kwong Y-L, Kim WS, Maeda Y, Hashimoto C, Suh C, et al. Phase II study of SMILE chemotherapy for newly diagnosed stage IV, relapsed, or refractory extranodal natural killer (NK)/T-cell lymphoma, nasal type: the NK-Cell Tumor Study Group study. J Clin Oncol. 2011;29:4410–6.
22. Jaccard A, Gachard N, Marin B, Rogez S, Audrain M, Suarez F, et al. Efficacy of L-asparaginase with methotrexate and dexamethasone (AspaMetDex regimen) in patients with refractory or relapsing extranodal NK/T-cell lymphoma, a phase 2 study. Blood. 2011;117:1834–9.
23. Cheung M, Chan J, Lau W. Primary non-Hodgkin's lymphoma of the nose and nasopharynx: clinical features, tumor immunophenotype, and treatment outcome in 113 patients. J Clin Oncol. 1998;16:70–7.
24. Takahara M, Kishibe K, Bandoh N, Nonaka S, Harabuchi Y. P53, N- and K-Ras, and β-catenin gene mutations and prognostic factors in nasal NK/T-cell lymphoma from Hokkaido. Japan Hum Pathol. 2004;35:86–95.
25. Sangueza M, Plaza JA. Hydroa vacciniforme-like cutaneous T-cell lymphoma: clinicopathologic and immunohistochemical study of 12 cases. J Am Acad Dermatol. 2013;69:112–9.
26. Roschewski M, Wilson WH. Lymphomatoid granulomatosis. Cancer J. 2012;18:469–74.
27. Gaulard P, Berti E, Willemze R, Jaffe ES, et al. Primary cutaneous peripheral T-cell lymphomas, rare subtypes. In: Swerdlow SH, Campo E, Harris NL, Jaffe ES, Pileri SA, Stein H, editors. WHO classification of tumors of haematopoietic and lymphoid tissues. Lyon: International Agency for Research on Cancer; 2008. p. 302–5.
28. Naeim F, Rao PN, Song SX, Grody WW. Disorders of dendritic cells. In: Naeim F, Rao PN, Song SX, Grody WW, editors. Atlas of hematopathology: morphology, immunophenotype, cytogenetics, and molecular approaches. San Diego: Academic; 2013. p. 649–61.
29. Ruocco E, Sangiuliano S, Gravina AG, Miranda A, Nicoletti G. Pyoderma gangrenosum: an updated review. J Eur Acad Dermatol Venerol. 2009;23:1008–17.

10 CD30+ Primary Cutaneous Anaplastic Large Cell Lymphoma

Amrita Goyal, Joi B. Carter, Jeffrey A. Barnes, Nicole R. LeBoeuf, and Lyn McDivitt Duncan

Primary cutaneous anaplastic large cell lymphoma (pcALCL), a member of the spectrum of CD30+ lymphoproliferative diseases, has an excellent prognosis. This indolent lymphoma is the second most common of all cutaneous T-cell lymphomas. It typically presents with solitary cutaneous and subcutaneous erythematous-to-violaceous papules and nodules. Although relapse after treatment is very common, patients are typically asymptomatic, and the vast majority do not experience extracutaneous spread.

A. Goyal, M.D.
Harvard-MIT Division of Health Sciences and Technology, Harvard Medical School, Boston, MA, USA

J.B. Carter, M.D.
Department of Dermatology, Massachusetts General Hospital, Harvard Medical School, Boston, MA, USA

J.A. Barnes, M.D., Ph.D.
Comprehensive Cutaneous Lymphoma Program, Department of Medicine, Massachusetts General Hospital Cancer Center, Boston, MA, USA

N.R. LeBoeuf, M.D.
Department of Dermatology, Brigham and Women's Hospital, Harvard Medical School, Boston, MA, USA

L.M. Duncan, M.D. (✉)
Dermatopathology Service, Department of Pathology, Massachusetts General Hospital, Harvard Medical School, Boston, MA, USA
e-mail: duncan@helix.mgh.harvard.edu

J.B. Carter et al. (eds.), *Atlas of Cutaneous Lymphomas: Classification and Differential Diagnosis*, DOI 10.1007/978-3-319-17217-0_10

10.1 Clinical Information

10.1.1 Clinical Presentation

CD30+ pcALCL is the second most common type of cutaneous T-cell lymphoma [1]. pcALCL accounts for 10 % of all cutaneous T-cell lymphomas and 25–40% of CD30+ lymphoproliferative disorders [2, 3]. This indolent lymphoma falls on the spectrum of CD30+ lymphoproliferative T-cell diseases and is closely related to lymphomatoid papulosis [2–6]. The mean age of patients at onset is 60 years [2–4]. pcALCL is more than twice as common in women than in men [1, 2]. Unlike systemic forms of ALCL, pcALCL has an extremely favorable prognosis. This lymphoma remains skin-limited in the vast majority of patients, and only 10 % experience extracutaneous dissemination, most frequently to the lymph nodes [3].

pcALCL typically presents with asymptomatic cutaneous or subcutaneous red-violet nodules, tumors, and occasional papules [2–5, 7]. These may range in size from 2 to 10 cm and approximately half show ulceration (see Figs. 10.1, 10.2, and 10.3) [4]. pcALCL has no specific location predilection and may occur on the face, trunk, extremities, or buttocks [2, 4]. While the vast majority of patients present with solitary lesions or multiple in a circumscribed area, 20 % may have multifocal lesions [2, 3]. Partial or complete regression is possible both with and without treatment, but when regression does occur, relapse is exceedingly common [2]. Patients are typically otherwise asymptomatic and rarely experience constitutional symptoms [3].

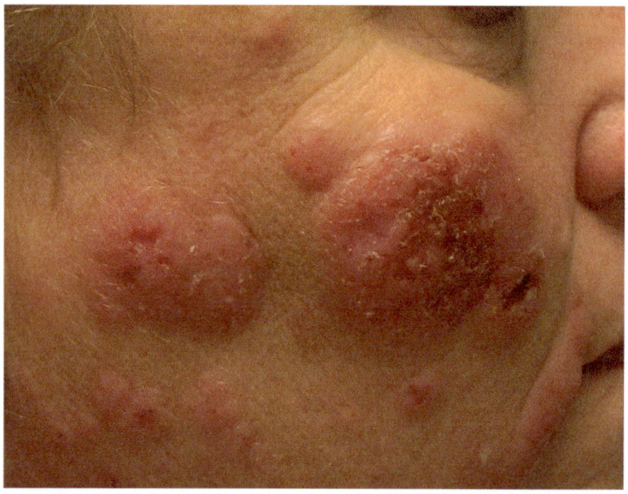

Fig. 10.1 On the right cheek of a woman in her 50s are two 3- to 4-cm erythematous, eroded, indurated plaques and several similar 0.5- to 1-cm nodules

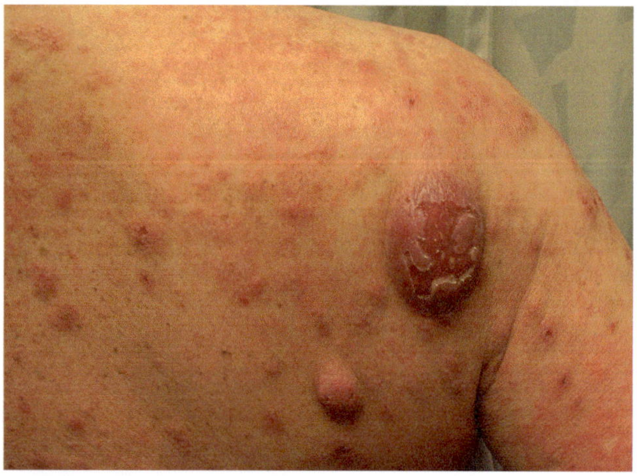

Fig. 10.2 On the right shoulder of a woman in her 50s is a 5-cm erythematous, ulcerated, exophytic tumor, a similar 2-cm tumor, and numerous 0.5- to 2-cm nodules and poorly demarcated plaques, with and without ulceration. These are similar to the lesions on her face (*see* Fig. 10.1)

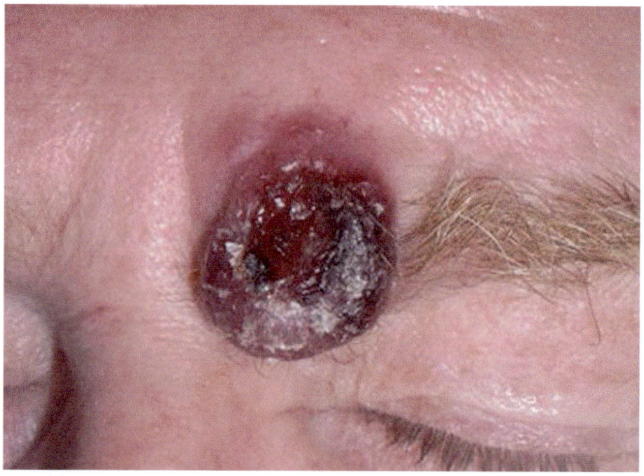

Fig. 10.3 CD30+ primary cutaneous anaplastic large cell lymphoma (pcALCL) (case 10.1). In the left medial eyebrow of a 55-year-old man is a 2.5 × 1.8 cm exophytic ulcerated nodule with overlying scale and hemorrhagic crust

10.1.2 Prognosis and Treatment

pcALCL has an extremely favorable prognosis, with a 10-year disease-specific survival of 90–100 % [1–3, 5]. Multifocality, lymph node involvement, and anaplastic phenotype have no statistically significant impact on survival outcome [2, 4].

Spontaneous remission with complete or partial clearance of skin lesions has been observed in up to 40 % of patients [3]. However, the vast majority of patients relapse and develop new cutaneous lesions repeatedly over the course of their lifetimes with an average disease-free period of 16–23 months [3, 4, 6]. Relapsed disease is not more aggressive than initial disease [8]. Given the tendency of this condition to spontaneously resolve, a 1- to 2-month waiting period of observation prior to treatment is a key element in clinical therapy in order to avoid misdiagnosis and overtreatment [3, 8, 9]. Solitary or localized lesions can be treated successfully with skin-directed therapies including radiation, excision, topical imiquimod, and intralesional methotrexate, among others [3, 8, 10, 11]. It is important to monitor patients for extracutaneous disease dissemination.

Approximately 10 % of patients develop extracutaneous disease at 5 years. Patients with multifocal skin lesions are more likely to develop progression to extracutaneous disease and to relapse after systemic chemotherapy [3, 4, 9]. Systemic chemotherapy is reserved for patients with multifocal or disseminated disease [1, 4, 9, 10]. There are no standard systemic treatments, but methotrexate, interferon [11], bexarotene [12], etoposide [8], and doxorubicin [9] have been used successfully.

10.2 Pathology

10.2.1 Histopathology

Neoplastic cells are likely derived from activated skin-homing lymphocytes [2]. There is a diffuse, dense, nonepidermotropic dermal to subcutaneous infiltrate of large lymphocytes (see Figs. 10.4 and 10.5) [2, 4, 9]. More than 75 % of these cells must be CD30+ (see Fig. 10.6) [1, 2, 9].

The neoplastic cells are large and anaplastic, although nonanaplastic (either pleomorphic or blastic) variants are possible [2, 4]. Nuclei are pleomorphic and can range from round or oval to irregular, with prominent eosinophilic staining [2, 4]. Abundant cytoplasm is common, and there may be areas of pale staining adjacent to eccentrically placed nuclei [4].

The sheets of neoplastic cells are often ringed with reactive lymphocytes, histiocytes, eosinophils, and neutrophils at their periphery [2, 4, 9]. In cases where there is substantial inflammation, epidermal hyperplasia may be marked [2].

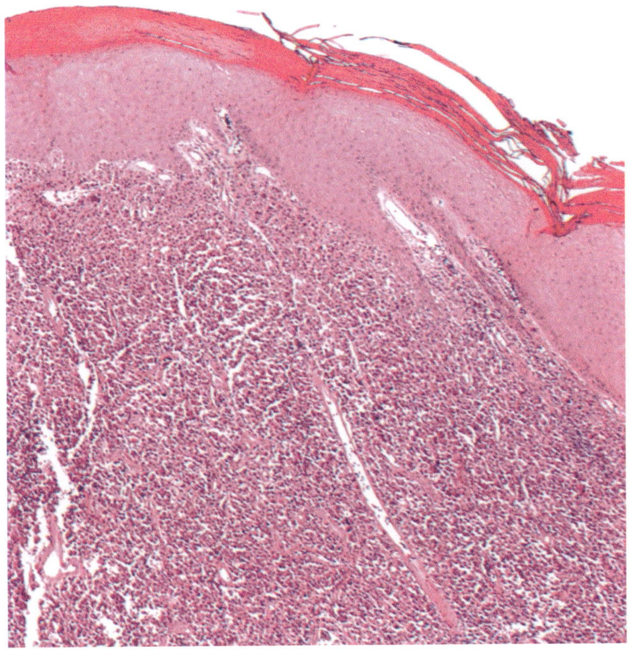

Fig. 10.4 CD30+ primary cutaneous anaplastic large cell lymphoma (pcALCL), (case 10.1) histopathology. The dermis is occupied by a dense, diffuse, non-epidermotropic sheet-like infiltrate of large lymphocytes (H&E, low power)

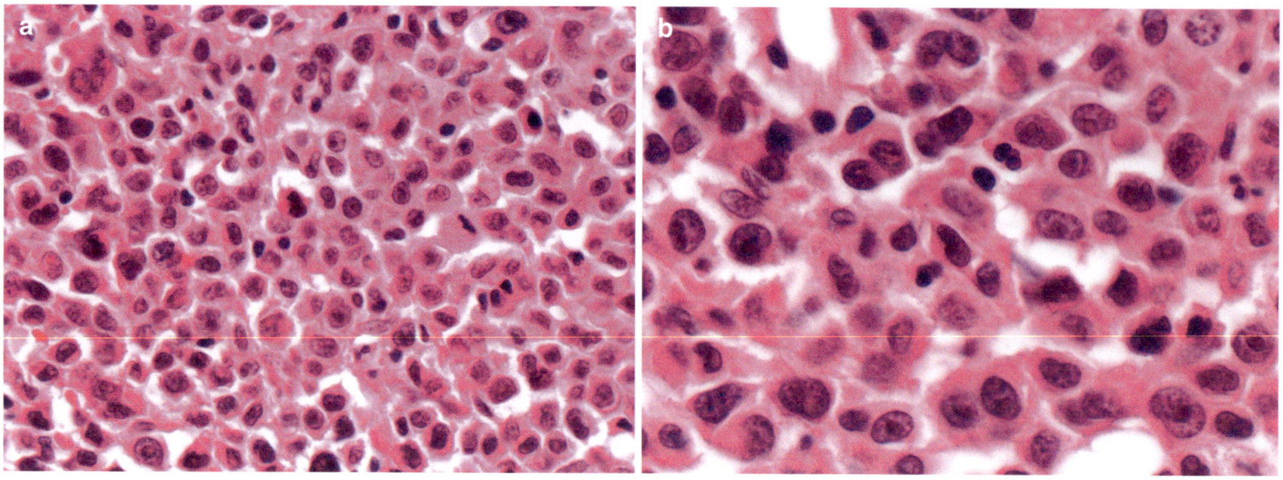

Fig. 10.5 CD30+ primary cutaneous anaplastic large cell lymphoma (pcALCL), (case 10.1) histopathology. (**a**) The neoplastic cells filling the dermis are large and anaplastic (H&E, medium power). (**b**) The nuclei of the tumor cells are pleiomorphic and range in shape from round to oval to entirely irregular. The nuclei are eccentrically located and perinuclear cytoplasm may be pale, resulting in the appearance of perinuclear clearing (H&E, high power). (See Fig. 10.2 for low-power image)

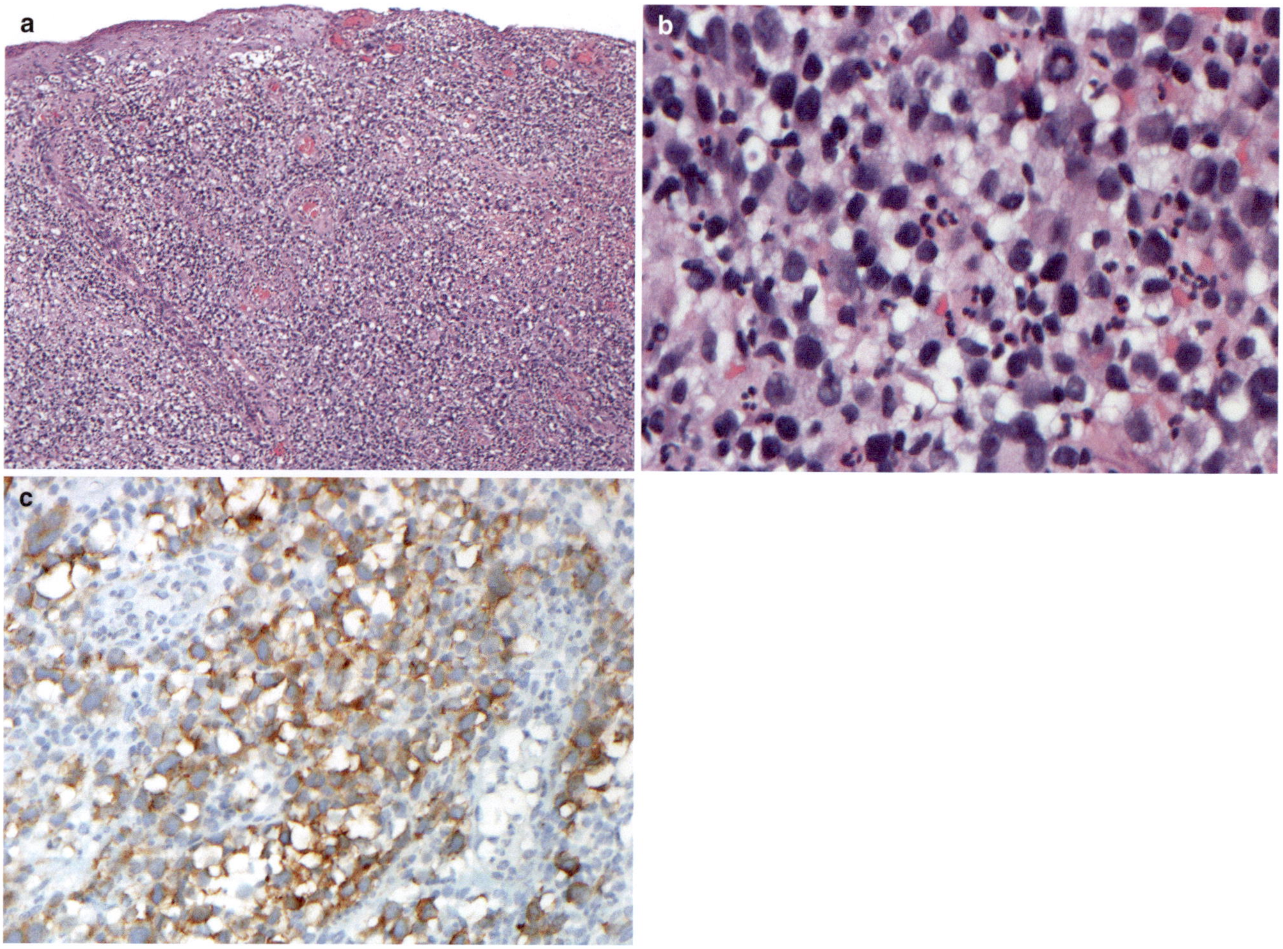

Fig. 10.6 CD30+ primary cutaneous anaplastic large cell lymphoma (pcALCL), histopathology and immunohistochemistry (case 10.1). (**a**) The dermis is filled with sheets of large, atypical lymphocytes. There is an overlying ulceration (H&E, 10×). (**b**) The atypical lymphocytes are large with irregularly shaped nuclei. Numerous neutrophils are present secondary to proximity to an overlying cutaneous ulcer; this is not an example of a neutrophil-rich variant of pcALCL (H&E, 40×). (**c**) More than 70 % of the large cells stain positively for CD30, consistent with a diagnosis of pcALCL (CD30, 20×)

10.2.2 Immunophenotype and Molecular Findings

The neoplastic cells are activated CD4+ cells and have variable loss of CD2, CD3, and CD5; 75 % of the neoplastic cells are CD30+. Cells are frequently positive for granzyme, TIA-1, and perforin. Neoplastic cells are CLA+, ALK−, and EMA− [2].

There are no commonly associated genetic abnormalities [2]. The T-cell receptor (TCR) may be clonal but is often not expressed [2]. Notably, in comparison to systemic ALCL, the t(2;5) translocation that results in anaplastic lymphoma kinase (ALK) expression is absent [2, 13]. Cells are Epstein-Barr virus negative [2, 3, 7].

10.3 Differential Diagnosis

10.3.1 Diagnostic Considerations

Diagnosis is based on clinical presentation and immunohistochemical analysis of biopsy specimens. Diagnosis depends on a combination of assessment of clinical lesions, clinical time course, and histopathology. Immunohistochemistry can be extremely valuable: the pattern of CD30 positivity and lack of ALK expression found in pcALCL can be key to diagnosis [1–3, 5].

10.3.2 Differential Diagnosis

10.3.2.1 Lymphomatoid Papulosis (LyP)

LyP and pcALCL fall on the spectrum of CD30+ cutaneous lymphoproliferative diseases. Differentiating them can be extremely challenging, both clinically for all subtypes of LyP and histopathologically for LyP, type C. In general, the lesions of pcALCL tend to be larger nodules and tumors as compared with the papules of LyP [3, 7]. Although regression of lesions sometimes occurs in pcALCL, it always occurs in LyP [2–4]. pcALCL has a tendency to be localized, whereas LyP is often regional or generalized [7]. Finally, patients with systemic ALCL may present with constitutional symptoms, while in LyP they will not [2]. Histopathologically the two diseases can be remarkably similar, and it may be impossible to distinguish LyP type C from pcALCL without clinical correlation. Both LyP type C and pcALCL are composed of CD4+ neoplastic cells, the majority of which are CD30+. In LyP type C, the lesions are composed of a diffuse dermal infiltrate of large CD30+ T cells. Immunohistochemistry analysis may not be helpful, given that cells of both disorders are CLA+, ALK−, and EMA−.

10.3.2.2 CD30+ Large Cell Transformation of Mycosis Fungoides (MF)

It is possible for MF to undergo CD30+ large cell transformation; the cells of transformed MF may appear quite similar to those of pcALCL. However, MF and pcALCL have very different natural histories: while MF typically progresses sequentially through patch, plaque, and tumor stages, pcALCL generally presents with nodules or tumors that may undergo spontaneous regression. Clinical pathologic correlation is key in differentiating these two conditions [1]. MF with large-cell transformation is more commonly positive for BCL-2 and is without staining for CD25 and perforin; this contrasts with pcALCL, which often is BCL-2 negative and usually stains for CD25 and perforin.

10.3.2.3 Systemic ALCL

Differentiating primary cutaneous ALCL from secondary cutaneous systemic ALCL can be challenging but is critically important clinically—systemic ALCL requires immediate systemic treatment, whereas pcALCL generally requires minimal treatment. Systemic ALCL typically demonstrates the t(2;5) translocation that results in ALK expression; this translocation is notably absent in pcALCL. Thus, assaying ALK expression can be very useful: ALK expression favors but is not diagnostic of systemic or nodal ALCL over cutaneous ALCL [1, 13]. In some cases, immunohistochemistry may be helpful in differentiating these diseases, given that pcALCL cells are usually CLA+, EMA−, ALK−, BCL-2−, whereas systemic ALCL cells are generally CLA−, EMA+, ALK+/−, BCL-2+ [2].

10.3.2.4 Primary Cutaneous Diffuse Large Cell B Cell Lymphoma, Leg Type (DLBCL)

One of the major histopathologic characteristics of pcALCL is that the atypical cells are large and blast-like. Primary cutaneous diffuse large B-cell lymphoma has similar cytomorphology and may be included in the differential diagnosis for pcALCL. Clinically DLBCL tends to present as red to bluish nodules occurring on the lower legs; pcALCL lesions may also manifest as red-violet nodules or papules but can occur anywhere on the body. Although both DLBCL and pcALCL demonstrate large blast-like cells, they are very distinct diseases and can easily be distinguished immunohistochemically. pcALCL is composed of CD30+ neoplastic T cells, while DLBCL is defined by the presence of CD20+ B cells.

10.4 Clinical Case

Case 10.1

A 50-year-old man presented with a 4- to 6-week history of a "pimple" on his left eyebrow that rapidly enlarged to form a 2-cm eroded exophytic nodule (see Fig. 10.3). This large nodule was accompanied by a smaller papule less than 1 cm under the left eye.

Biopsy of the nodule revealed an infiltrate of large CD30+ ALK- cells (see Figs. 10.4, 10.5, and 10.6). A PET-CT scan and blood work were performed and showed evidence of regional lymph node involvement. The patient was diagnosed with pcALCL and multifocal involvement.

The patient underwent systemic chemotherapy and local radiation therapy with excellent regression of both lesions. Five years after his initial diagnosis, he remains well and has had no recurrence of his lymphoma.

Commentary This case highlights the striking clinical findings associated with pcALCL. This patient was treated with systemic chemotherapy given that his disease was multifocal and involved regional lymph nodes. Of note, given the multifocality of his disease, this patient is prone to progression and relapse and must be monitored closely for signs of recurrent cutaneous or extracutaneous disease. Although not pictured, this patient's biopsies demonstrated the histologic appearance classic for pcALCL, with >70 % large CD30+ ALK-lymphocytes.

References

1. Liu HL, Hoppe RT, Kohler S, Harvell JD, Reddy S, Kim YH. CD30+ cutaneous lymphoproliferative disorders: the Stanford experience in lymphomatoid papulosis and primary cutaneous anaplastic large cell lymphoma. J Am Acad Dermatol. 2003;49:1049–58.
2. Ralfkiaer E, Willemze R, Paulli M, Kadin ME, et al. Primary cutaneous CD30-positive T-cell lymphoproliferative disorders. In: Swerdlow SH, Campo E, Harris NL, Jaffe ES, Pileri SA, Stein H, et al., editors. WHO classification of tumors of hematopoietic and lymphoid tissues. Lyon: International Agency for Research on Cancer; 2008. p. 300–1.
3. Bekkenk MW, Geelen AMJ, Vader PCVV, Heule F, Geerts M, van Vloten WA, et al. Primary and secondary cutaneous CD30 lymphoproliferative disorders: a report from the Dutch Cutaneous Lymphoma Group on the long-term follow-up data of 219 patients and guidelines for diagnosis and treatment. Blood. 2000;95:3653–61.
4. Beljaards RC, Kaudewitz P, Berti E, Gianotti R, Neumann C, Rosso R, et al. Primary cutaneous CD30-positive large cell lymphoma: definition of a new type of cutaneous lymphoma with a favorable prognosis. A European Multicenter Study of 47 patients. Cancer. 1993;71:2097–104.
5. Berge RL, Oudejans JJ, Ossenkoppele GJ, Pulford K, Willemze R, Falini B, et al. ALK expression in extranodal anaplastic large cell lymphoma favours systemic disease with (primary) nodal involvement and a good prognosis and occurs before dissemination. J Clin Pathol. 2000;53:445–50.
6. Savage KJ, Harris NL, Vose JM, Ullrich F, Jaffe ES, Connors JM, et al. ALK- anaplastic large-cell lymphoma is clinically and immunophenotypically different from both ALK+ ALCL and peripheral T-cell lymphoma, not otherwise specified: report from the International Peripheral T-Cell Lymphoma Project. Blood. 2008;111:5496–504.
7. Stein H, Foss H, Dürkop H, Marafioti T, Delsol G, Pulford K, et al. Review article. CD30(+) anaplastic large cell lymphoma: a review of its histopathologic, genetic, and clinical features. Blood. 2013;96(12):3681–95.
8. Drews R, Samel A, Kadin ME. Lymphomatoid papulosis and anaplastic large cell lymphomas of the skin. Semin Cutan Med Surg. 2000;19:109–17.
9. Shehan JM, Kalaaji AN, Markovic SN, Ahmed I. Management of multifocal primary cutaneous CD30 anaplastic large cell lymphoma. J Am Acad Dermatol. 2004;51:103–10.
10. Yu JB, McNiff JM, Lund MW, Wilson LD. Treatment of primary cutaneous CD30+ anaplastic large-cell lymphoma with radiation therapy. Int J Radiat Oncol Biol Phys. 2008;70:1542–5.
11. Blume JE, Stoll HL, Cheney RT. Treatment of primary cutaneous CD30+ anaplastic large cell lymphoma with intralesional methotrexate. J Am Acad Dermatol. 2006;54:S229–30.
12. Oliveira A, Fernandes I, Alves R, Lima M, Selores M. Primary cutaneous CD30 positive anaplastic large cell lymphoma – report of a case treated with bexarotene. Leuk Res. 2011;35:e190–2.
13. Kutok JL. Molecular biology of anaplastic lymphoma kinase-positive anaplastic large-cell lymphoma. J Clin Oncol. 2002;20:3691–702.

11 Lymphomatoid Papulosis

Amrita Goyal, Joi B. Carter, and Lyn McDivitt Duncan

Lymphomatoid papulosis (LyP) is a benign CD30+ lymphoproliferative disease that presents as recurrent, spontaneously healing crops of papules and nodules. There are four histologic variants of this lymphoma: types A, B, C, and D. Types B, C, and D resemble more aggressive lymphomas and can be difficult to differentiate from mycosis fungoides (MF), anaplastic large-cell lymphoma (ALCL), and CD8+ aggressive epidermotropic T-cell lymphoma (CD8+ AECTCL). Although LyP is benign and requires minimal treatment, it is occasionally associated with the development of malignant lymphomas, including MF, primary cutaneous ALCL, and Hodgkin lymphoma, thus mandating careful surveillance of patients with LyP. This chapter addresses the clinical presentation, prognosis, and treatment of LyP, followed by a discussion of the immunohistochemical, histopathologic, and molecular characteristics of the four subtypes. It closes with a clinical case.

A. Goyal, M.D.
Harvard-MIT Division of Health Sciences and Technology, Harvard Medical School, Boston, MA, USA

J.B. Carter, M.D.
Department of Dermatology, Massachusetts General Hospital, Harvard Medical School, Boston, MA, USA

L.M. Duncan, M.D. (✉)
Dermatopathology Service, Department of Pathology, Massachusetts General Hospital, Harvard Medical School, Boston, MA, USA
e-mail: duncan@helix.mgh.harvard.edu

J.B. Carter et al. (eds.), *Atlas of Cutaneous Lymphomas: Classification and Differential Diagnosis*,
DOI 10.1007/978-3-319-17217-0_11

11.1 Clinical Information

11.1.1 Clinical Presentation

LyP, a member of the family of CD30+ lymphoproliferative disorders, is a recurrent, self-healing, papulonodular skin eruption that is benign and chronic in nature [1]. Although LyP is most often found in adults with a median age of 45 years [2], cases have been reported in children under the age of 12 [3]. LyP affects men three times more often than women [2].

The recurrent papules and nodules of LyP progress through a number of stages over the course of 3–12 weeks: they begin as small red papules that develop into larger papules or nodules (with or without central ulceration) (see Figs. 11.1, 11.2, and 11.3). As they regress, they turn brown-red and heal as varioliform scars. The lesions are typically multifocal and may exist in different stages simultaneously. The most notable clinical aspect of LyP is that although patients continue to develop new lesions, each one will heal spontaneously and completely [1, 2, 4].

This disease is skin-limited with no systemic involvement and most commonly is seen on the trunk and extremities; oral mucosal lesions are rare [1, 2, 4].

11.1.2 Prognosis and Treatment

LyP has an excellent prognosis, with a disease-specific survival of 100 % at 5 and 10 years [3]. However, in spite of excellent survival, the vast majority of patients continue to experience LyP eruptions irrespective of treatment. The disease may last from several months to over 40 years [3].

There is evidence that LyP is associated with the development of malignant lymphomas [5], particularly mycosis fungoides (MF) [6–8], primary cutaneous anaplastic large-cell lymphoma (pcALCL) [7, 9, 10], or very rarely Hodgkin lymphoma [7, 11, 12]. The rate of secondary malignancy is generally cited as 10–20 % [13, 14], but studies have reported a rate of up to 40 % [15]. Lymph node involvement is rare but not unheard of; such cases may be difficult to distinguish from Hodgkin lymphoma with cutaneous involvement [16].

Patients with LyP can be treated with topical steroids, ultraviolet light phototherapy, and low-dose methotrexate; however, complete remission from the disease is rare [17]. Other reported treatments include topical bexarotene [18] and imiquimod [19]. Given the high likelihood of secondary neoplasms, vigilant patient surveillance is necessary. There is no evidence that early intense therapy is associated with a lower rate of disease progression [17].

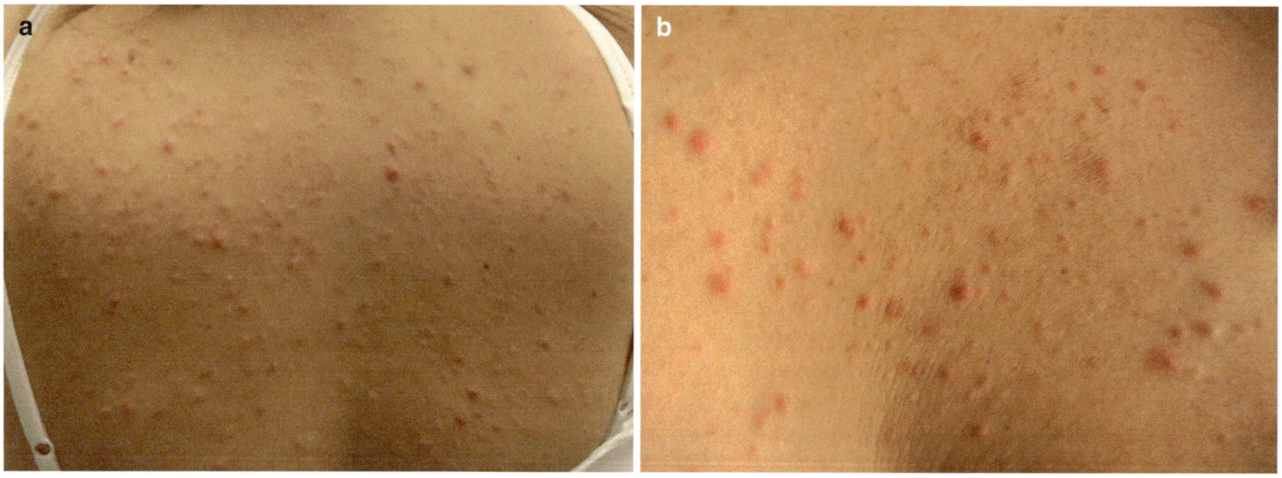

Fig. 11.1 Clinical presentation of LyP (case 11.1). (**a**) Numerous 0.5- to 1-cm erythematous, dermal papules and nodules in various stages of development (all without ulceration) on the back of a 56-year-old woman with a 26-year history of LyP. Also present are scattered atrophic and/or hypopigmented scars from prior relapses of LyP. (**b**) Similar pink-to-erythematous papules across her chest

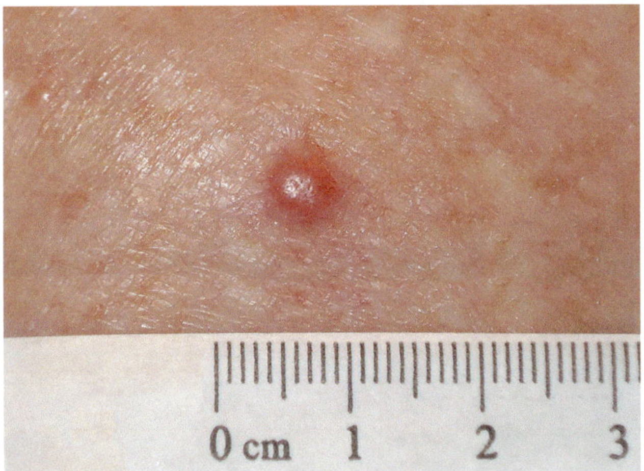

Fig. 11.2 Clinical presentation of LyP: 5 mm, pink-orange, smooth papule on the shoulder of a 72-year-old woman with LyP

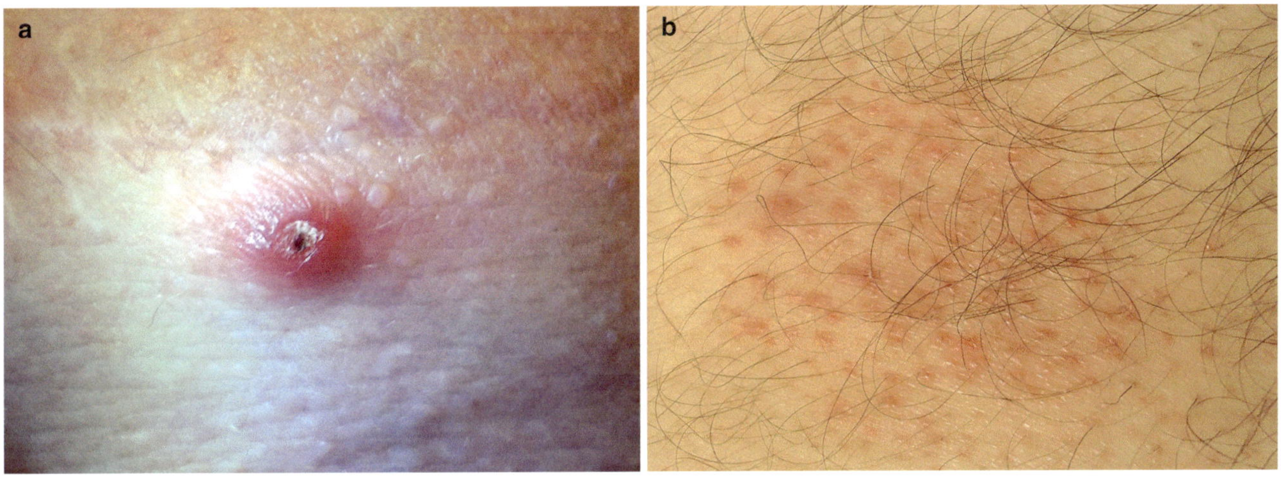

Fig. 11.3 Clinical presentation of LyP. (**a**) A 5-mm erythematous papule with central ulceration and a punctum of hemorrhagic crust located in the antecubital fossa. (**b**) A grouping of numerous non-follicularly based papules on a base of faint erythema located on the buttock

11.2 Pathology

11.2.1 Histopathology

The catch phrase used to describe LyP is that it is "*clinically benign but histologically malignant*," meaning that even though the histologic appearance of biopsies of LyP may be markedly atypical and may raise concern for malignancy, LyP is in fact a benign condition [1]. There are four major histologic variants of LyP (see Fig. 11.4), although different lesions biopsied from the same patient may demonstrate variation in histologic type [2, 4, 20].

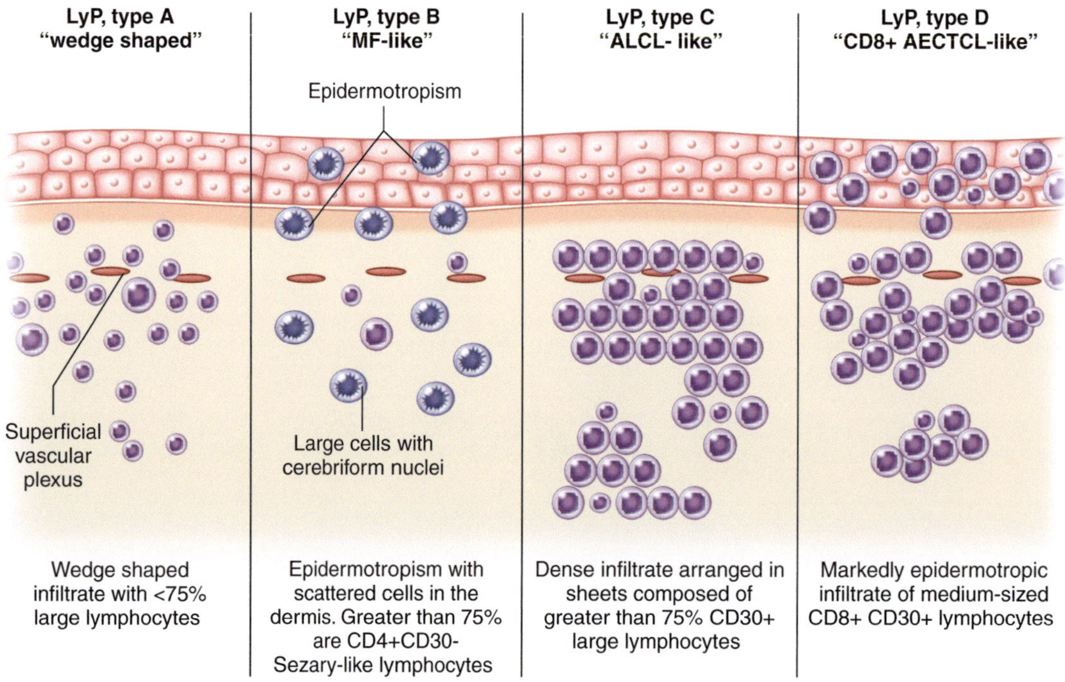

Fig. 11.4 Histology of lymphomatoid papulosis (LyP) types A, B, C, and D. LyP, type A (*left*), is often composed of a wedge-shaped infiltrate with fewer than 75 % large cells. LyP, type B (*second from left*) is "MF-like" and presents with epidermotropism and scattered cells in the dermis. More than 75 % of the cells are CD4+ CD30– Sézary-like cells. LyP, type C (*second from right*), is "ALCL-like," presenting with a dense infiltrate of lymphocytes arranged in sheets. There are more than 75 % CD30+ large cells. LyP, type D (*right*), is likened to CD8+ aggressive epidermotropic T-cell lymphoma (CD8+ AECTCL), with a markedly epidermotropic infiltrate of medium-sized CD8+ CD30+ cells

11.2.1.1 Type A

This is the most common form of LyP and manifests with a classic wedge-shaped dermal infiltrate. Ulceration, spongiosis, or exocytosis may be present, depending on the stage of the lesion. The infiltrate is composed of medium-to-large pleomorphic or anaplastic CD30+ lymphocytes [2, 4, 20]. These are sometimes multinucleated or resemble Reed-Sternberg cells [2, 4]. The large CD30+ cells have abundant cytoplasm, vesicular nuclei, clumped chromatin, and prominent nucleoli and may be scattered or clustered (Fig. 11.5) [2, 4]. Numerous mixed inflammatory cells, including histiocytes, lymphocytes, neutrophils, and eosinophils dominate the infiltrate [2, 4, 20]. Half of cases demonstrate overlying epidermal hyperplasia [20].

11.2.1.2 Type B

This form of LyP is the least common and is histopathologically very similar to (MF). LyP, type B, presents with a dense, bandlike infiltrate in the superficial reticular dermis, occasionally extending into the deep reticular dermis. This atypical lymphoid proliferation owes its MF-like appearance to its characteristic epidermotropic infiltrate of small-to-medium atypical CD4+ lymphocytes with Sézary-like, convoluted, cerebriform nuclei [2, 4].

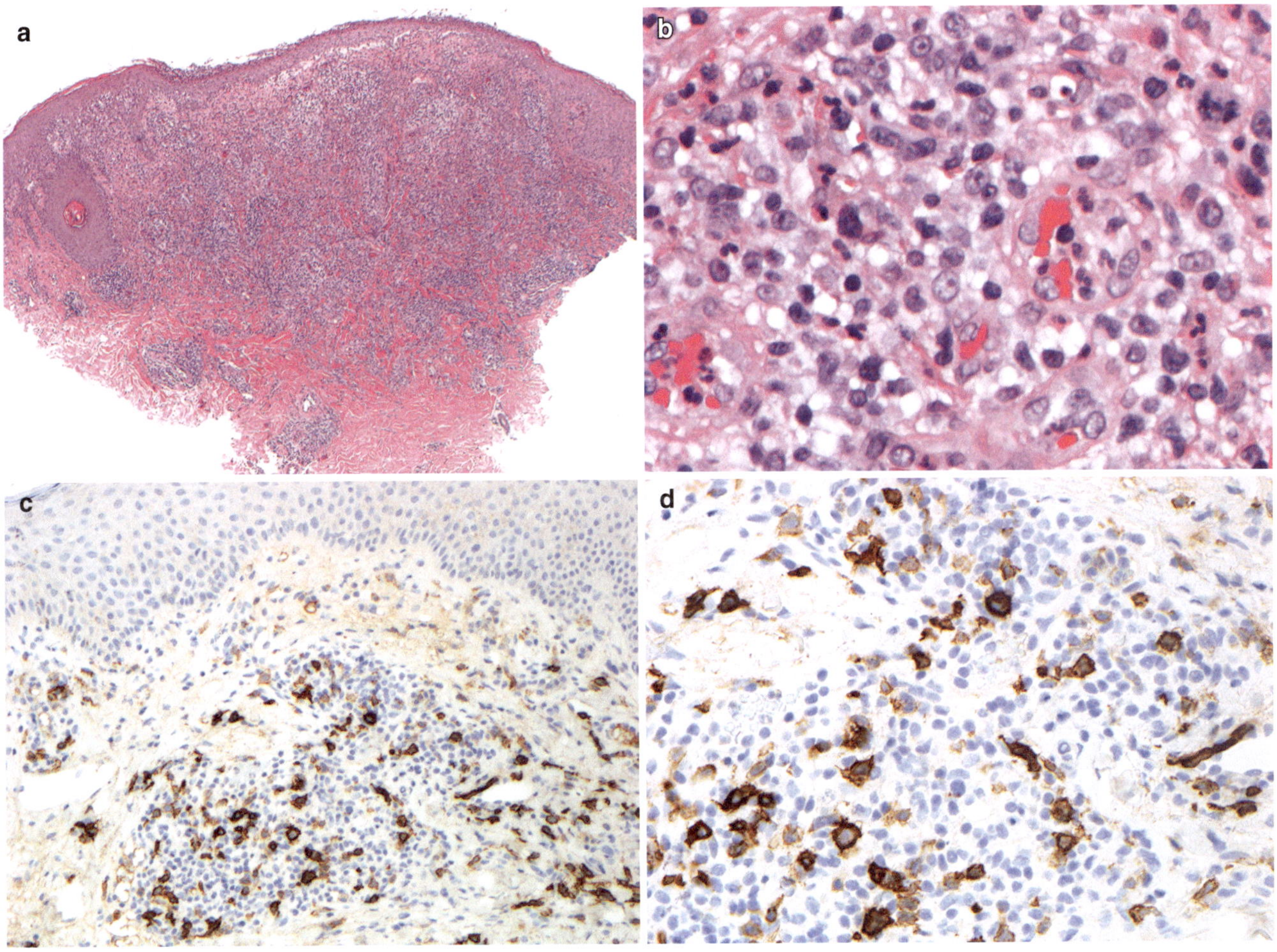

Fig. 11.5 Histopathology and immunohistochemistry of LyP, type A. (**a**) Wedge-shaped lymphocytic infiltrate occupies the superficial and deep dermis with some epidermal spongiosis and subepidermal vesicle formation (H&E, 2×). (**b**) The infiltrate is composed of large atypical lymphocytes with irregular nuclear contours, vesicular nuclei, prominent nucleoli, and clumped and irregular chromatin. Mitoses are common (*top right corner*). Numerous histiocytes are also present (H&E, 40×). (**c**) The majority of the large atypical lymphocytes in the dermal infiltrate are CD30+ (CD30, 20×). (**d**) The CD30+ cells are large and irregular with substantial amounts of cytoplasm and nuclear atypia. Surrounding reactive lymphocytes and histiocytes do not stain for CD30 (CD30, 40×)

11.2.1.3 Type C

This variant of LyP is considered to be histologically identical to pcALCL, another member of the spectrum of CD30+ lymphoproliferative disorders. Like pcALCL, it is characterized by a dense, diffuse, superficial and deep dermal proliferation of medium-to-large atypical CD30+ cells. By definition, large CD30+ cells must comprise more than 75 % of the cellular infiltrate [2, 4] (Fig. 11.6). Admixed eosinophils and neutrophils are common [20].

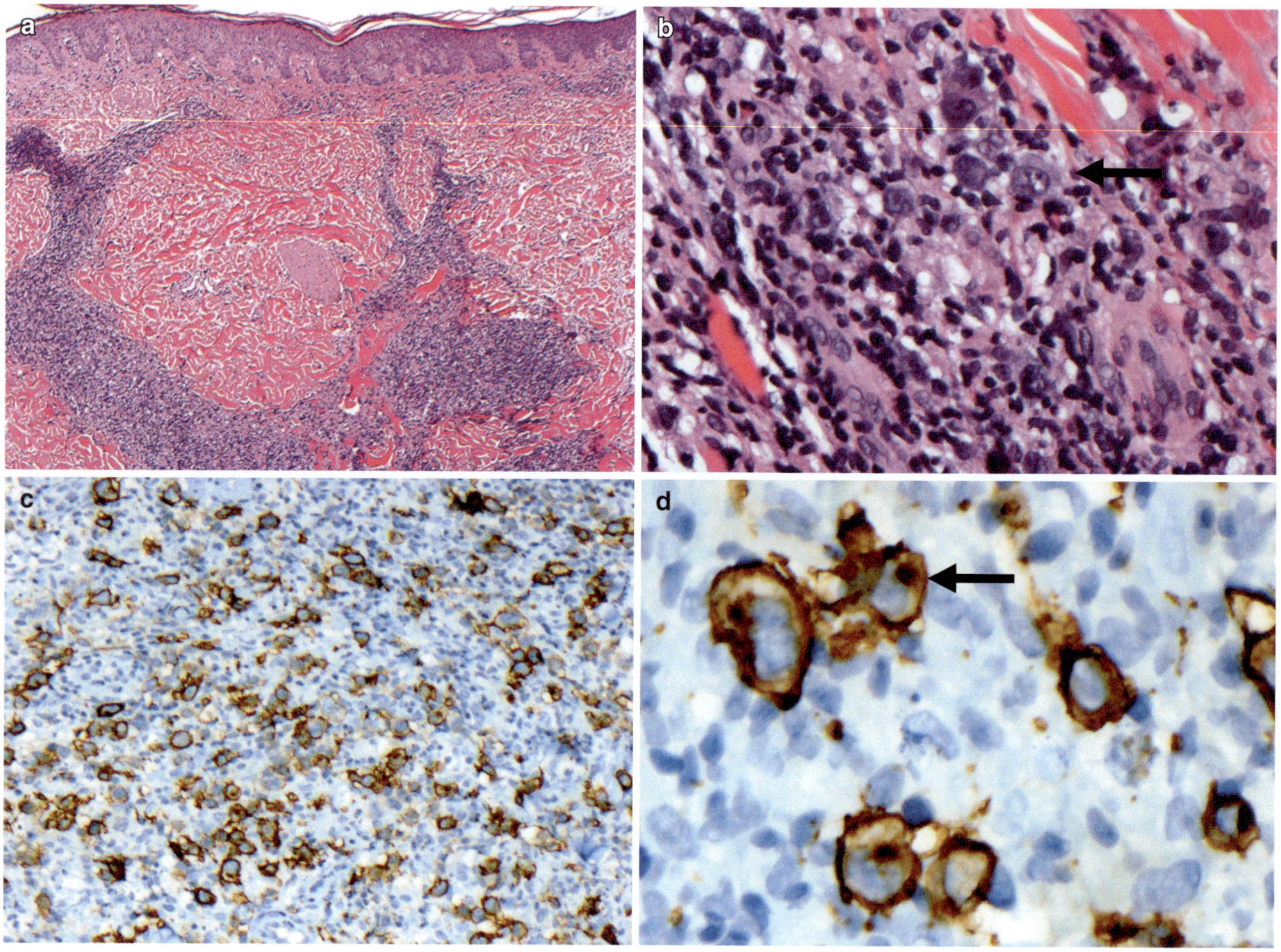

Fig. 11.6 Histopathology and immunohistochemistry of LyP, type C, clinical case 11.1. (**a**) Dense, non–epidermotropic superficial and deep perivascular lymphoid infiltrate (H&E, 4×). (**b**) The neoplastic T cells are large and anaplastic. Nuclei are prominent and range from round to irregular in shape. The infiltrate contains Reed-Sternberg-like cells (*arrow*) (H&E, 40×). (**c**) More than 75 % of the large atypical cells express CD30. There are numerous small, round, reactive lymphocytes that do not express CD30 (CD30, 40×). (**d**) Higher magnification reveals a dot-like pattern of perinuclear staining and peri-golgi zone accentuation (*black arrow*) (CD30, 60×)

11.2.1.4 Type D

This form of LyP is not formally recognized by the WHO/EORTC classification system. It is characterized by an epidermotropic infiltrate of CD8+ CD30+ medium-to-large sized lymphocytes with hyperchromatic, irregular nuclei. The epidermal infiltrate is accompanied by sheets of atypical cells in the dermis [2, 4, 21]. Some have described the degree of epidermotropism as "massive," in some cases approaching complete replacement of the epidermis [22]. Spongiosis and parakeratosis are often present, as is perivascular accentuation [23]. The epidermotropism and epidermal infiltration of LyP, type D, is more striking than that of type B [21]. Type D may be very difficult to distinguish from the extremely aggressive CD8+ epidermotropic cytotoxic T-cell lymphoma (CD8+ AECTCL) [2, 4, 21, 24].

11.2.2 Immunophenotype and Molecular Findings

The infiltrating cells in LyP types A and C are CD30+ with variable loss of CD2, CD5, and/or CD3. Although they are CD4+, they commonly express cytotoxic proteins, including granzyme B, TIA1, and perforin. These cells are often CD25+ with a high Ki-67 fraction. They are characteristically ALK– and CD15– [2].

The infiltrating cells of type B LyP are markedly different from the CD30+ cells in other types of LyP: they are CD30–, CD3+ CD4+ CD8– [2, 20].

The cells of LyP, type D, have a cytotoxic phenotype and express CD8, CD30, TIA-1, and granzyme B. They are also CD3+, betaF1+, and CD4– (Table 11.1) [25].

Clonally rearranged T-cell receptor genes are present in over half of LyP lesions [2]. Several case reports have demonstrated the presence of the same T-cell receptor (TCR) rearrangement in multiple lesions from the same patient; this has been taken as evidence that LyP is a monoclonal disease [26, 27].

The t(2;5) translocation that is often present in systemic ALCL is absent in LyP [28]. There are no consistent genetic abnormalities, but rearrangements of the 6p25.3 locus have been implicated in some cases [29].

Table 11.1 Immunohistochemical staining patterns of the subtypes of LyP

	CD3	CD4	CD8	CD2/CD5	CD30	Cytotoxic	ALK
Type A	±	+	–	±	+	±	–
Type B	±	+	–	±	–	–	–
Type C	±	+	–	±	+	±	–
Type D	+	–	+	±	+	+	–

11.3 Differential Diagnosis

11.3.1 Diagnostic Considerations

LyP is diagnosed based on a combination of the time course of clinical presentation, the morphology of skin lesions, and the histopathology seen on skin biopsies. Clinical pathologic correlation is required for accurate diagnosis.

11.3.2 Differential Diagnosis

11.3.2.1 Primary Cutaneous Anaplastic Large Cell Lymphoma (pcALCL)

LyP and pcALCL both belong to the spectrum of primary cutaneous CD30+ lymphoproliferative disorders [30, 31]. The histopathology of pcALCL and type C LyP can be indistinguishable: both are characterized by a dense dermal proliferation of large atypical CD30+ cells. Because of this histopathologic overlap between LyP and pcALCL, diagnosis rests on the clinical course of the lesions; if all of the lesions are spontaneously resolving papules, the patient likely has LyP. If the lesions are greater than 2 cm and do not heal, pcALCL is more likely [2, 4, 32]. The presence of the *IRF4* translocation favors the diagnosis of pcALCL over LyP (and, interestingly, over systemic ALCL), and assessment for this translocation may be a helpful diagnostic tool [33].

11.3.2.2 Systemic ALCL (sALCL) with Secondary Cutaneous Involvement

Given the difficulty of differentiating primary cutaneous and systemic ALCL, the differential diagnosis for LyP also includes systemic ALCL with secondary cutaneous involvement. Clinical presentation is often invaluable: patients with systemic ALCL generally present with B symptoms and lymphadenopathy, whereas LyP patients never show systemic symptoms [2]. Immunohistochemistry can be helpful in that while LyP cells are EMA- and ALK-, the neoplastic cells of sALCL cells may be EMA+ and often ALK+. Of note, regardless of ALK positivity or negativity, all patients with suspected ALCL should be evaluated for systemic disease.

11.3.2.3 Primary Cutaneous Aggressive Epidermotropic CD8+ Cytotoxic T-Cell Lymphoma (CD8+ AECTCL)

This very aggressive T-cell lymphoma can be difficult to differentiate histologically from LyP, type D, given that both are characterized by an epidermotropic CD8+ cytotoxic T-cell infiltrate [25]. However, these diseases follow very different clinical courses. While patients with LyP experience a benign course of recurrent self-healing crops of papules and nodules, the nodules and ulcers of CD8+ AECTCL do not heal [34]. In contrast to the excellent 5-year survival rate of patients with LyP, patients with CD8+ AECTCL have an average 5-year survival rate of 18 % [35]. Immunohistochemistry may be useful in differentiating these conditions. While LyP, type D, is nearly always CD30+, CD8+, AECTCL generally lacks CD30. However, there are reports of occasional cases of CD8+ AECTCL that are CD30+ [24].

11.3.2.4 Mycosis Fungoides (MF)

MF and LyP, type B, mimic one another histopathologically: both present with marked epidermotropism of CD4+ T cells that lack CD30 expression. Clinically, the lesions of tumor stage MF can be similar to the ulcerated papules of LyP. However, MF tends to progress through patch, plaque, and tumor stages whereas LyP does not. Additionally, the papules of LyP spontaneously regress, while the tumors of MF do not. A complicating factor in parsing this differential is that patients with LyP are at higher risk of developing secondary malignancies, *including* MF [15]. The co-occurrence of LyP and MF is not uncommon, and lesions of LyP may be present in nearly 5 % of patients with MF [36].

11.3.2.5 CD30+ Variants of Pityriasis Lichenoides et Varioliformis Acuta (PLEVA)

This non-neoplastic cutaneous inflammatory disease manifests as erythematous scaly papules that become vesicular, hemorrhagic, then necrotic and ulcerative in rapid sequence. Clinically, these may closely resemble the ulcerative papulonodules of LyP, with the exception of the finding that the lesions of LyP wax and wane spontaneously while those of PLEVA do not [37]. Differentiating PLEVA and LyP can be complicated by the observation that biopsies of PLEVA may be rich in CD30+ lymphocytes [37] and that clonal T-cell receptor gene rearrangements are not uncommon [38]. Some authors have suggested that PLEVA and LyP may in fact belong to the same spectrum of T-cell lymphoproliferative disorders [37, 38]. Histopathology can be helpful in differentiating these clinically similar conditions: PLEVA more often displays a constellation of findings that includes parakeratosis, spongiosis, mild-to-moderate acanthosis, keratinocyte necrosis, erythrocyte extravasation, and perivascular lymphocytic infiltrate of memory cytotoxic T cells that may obscure the dermoepidermal junction [37].

11.4 Clinical Case

Case 11.1

A 56-year-old woman presented with a 20-plus years history of recurrent crops of papules over her arms, legs, back, abdomen, breasts, and buttocks. She also had a distant history of Hodgkin lymphoma, now in remission. The papules were slightly pruritic and ranged in size from 0.5 to 1.5 cm. (see Fig. 11.1). The papules would resolve spontaneously after 3–4 weeks. These were initially thought to be acne.

A biopsy of a papule from her neck showed a superficial and deep dermal nodular to diffuse lymphocytic infiltrate with admixed eosinophils, neutrophils, and scattered large atypical cells with vesicular nuclei and prominent nucleoli (see Fig. 11.6). The large cells were positive for CD30 and CD15 and negative for CD20, CD2, CD3, CD4, and CD5. The patient was diagnosed with a CD30+ lymphoproliferative disorder. Given her history of recurrent crops of self-resolving papules, this was most consistent with lymphomatoid papulosis.

Since her diagnosis, she has undergone numerous treatments, including psoralen plus ultraviolet A therapy, steroids, interferon, bexarotene, and nitrogen mustard, all with poor efficacy and poor tolerance. Methotrexate did decrease the frequency of her flares. Because her disease was refractory to all standard treatments, after 3 years of somewhat unsuccessful treatment with methotrexate she began brentuximab (an anti-CD30 antibody–drug conjugate). Although this medication led to dramatic clearing of her skin, she was forced to discontinue it after only a few cycles because of severe drug-induced neuropathy. She was restarted on methotrexate and intermittent steroid tapers to treat disease flares. Her disease remains recalcitrant to treatment, and she continues to develop new crops of papules all over her body.

Commentary This clinical case demonstrates several important points about LyP. First, the lesions are recurrent and self-resolving, as is classic for LyP. Second, this case demonstrates the association of LyP with other lymphomas, i.e., in this patient's case, Hodgkin disease. Third, patients with LyP frequently have life-long disease. LyP can be very difficult to treat, and this patient exhausted all standard treatments. Finally, it is notable that LyP is exquisitely responsive to brentuximab owing to the expression of CD30 by the atypical cells. In spite of this efficacy, treatment is limited by side effects.

References

1. Macaulay WL. Lymphomatoid papulosis: a continuing self healing eruption, clinically benign — histologically malignant. Arch Dermatol. 1968;97:23–30.
2. Ralfkiaer E, Willemze R, Paulli M, Kadin ME. Primary cutaneous CD30-positive T-cell lymphoproliferative disorders. In: Swerdlow SH, Campo E, Harris NL, Jaffe ES, Pileri SA, Stein H, et al., editors. WHO classification of tumors of hematopoietic and lymphoid tissues. Lyon: International Agency for Research on Cancer; 2008. p. 300–1.
3. Bekkenk MW, Geelen AMJ, Vader PCVV, Heule F, Geerts M, Van Vloten WA, et al. Primary and secondary cutaneous CD30(+) lymphoproliferative disorders: a report from the Dutch Cutaneous Lymphoma Group on the long-term follow-up data of 219 patients and guidelines for diagnosis and treatment. Blood. 2000;95:3653–61.
4. Duvic M. CD30+ neoplasms of the skin. Curr Hematol Malig Rep. 2011;6:245–50.
5. Kadin ME. Lymphomatoid papulosis and associated lymphomas. How are they related? Arch Dermatol. 1993;129:351–3.
6. Zackheim HS, Jones C, Leboit PE, Kashani-Sabet M, McCalmont TH, Zehnder J. Lymphomatoid papulosis associated with mycosis fungoides: a study of 21 patients including analyses for clonality. J Am Acad Dermatol. 2003;49:620–3.
7. Beljaards RC, Willemze R. The prognosis of patients with lymphomatoid papulosis associated with malignant lymphomas. Br J Dermatol. 1992;126:596–602.
8. De Souza A, El-Azhary RA, Camilleri MJ, Wada DA, Appert DL, Gibson LE. In search of prognostic indicators for lymphomatoid papulosis: a retrospective study of 123 patients. J Am Acad Dermatol. 2012;66:928–37.
9. LeBoit PE. Lymphomatoid papulosis and cutaneous CD30+ lymphoma. Am J Dermatopathol. 1996;18:221–35.
10. McCarty MJ, Vukelja SJ, Sausville EA, Perry JJ, James WD, Jaffe ES, et al. Lymphomatoid papulosis associated with Ki-1-positive anaplastic large cell lymphoma. A report of two cases and a review of the literature. Cancer. 1994;74:3051–8.
11. Zackheim HS, LeBoit PE, Gordon BI, Glassberg AB. Lymphomatoid papulosis followed by Hodgkin's lymphoma. Differential response to therapy. Arch Dermatol. 1993;129:86–91.
12. Davis TH, Morton CC, Miller-Cassman R, Balk SP, Kadin ME. Hodgkin's disease, lymphomatoid papulosis, and cutaneous T-cell lymphoma derived from a common T-cell clone. N Engl J Med. 1992;326:1115–22.
13. Wang HH, Myers T, Lach LJ, Hsieh CC, Kadin ME. Increased risk of lymphoid and nonlymphoid malignancies in patients with lymphomatoid papulosis. Cancer. 1999;86:1240–5.
14. Cabanillas F, Armitage J, Pugh WC, Weisenburger D, Duvic M. Lymphomatoid papulosis: a T-cell dyscrasia with a propensity to transform into malignant lymphoma. Ann Intern Med. 1995;122:210–7.

15. Kunishige JH, McDonald H, Alvarez G, Johnson M, Prieto V, Duvic M. Lymphomatoid papulosis and associated lymphomas: a retrospective case series of 84 patients. Clin Exp Dermatol. 2009;34:576–81.
16. Eberle FC, Song JY, Xi L, Raffeld M, Harris NL, Wilson WH, et al. Nodal involvement by cutaneous CD30-positive T-cell lymphoma mimicking classical Hodgkin lymphoma. Am J Surg Pathol. 2012;36:716–25.
17. Kempf W, Pfaltz K, Vermeer MH, Cozzio A, Ortiz-Romero PL, Bagot M, et al. EORTC, ISCL, and USCLC consensus recommendations for the treatment of primary cutaneous CD30-positive lymphoproliferative disorders: lymphomatoid papulosis and primary cutaneous anaplastic large-cell lymphoma. Blood. 2011;118:4024–35.
18. Krathen RA, Ward S, Duvic M. Bexarotene is a new treatment option for lymphomatoid papulosis. Dermatology. 2003;206:142–7.
19. Hughes PSH. Treatment of lymphomatoid papulosis with imiquimod 5 % cream. J Am Acad Dermatol. 2006;54:546–7.
20. El Shabrawi-Caelen L, Kerl H, Cerroni L. Lymphomatoid papulosis: reappraisal of clinicopathologic presentation and classification into subtypes A, B, and C. Arch Dermatol. 2004;140:441–7.
21. Plaza JA, Feldman AL, Magro C. Cutaneous CD30-positive lymphoproliferative disorders with CD8 expression: a clinicopathologic study of 21 cases. J Cutan Pathol. 2013;40:236–47.
22. Bertolotti A, Pham-Ledard AL, Vergier B, Parrens M, Bedane C, Beylot-Barry M. Lymphomatoid papulosis type D: an aggressive histology for an indolent disease. Br J Dermatol. 2013;169:1157–9.
23. McQuitty E, Curry JL, Tetzlaff MT, Prieto VG, Duvic M, Torres-Cabala C. The differential diagnosis of CD8-positive ("type D") lymphomatoid papulosis. J Cutan Pathol. 2014;41:88–100.
24. Magro CM, Morrison C, Merati K, Porcu P, Wright ED, Crowson AN. CD8+ lymphomatoid papulosis and its differential diagnosis. Am J Clin Pathol. 2006;125:490–501.
25. Saggini A, Gulia A, Argenyi Z, Fink-Puches R, Lissia A, Magaña M, et al. A variant of lymphomatoid papulosis simulating primary cutaneous aggressive epidermotropic CD8+ cytotoxic T-cell lymphoma. Description of 9 cases. Am J Surg Pathol. 2010;34:1168–75.
26. Steinhoff M, Hummel M, Anagnostopoulos I, Kaudewitz P, Seitz V, Assaf C, et al. Single-cell analysis of CD30+ cells in lymphomatoid papulosis demonstrates a common clonal T-cell origin. Blood. 2002;100:578–84.
27. Chott A, Vonderheid EC, Olbricht S, Miao NN, Balk SP, Kadin ME. The dominant T cell clone is present in multiple regressing skin lesions and associated T cell lymphomas of patients with lymphomatoid papulosis. J Invest Dermatol. 1996;106:696–700.
28. DeCoteau JF, Butmarc JR, Kinney MC, Kadin ME. The t(2;5) chromosomal translocation is not a common feature of primary cutaneous CD30+ lymphoproliferative disorders: comparison with anaplastic large-cell lymphoma of nodal origin. Blood. 1996;87:3437–41.
29. Karai LJ, Kadin ME, Hsi ED, Sluzevich JC, Ketterling RP, Knudson RA, et al. Chromosomal rearrangements of 6p25.3 define a new subtype of lymphomatoid papulosis. Am J Surg Pathol. 2013;37:1173–81.
30. Paulli M, Berti E, Rosso R, Boveri E, Kindl S, Klersy C, et al. CD30/Ki-1-positive lymphoproliferative disorders of the skin—clinicopathologic correlation and statistical analysis of 86 cases: a multicentric study from the European Organization for Research and Treatment of Cancer Cutaneous Lymphoma Project Group. J Clin Oncol. 1995;13:1343–54.
31. Demierre MF, Goldberg LJ, Kadin ME, Koh HK. Is it lymphoma or lymphomatoid papulosis? J Am Acad Dermatol. 1997;36:765–72.
32. Kempf W. CD30+ lymphoproliferative disorders: histopathology, differential diagnosis, new variants, and simulators. J Cutan Pathol. 2006;33 Suppl 1:58–70.
33. Wada DA, Law ME, Hsi ED, Dicaudo DJ, Ma L, Lim MS, et al. Specificity of IRF4 translocations for primary cutaneous anaplastic large cell lymphoma: a multicenter study of 204 skin biopsies. Mod Pathol. 2011;24:596–605.
34. Liu V, Cutler C, Young AZ. Case 38–2007: a 44-year-old woman with generalized, painful, ulcerated skin lesions. N Engl J Med. 2007;357:2496–505.
35. Nofal A, Abdel-Mawla MY, Assaf M, Salah E. Primary cutaneous aggressive epidermotropic CD8+ T-cell lymphoma: proposed diagnostic criteria and therapeutic evaluation. J Am Acad Dermatol. 2012;67:748–59.
36. Agar NS, Wedgeworth E, Crichton S, Mitchell TJ, Cox M, Ferreira S, et al. Survival outcomes and prognostic factors in mycosis fungoides/Sézary syndrome: validation of the revised International Society for Cutaneous Lymphomas/European Organisation for Research and Treatment of Cancer Staging Proposal. J Clin Oncol. 2010;28:4730–9.
37. Kempf W, Kazakov DV, Palmedo G, Fraitag S, Schaerer L, Kutzner H. Pityriasis lichenoides et varioliformis acuta with numerous CD30(+) cells: a variant mimicking lymphomatoid papulosis and other cutaneous lymphomas. A clinicopathologic, immunohistochemical, and molecular biological study of 13 cases. Am J Surg Pathol. 2012;36:1021–9.
38. Dereure O, Levi E, Kadin ME. T-cell clonality in pityriasis lichenoides et varioliformis acuta: a heteroduplex analysis of 20 cases. Arch Dermatol. 2000;136:1483–6.

12 Primary Cutaneous CD8+ Aggressive Epidermotropic Cytotoxic T-Cell Lymphoma

Amrita Goyal, Joi B. Carter, Daniela Kroshinsky, Jeffrey A. Barnes, Aliyah R. Sohani, and Lyn McDivitt Duncan

Primary cutaneous CD8+ aggressive epidermotropic cytotoxic T-cell lymphoma (CD8+ AECTCL) is a rare, aggressive cutaneous T-cell lymphoma with a poor prognosis. Although CD8+ AECTCL typically initially presents on the skin, visceral dissemination is common. Given the rarity of this condition, it is considered a provisional entity in the fourth edition of the World Health Organization/European Organization for Research and Treatment of Cancer (WHO/EORTC) classification guidelines. In this chapter we discuss the clinical presentation, prognosis, treatment, histopathology, immunohistochemistry, molecular characteristics, and differential diagnosis of CD8+ AECTCL. The chapter closes with a clinical case.

A. Goya, M.D.
Harvard-MIT Division of Health Sciences and Technology, Harvard Medical School, Boston, MA, USA

J.B. Carter, M.D. • D. Kroshinsky, M.D.
Department of Dermatology, Massachusetts General Hospital, Harvard Medical School, Boston, MA, USA

J.A. Barnes, M.D., Ph.D.
Comprehensive Cutaneous Lymphoma Program, Department of Medicine, Massachusetts General Hospital Cancer Center, Boston, MA, USA

A.R. Sohani, M.D.
Hematopathology Service, Department of Pathology Massachusetts General Hospital, Harvard Medical School, Boston, MA, USA

L.M. Duncan, M.D. (✉)
Dermatopathology Service, Department of Pathology, Massachusetts General Hospital, Harvard Medical School, Boston, MA, USA
e-mail: duncan@helix.mgh.harvard.edu

J.B. Carter et al. (eds.), *Atlas of Cutaneous Lymphomas: Classification and Differential Diagnosis*, DOI 10.1007/978-3-319-17217-0_12

12.1 Clinical Information

12.1.1 Clinical Presentation

CD8+ AECTCL is very rare, accounting for less than 1 % of all cutaneous T-cell lymphomas. It is seen mostly in males, but there are no known predisposing factors [1].

The most common presentation of CD8+ AECTCL is widely disseminated ulcerative and necrotic papules and/or nodules ranging from 3 to 6 cm in diameter (see Fig. 12.1) [2–5]. Patients may also present with superficial hyperkeratotic plaques and patches [2–4]. Although any site may be involved, lesions are commonly found on mucosal surfaces, palms, and soles, with acral accentuation [3, 4]. Lesions can be exceptionally painful, and patients may require narcotic pain medication. Superinfection of ulcerated, cracked, or necrotic lesions may occur [5].

Patients typically experience extremely rapid progression of their disease over the course of months. Although CD8+ AECTCL frequently disseminates to viscera, including the lung, testes, central nervous system, and oral mucosa, lymph nodes are typically spared [1, 3, 6, 7]. Factors associated with visceral involvement include the presence of disseminated ulcerative plaques and nodules, involvement of most of the body surface area, and rapid onset of lesions [4]. Extracutaneous involvement portends a worse prognosis [4].

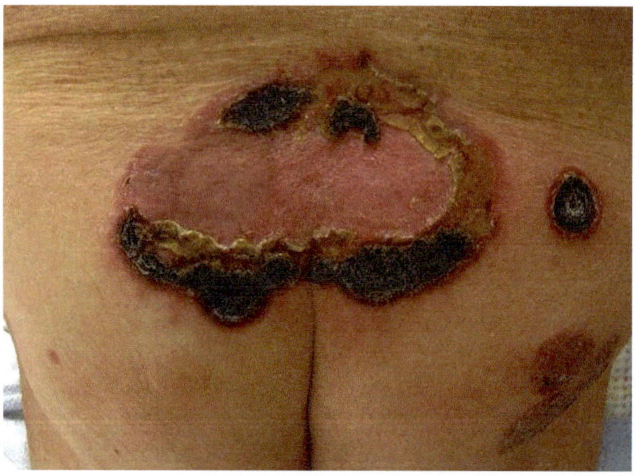

Fig. 12.1 CD8+ aggressive epidermotropic cytotoxic T-cell lymphoma, clinical image (case 12.1). On the patient's lower back and buttocks are numerous large ulcerated plaques, ranging from 2 to 15 cm in diameter, in various stages of healing

12.1.2 Prognosis and Treatment

The median survival for CD8+ AECTCL ranges from 23 to 32 months, with a median 5-year survival of 18 % [2, 4, 8]. These extremely poor outcomes are attributable to the disease's rapid rate of dissemination, its intractable resistance to chemotherapy, and the high rate of relapse [4].

Treatment is extremely challenging. As a consequence of the rarity of CD8+ AECTCL, no randomized controlled trials have been possible and there are no standardized treatments. Numerous treatments have been attempted, including localized radiotherapy, oral bexarotene, multiagent chemotherapy, bone marrow transplantation, and targeted biologics, but they have all been met with minimal success. Patients who do experience some improvement with treatment almost universally relapse once treatment is discontinued. Notably, the skin-directed therapies often used for mycosis fungoides (including topical steroids, topical chemotherapy, topical retinoids, and phototherapy) are often ineffective. Interferon-alpha may actually worsen the disease [4].

12.2 Pathology

12.2.1 Histopathology

CD8+ AECTCL characteristically displays a lichenoid and epidermotropic infiltrate of CD8+ T cells with subepidermal edema. Deep nodular infiltrates may be present. Biopsies may demonstrate epidermal acanthosis or atrophy, necrosis, ulceration, and/or subepidermal bullae (see Fig. 12.2a, b) [1].

The tumor cells range from small-medium to medium-large in size. These T cells may have blastic or pleomorphic nuclei (see Fig. 12.2c). The neoplastic infiltrate may display angiocentricity and angioinvasion, and adnexal structure invasion and destruction are common [1].

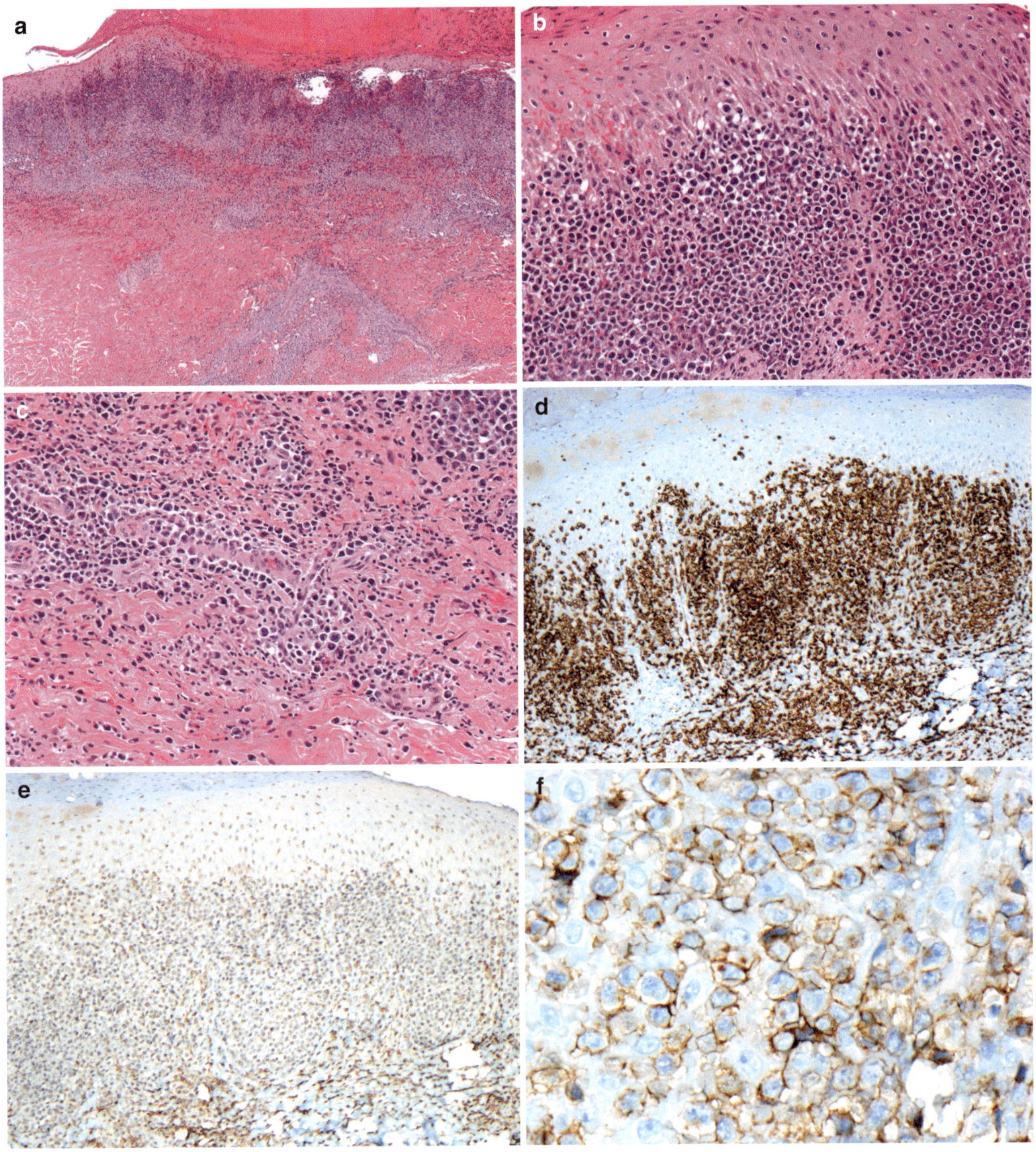

Fig. 12.2 CD8+ aggressive epidermotropic cytotoxic T-cell lymphoma, histopathology (case 12.1). (**a**) Dense sheet-like and nodular infiltrate of large atypical lymphoid cells along the dermal-epidermal junction and in the superficial dermis. The epidermis is largely eroded with overlying scale crust (H&E, 10×). (**b**) The infiltrate demonstrates marked epidermotropism, a primary characteristic of CD8+ AECTCL (H&E, 20×). (**c**) The neoplastic infiltrate is composed of large atypical cells with scant cytoplasm. Nuclei have markedly irregular contours, vesicular chromatin, and prominent nucleoli (H&E, 20×). (**d**) The atypical large T cells stain positively for CD3 (CD3, 10×). (**e**) Although some non-neoplastic small CD4+ cells and CD4+ histiocytes are present in the background, the majority of the large atypical cells do not express CD4 (CD4, 20×). (**f**) The atypical large cells express CD8 (CD8, 40×).

12.2.2 Immunophenotype and Molecular Findings

The CD8+ T cells also typically express betaF1, CD3, granzyme B, perforin, and TIA-1 (Fig. 12.2d–f). The latter three are cytotoxic granule proteins, demonstrating the cytotoxic nature of this neoplasm. The T cells are CD4- and may display loss of the pan-T cell antigens CD2 and CD5 [1, 2]. This tumor is not associated with Epstein-Barr virus (EBV) infection [1] (Table 12.1).

While clonal TCR rearrangement is often detected, no specific genetic or chromosomal abnormalities have been identified [1].

Table 12.1 Summary of immunohistochemical staining patterns in CD8+ AECTCL

Positive	Negative
CD3	CD2 (variable)
CD8	CD4
BetaF1	CD5 (variable)
Granzyme B	EBER
Perforin	
TIA-1	

12.3 Differential Diagnosis

12.3.1 Diagnostic Considerations

Diagnosis is based on a synthesis of histologic features, presentation, and clinical behavior, including time-course and response to therapy. The most striking and helpful diagnostic finding is the epidermotropic infiltrate of atypical CD8+ cytotoxic T cells [1]. The clinical differential diagnosis may include other processes that appear as large ulcerated plaques, such as pyoderma gangrenosum, non–melanoma skin cancers, hypersensitivity reaction, and other types of cutaneous lymphoma. Conditions characterized by an epidermotropic CD8+ T cell infiltrate are important considerations; these include CD8+ mycosis fungoides, lymphomatoid papulosis, type D, and hypersensitivity reactions.

12.3.2 Differential Diagnosis

12.3.2.1 Mycosis Fungoides (MF), CD8+ Variant

Both CD8+ MF and CD8+ AECTCL present with an epidermotropic CD8+ lymphocytic infiltrate. However, CD8+ AECTCL lacks the tagging of the dermal-epidermal junction (DEJ) by atypical lymphocytes and the Pautrier microabscesses of MF. The epidermotropic component of CD8+ AECTCL is denser than that of MF and is distributed in a "shotgun"-like pattern throughout the epidermis. Finally, while the cells of MF have cerebriform nuclei, those of CD8+ AECTCL are large with irregular hyperchromatic nuclei (see Fig. 12.3). Clinical features usually allow the differentiation of CD8+ AECTCL from CD8+ MF: CD8+ AECTCL does not progress through the typical patch-plaque-tumor stages characteristic of MF [3, 5]. These two forms of CTCL also have dramatically different prognoses and responses to chemotherapy, given that MF is far more indolent and responsive to treatment than CD8+ AECTCL [1, 3, 4].

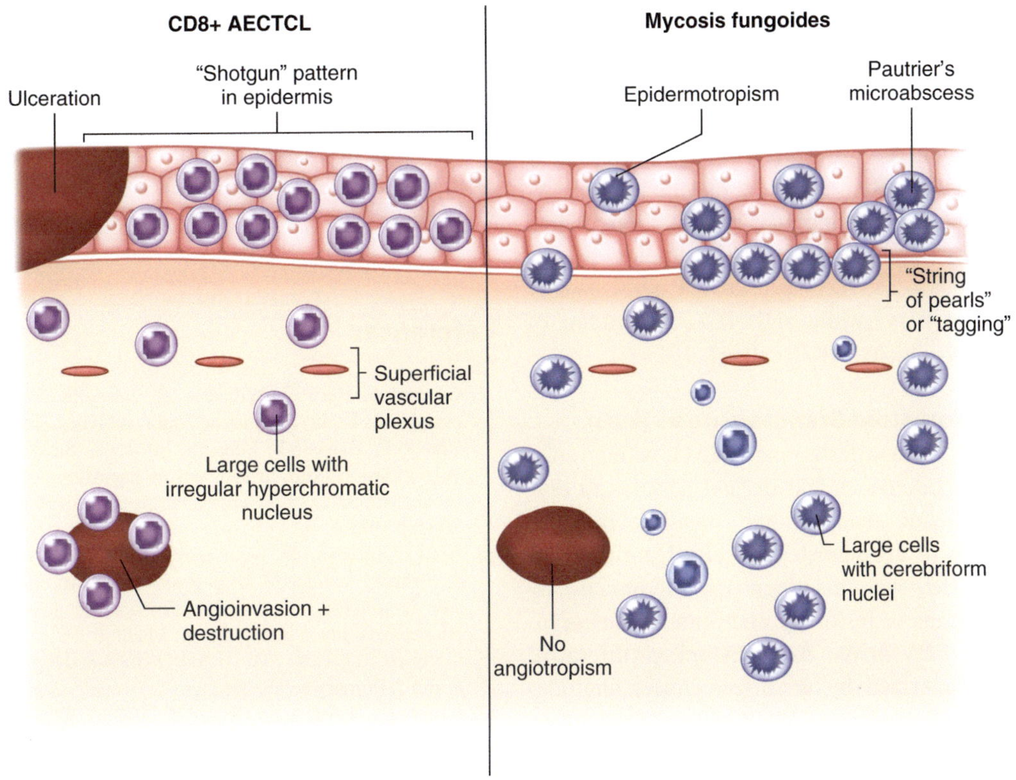

Fig. 12.3 Differentiating CD8+ AECTCL and MF. Although CD8+ MF is in the differential diagnosis of CD8+ AECTCL, these two neoplasms demonstrate very different histopathologic patterns. The neoplastic cells of CD8+ AECTCL are large, round, and have hyperchromatic irregular nuclei, while those of MF are large with cerebriform nuclei. Although both involve the epidermis, the neoplastic cells of CD8+ AECTCL are present in a shotgun pattern. Tagging of the dermal epidermal junction and Pautrier microabscesses are absent in CD8+ AECTCL. While angioinvasion, angiodestruction, and ulceration are common in CD8+ AECTCL, they are uncommon in MF

12.3.2.2 Hypersensitivity Reaction

The cutaneous infiltrate of a subset of hypersensitivity reactions may demonstrate a dominant intraepidermal population of CD8+ T cells. Whereas at first glance the differential diagnosis may include CD8+ AECTCL, several distinguishing features exist. In CD8+ AECTCL there is more lymphocytic atypia with a relatively monomorphic proliferation of enlarged CD8+ epidermotropic T cells. In a hypersensitivity reaction, epidermal dyskeratosis, spongiosis, and papillary dermal pigment–laden macrophages are commonly present, and the dermal CD4+ T cell infiltrate is more conspicuous.

12.3.2.3 Lymphomatoid Papulosis (LyP), Type D

This subtype of LyP also presents with a CD8+ epidermotropic infiltrate. Clinical findings usually allow LyP type D and CD8+ AECTCL to be distinguished. Lesions of LyP, type D tend to be smaller necrotic papules that regress, whereas those of CD8+ AECTCL are more likely to be larger, persistent, ulcerated plaques [5]. Immunohistochemistry may also be helpful, i.e., while the atypical cells in LyP, type D have a CD30+ CD8+ immunophenotype, the cells of CD8+ AECTCL usually do not express CD30 [10, 11].

12.3.2.4 Subcutaneous Panniculitis–Like T-Cell Lymphoma (SPTCL)

While CD8+AECTCL and SPTCL are both neoplasms of CD8+ cytotoxic T cells and either may present with papules and nodules, their patterns of histopathologic infiltration of the skin are distinctive. SPTCL exhibits lobular subcutaneous involvement with rare epidermotropism, while CD8+ AECTCL presents with marked epidermotropism and occasional deep nodular infiltrates [5].

12.3.2.5 Primary Cutaneous Gamma/Delta T-Cell Lymphoma (pcGDTCL)

This cytotoxic T-cell lymphoma may have a similar clinical presentation to that of CD8+ AECTCL. Additionally, pcGDTCL may display a predominantly epidermotropic infiltrate (although dermal nodules and subcutaneous tumors may also occur). Immunohistochemical stains allow the distinction of these tumors: pcGDTCL is composed of CD8- CD4- betaF1- T cells, while CD8+ AECTCL is a neoplasm of CD8+ CD4- betaF1 positive T cells. Rare cases of betaF1 silent CD8+ AECTCL may occur [1].

12.3.2.6 Extranodal NK/T Cell Lymphoma (eNK/ TCL)

When this aggressive tumor involves the skin, it manifests as painful dermal or subcutaneous nodules, with or without ulceration. eNK/TCL is histologically characterized by angiodestruction and angioinvasion and may be reminiscent of CD8+ AECTCL. These lymphomas may be differentiated on the basis of immunohistochemical studies: CD8+ AECTCL is composed of CD8+ cytotoxic T cells, usually lacking CD56 and EBV, while eNK/TCL is a tumor of CD56+ CD8− EBV-infected NK/T cells [1, 12].

12.3.2.7 Lymphomatoid Granulomatosis (LyG)

The varied cutaneous manifestations of LyG, which range from ulcerated subcutaneous and dermal nodules to erythematous, violaceous macules and papules, may be extremely difficult to distinguish clinically from those of CD8+ AECTCL. However, this diagnostic dilemma is easily resolved by means of histology and immunophenotyping. LyG, a rare, EBV-driven B-cell lymphoproliferative disorder, is characterized by an angiocentric, angiodestructive infiltrate of atypical EBV+ B cells and numerous reactive T cells [13]. In contrast, CD8+ AECTCL is a lymphoma of CD8+ T cells and has no association with EBV.

12.3.2.8 Pyoderma Gangrenosum (PG)

PG also presents clinically with large ulcerative lesions and is one of the first entities on the clinical differential. However, PG is a neutrophilic dermatosis with prominent edema and extremely dense neutrophilic inflammation as opposed to the CD8+ lymphocytic infiltrate of CD8+ AECTCL [4, 9].

12.4 Clinical Case

Case 12.4.1

A 65-year-old man presented with a 2- to 3-month history of ulcers, erythematous patches, and necrotic skin lesions on his back, abdomen, buttocks, and soles (see Fig. 12.1). The lesions started as small red macules that eroded and crusted over. Over the preceding 2 months he also noted increasing fatigue and a 20-lb weight loss.

A skin biopsy revealed an atypical CD8+ infiltrate of highly epidermotropic T cells. He was given a diagnosis of CD8+ aggressive epidermotropic T-cell lymphoma (see Fig. 12.2). The patient initially went into remission with combination chemotherapy followed by a matched unrelated donor allogeneic stem cell transplant. He experienced a relapse of his disease and died of sepsis 18 months after diagnosis.

Commentary This patient presented with lesions classic of CD8+ AECTCL, with widespread, large, ulcerative and necrotic patches and nodules. The timecourse and progression of his disease are typical for CD8+ AECTCL, with initial remission followed by a rapid relapse, even in the setting of combination chemotherapy and a bone marrow transplant.

References

1. Gaulard P, Berti E, Willemze R, Jaffe ES. Primary cutaneous peripheral T-cell lymphomas, rare subtypes. In: Swerdlow SH, Campo E, Harris NL, Jaffe ES, Pileri SA, Stein H, et al., editors. WHO classification of tumours of haematopoietic and lymphoid tissues. 4th ed. Lyon: International Agency for Research on Cancer; 2008. p. 302–5.
2. Berti E, Tomasini D, Vermeer MH, Meijer CJ, Alessi E, Willemze R. Primary cutaneous CD8-positive epidermotropic cytotoxic T cell lymphomas. A distinct clinicopathological entity with an aggressive clinical behavior. Am J Pathol. 1999;155:483–92.
3. Gormley RH, Hess SD, Anand D, Junkins-Hopkins J, Rook AH, Kim EJ. Primary cutaneous aggressive epidermotropic CD8+ T-cell lymphoma. J Am Acad Dermatol. 2010;62:300–7.
4. Nofal A, Abdel-Mawla MY, Assaf M, Salah E. Primary cutaneous aggressive epidermotropic CD8+ T-cell lymphoma: proposed diagnostic criteria and therapeutic evaluation. J Am Acad Dermatol. 2012;67:748–59.
5. Liu V, Cutler C, Young AZ. Case 38–2007: a 44-year-old woman with generalized, painful, ulcerated skin lesions. N Engl J Med. 2007;357:2496–505.
6. Diwan H, Ivan D. CD8-positive mycosis fungoides and primary cutaneous aggressive epidermotropic CD8-positive cytotoxic T-cell lymphoma. J Cutan Pathol. 2009;36:390–2.
7. Marzano AV, Ghislanzoni M, Gianelli U, Caputo R, Alessi E, Berti E. Fatal CD8+ epidermotropic cytotoxic primary cutaneous T-cell lymphoma with multiorgan involvement. Dermatology. 2005;211:281–5.
8. Santucci M, Pimpinelli N, Massi D, Kadin ME, Meijer CJLM, Müller-Hermelink HK, et al. Cytotoxic/natural killer cell cutaneous lymphomas. Report of EORTC Cutaneous Lymphoma Task Force Workshop. Cancer. 2003;97:610–27.
9. Ruocco E, Sangiuliano S, Gravina AG, Miranda A, Nicoletti G. Pyoderma gangrenosum: an updated review. J Eur Acad Dermatol Venerol. 2009;23:1008–17.
10. Saggini A, Gulia A, Argenyi Z, Fink-Puches R, Lissia A, Magaña M, et al. A variant of lymphomatoid papulosis simulating primary cutaneous aggressive epidermotropic CD8+ cytotoxic T-cell lymphoma. Description of 9 cases. Am J Surg Pathol. 2010;34:1168–75.
11. Kempf W, Kazakov DV, Ru A, Mentzel T, Paredes BE, Palmedo G, et al. Angioinvasive lymphomatoid papulosis. Am J Surg Pathol. 2013;37:1–13.
12. Chan J, Quintanilla-Martinez L, Ferry J, Peh S-C. Extranodal NK/T-cell lymphoma, nasal type. In: Swerdlow SH, Campo E, Harris NL, Jaffe ES, Pileri SA, Stein H, et al., editors. WHO classification of tumours of haematopoietic and lymphoid tissues. 4th ed. Lyon: International Agency for Research on Cancer; 2008. p. 285–8.
13. Roschewski M, Wilson WH. Lymphomatoid granulomatosis. Cancer J. 2012;18:469–74.

13 Primary Cutaneous Gamma-Delta T-Cell Lymphoma

Amrita Goyal, Joi B. Carter, Alexandra E. Kovach, Thomas S. Kupper, and Lyn McDivitt Duncan

Primary cutaneous gamma-delta T-cell lymphoma (pcGDTCL) is a rare but lethal lymphoma. Patients typically develop ulcerated cutaneous nodules, metastases to other extranodal sites, B (systemic) symptoms, and hemophagocytic syndrome. It is highly treatment-resistant and has a very poor prognosis. This condition is considered a provisional entity in the fourth edition of the WHO/EORTC guidelines [1]. This chapter will discuss the clinical presentation, prognosis, treatment, histopathology, immunophenotype, and differential diagnosis of pcGDTCL. It closes with two clinical cases, including clinical images and histopathology.

A. Goyal, M.D.
Harvard-MIT Division of Health Sciences and Technology, Harvard Medical School, Boston, MA, USA

J.B. Carter, M.D.
Department of Dermatology, Massachusetts General Hospital, Harvard Medical School, Boston, MA, USA

A.E. Kovach, M.D.
Department of Pathology, Boston Children's Hospital, Boston, MA, USA

T.S. Kupper, M.D., Ph.D.
Department of Dermatology, Brigham and Women's Hospital, Harvard Medical School, Boston, MA, USA

L.M. Duncan, M.D. (✉)
Dermatopathology Service, Department of Pathology, Massachusetts General Hospital, Harvard Medical School, Boston, MA, USA
e-mail: duncan@helix.mgh.harvard.edu

J.B. Carter et al. (eds.), *Atlas of Cutaneous Lymphomas: Classification and Differential Diagnosis*, DOI 10.1007/978-3-319-17217-0_13

13.1 Clinical Information

13.1.1 Clinical Presentation

pcGDTCL is an uncommon, highly aggressive skin lymphoma, a clonal proliferation of mature, activated γδ cytotoxic T cells [1–3]. pcGDTCL accounts for less than 1 % of all cutaneous T-cell lymphomas [4]. The median age of patients at presentation is 40 years, and this tumor occurs with the same frequency in men and women [1, 5]. pcGDTCL has a markedly poor prognosis because it is generally refractory to treatment [2, 4].

pcGDTCL patients typically present with erythematous to violaceous patches, plaques, and deep-seated dermal or subcutaneous nodules with ulceration and overlying epidermal necrosis (see Figs. 13.1 and 13.2) [1, 3]. Tumors can occur anywhere on the body but have a predilection for the extremities, thighs, and buttocks [3, 5]. Patients nearly always have systemic symptoms (B symptoms) at diagnosis, including fever, night sweats, weight loss, and malaise [1]. While dissemination to mucosal and extranodal sites is common and metastasis to the testes in men and the central nervous system has also been reported, involvement of lymph nodes, bone marrow, and spleen is uncommon [1, 6–8]. Hemophagocytic syndrome can occur and portends an especially negative prognosis [8, 9].

It is important to note is that the mere presence of T cells with a $\gamma\delta^+$ T-cell receptor (TCR) in a cutaneous lymphoma does not necessarily define pcGDTCL or correlate with a poor prognosis. Rather, evidence suggests that there is some heterogeneity within the group of lymphomas of $\gamma\delta^+$ T-cells [7, 10–12].

13.1.2 Prognosis and Treatment

pcGDTCL is extremely aggressive, with a median survival of 15 months [2]. Patients with subcutaneous involvement have a dramatically worse prognosis compared with patients with only epidermotropic or dermal involvement [1, 3]. Additional negative prognostic indicators include patient age over 40 years, associated cytopenias, tumor ulceration, and neoplastic cells with a CD8–, CD95(Fas)+, and/or CD56+ immunophenotype [13].

Few if any effective treatments exist for pcGDTCL. This lymphoma is highly resistant to both radiation therapy and chemotherapy [2, 4]. There have been case reports of successful treatment with allogenic stem-cell transplantation [2], etretinate or methotrexate combined with narrow-band ultraviolet B treatment [7, 14], and bexarotene [15]. There have also been recent case reports of more indolent cases of pcGDTCL that responded well to administration of systemic corticosteroids [16].

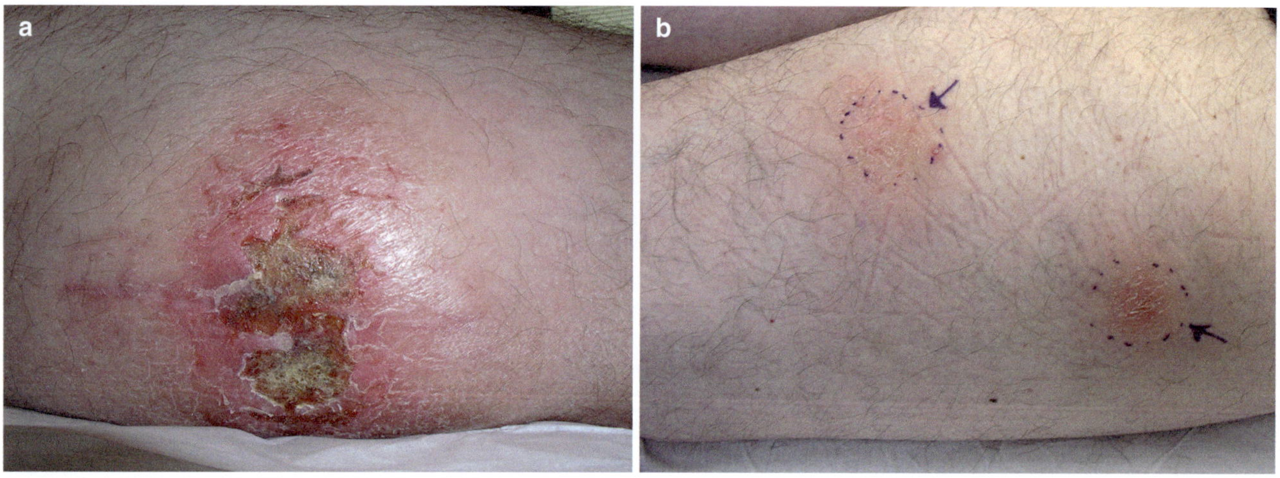

Fig. 13.1 Primary cutaneous gamma delta T-cell lymphoma, clinical photos, Case 13.1. (**a**) On the patient's right thigh is a 10-cm ulcerated subcutaneous tumor with hemorrhagic crust and surrounding erythema. (**b**) On the patient's left upper thigh are two 1–2 cm subcutaneous nodules with overlying erythema, outlined in blue marker

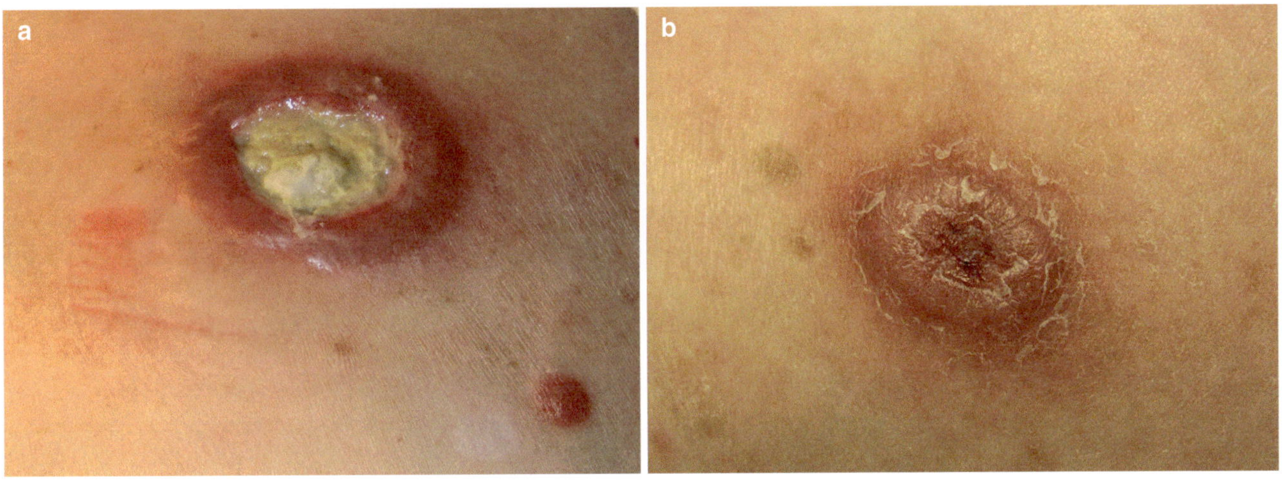

Fig. 13.2 Primary cutaneous gamma delta T-cell lymphoma, clinical photos, Case 13.2. (**a**) On the patient's left upper abdomen is a 5-cm ulcer with a raised violaceous border and fibrinous base. Inferiorly and laterally from the ulcer is a 1-cm pink nodule. (**b**) On the patient's right hip is a pink-orange nodule with central ulceration, a collarette of scale, and surrounding erythema

13.2 Pathology

13.2.1 Histopathology

The histology of pcGDTLC can vary widely among patients and among lesions from a single patient [2]. Although pcGDTCL commonly involves the subcutaneous tissue, the epidermis and dermis are often also invaded by neoplastic cells (see Figs. 13.3 and 13.4) [1, 5]. Angioinvasion, angiodestruction, and fibrinoid tissue necrosis are often seen [1, 6]. Epidermal involvement can range from mild epidermotropism of neoplastic cells to dramatic pagetoid reticulosis-like infiltration [1]. Subcutaneous tissue involvement typically demonstrates lobular and focal septal infiltration [1, 5]. Additionally, as with other lymphomas involving the subcutis, rimming of adipocytes by neoplastic cells is characteristic but not specific [5]. The neoplastic cells tend to be large, with coarse chromatin. Occasionally, large blast-like cells with vesicular nuclei and prominent nucleoli are present [1].

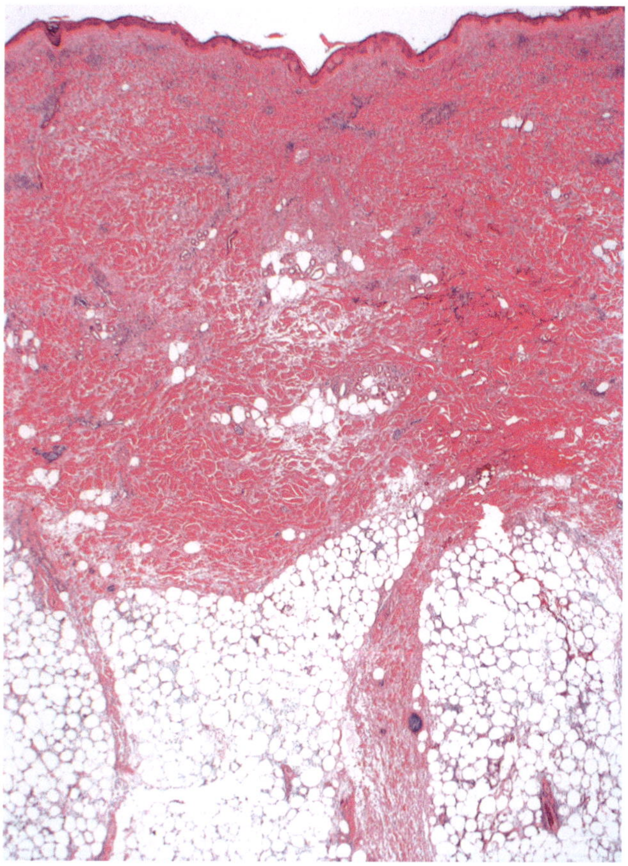

Fig. 13.3 Primary cutaneous gamma-delta T-cell lymphoma. Histopathology. The neoplastic infiltrate is primarily a subtle subcutaneous lobular infiltrate with focal septal involvement. Adipocyte rimming is present. Angioinvasion is seen in a vessel in the fibrous septum of the subcutis. There is minimal dermal or epidermal involvement in this case (H&E, 2×)

13.2.2 Immunophenotype and Molecular Findings

In pcGDTCL, the neoplastic cells are mature, activated cytotoxic T cells, typically positive for CD2, CD3, and CD56. They also lack expression of CD4, CD8, CD30, βF1, and CD5 [1]. Lack of TCRβ expression is sometimes used to infer a γδ phenotype in lieu of TCR gamma staining [17]. By definition, the cells demonstrate expression of TCRδ by immunohistochemistry and flow cytometry. Consistent with their cytotoxic phenotype, the cells typically produce cytotoxic enzymes, including TIA-1 and granzyme B.

The neoplastic cells demonstrate clonal rearrangement of the TCRγ and TCRδ genes. Epstein-Barr virus is absent [1]. Complex cytogenetic rearrangements may be present, but no characteristic mutations have been identified [18].

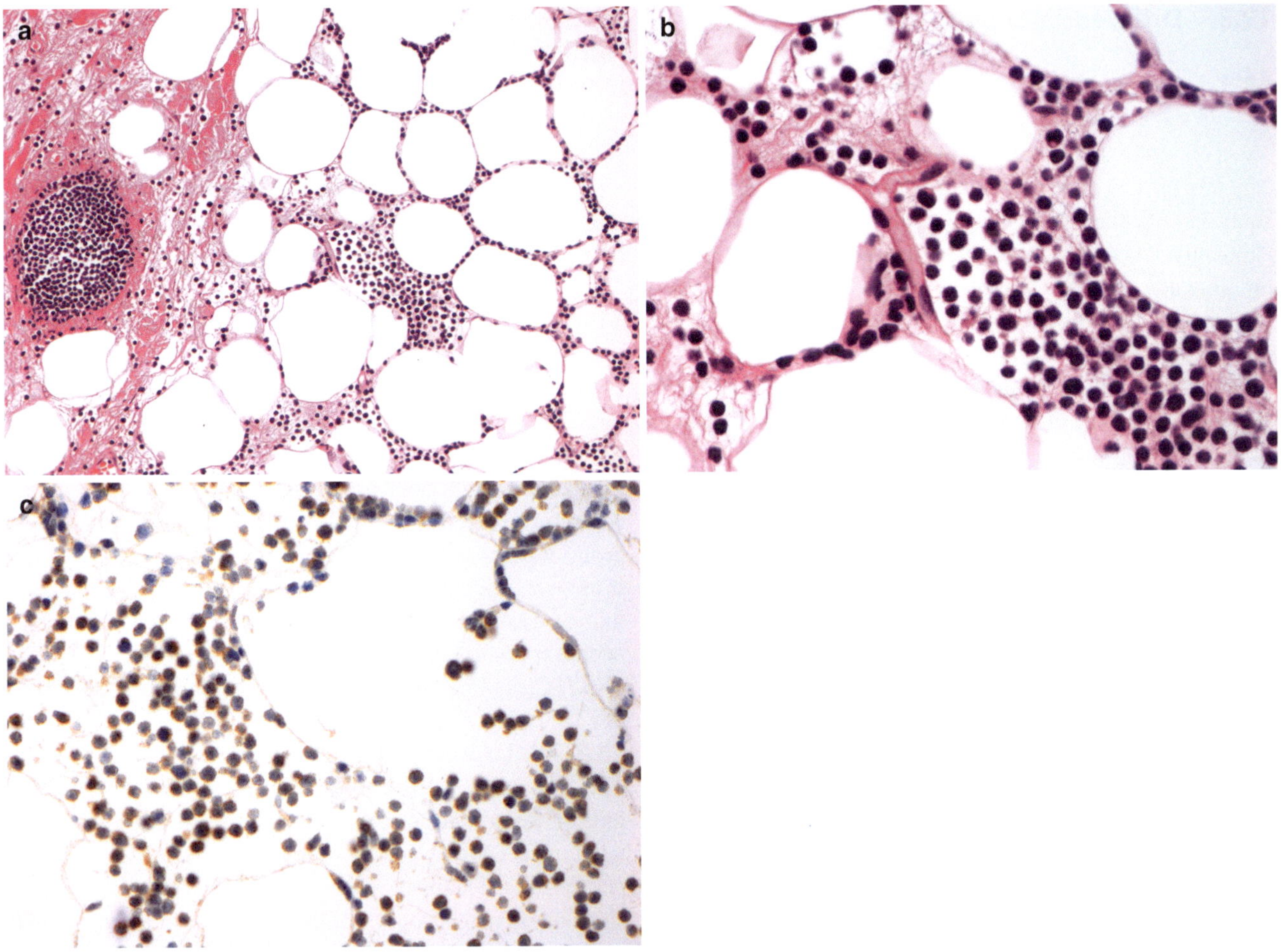

Fig. 13.4 Primary cutaneous gamma-delta T-cell lymphoma. Histopathology and immunohistochemistry. (**a**) A higher power view of one of the septae seen in Fig. 13.3. Neoplastic cells are present in the fibrous septum in a vessel within the septum and between the fat lobules. Rimming of the fat spaces by neoplastic cells is present (H&E, 20×). (**b**) The neoplastic cells are large with irregular nuclear contours and coarse chromatin (H&E, 40×). (**c**) The tumor cells stain positively for TCR gamma, identifying the atypical cells as gamma/delta T-cells (TCR gamma, 20×)

13.3 Differential Diagnosis

13.3.1 Diagnostic Considerations

As with other cutaneous lymphomas, accurate diagnosis depends on a synthesis of clinical presentation, pathologic analysis of the skin biopsy, and immunophenotype. Clinically, it is important to assess the distribution of lesions, the time course of the presentation, and any extracutaneous manifestations and systemic symptoms. Immunophenotypic identification of the T-cell receptor subunits may be critical. The difficulty inherent in diagnosing pcGDTCL is highlighted in the clinical cases below. Both patients were initially misdiagnosed.

13.3.2 Differential Diagnosis

13.3.2.1 Subcutaneous Panniculitis-Like T-Cell Lymphoma (SPTCL)

Until recently pcGDTCL and SPTCL were grouped under the heading of SPTCL. However, they recently have been shown to have markedly different prognoses and time courses and are now considered separate entities. Both may present with violaceous subcutaneous nodules or plaques. Histopathologically, both SPTCL and pcGDTCL may show a lobular panniculitis-like morphology with an infiltrate composed of cytotoxic T cells [1, 3, 19]. However, while SPTCL has an excellent prognosis, pcGDTCL is nearly always fatal, with a median survival of 15 months [1]. The most rapid method of differentiating these two neoplasms is via immunohistochemistry. Both SPTCL and extranodal NK/T-cell lymphoma (eNK/TCL, see below) express alpha and beta subunits as opposed to the gamma and delta subunits of pcGDTCL [1, 3, 9]. Expression of the alpha/beta TCR and gamma/delta TCR are mutually exclusive as a result of normal T-cell development and gene rearrangement [4]. Clonal expression of gamma delta TCR genes is seen in pcGDTCL but not in SPTCL. In addition to the differences in TCR subunits, the neoplastic cells of SPTCL have a CD4–, CD8+, and CD56– phenotype, whereas pcGDTCL tumor cells have a CD4–, CD8–, CD56+ phenotype [9]. Finally, although both SPTCL and pcGDTCL typically display rimming of fat cells, pcGDTCL is more likely to demonstrate dermal or epidermal involvement.

13.3.2.2 Extranodal NK/T-Cell Lymphoma, Nasal Type (eNK/TCL)

Differentiating eNK/TCL from pcGDTCL can be difficult both clinically and histopathologically. Both of these T-cell lymphomas can manifest as ulcerated nodules, and both are associated with a poor prognosis. Histopathologic findings common to eNK/TCL and pcGDTCL include panniculitis, prominent angiodestruction, and marked angioinvasion. Immunohistochemistry may or may not be helpful given that of cases of eNK/TCL with a gamma delta TCR have been reported [20]. However, in contrast to pcGDTCL, eNK/TCL is Epstein-Barr virus–positive (EBV).

13.3.2.3 Lupus Erythematosus Profundus (LEP)

This autoimmune panniculitis also presents with erythematous or violaceous dermal and subcutaneous nodules, with or without ulceration, and can be difficult to distinguish from pcGDTCL [21]. Histologically, both LEP and pcGDTCL can show epidermal changes, hyaline fat necrosis, lobular panniculitis, rimming of fat cells by lymphocytes, and karryorhexis [1, 5, 21]. In contrast, reactive lymphoid follicles are usually seen in lupus profundus and not in pcGDTCL. Although the cells of LEP generally appear more cytologically bland than those of pcGDTCL [5, 16], repeated excisional biopsies may be required to differentiate the two entities convincingly [21]. Expression of the gamma and delta T-cell receptor subunits as opposed to the alpha and beta subunits is tremendously helpful in making the diagnosis of pcGDTCL [21].

13.4 Clinical Cases

Case 13.1

A 46-year-old man presented with a 4-month history of a nodule on his left ankle, followed by the development of several waxing and waning nodules on his bilateral thighs (Fig. 13.1a). He did not report any fevers, chills, night sweats, or weight loss. A biopsy of one of the nodules was performed and was diagnosed differently at two institutions as CD30+ lymphoproliferative disorder and SPTCL.

Over the next several weeks the patient developed a large, painful, erythematous mass over his right lateral thigh (Fig. 13.1b). This was biopsied and revealed an atypical T-cell infiltrate composed of neoplastic T-cells positive for CD3, CD2, CD56, TIA-1, granzyme, perforin, and TCR-gamma/delta, with loss of CD5 and CD7. Polymerase chain reaction testing revealed a clonal TCR rearrangement. A diagnosis of pcGDTCL was made.

In spite of undergoing six cycles of chemotherapy with cyclophosphamide, doxorubicin, vincristine, and prednisone (CHOP), the patient experienced rapid recurrence of the cutaneous lesions. He underwent a matched allogeneic hematopoietic stem-cell transplant complicated by multiorgan failure and invasive fungal infection. He died 22 days after transplant, less than 9 months after his initial presentation.

Comment This patient's disease presented on the lower extremity and thighs, a distribution classic for pcGDTCL. This case highlights the difficulties commonly encountered in diagnosing pcGDTCL. Given the marked variation in histology commonly seen in pcGDTCL, it took numerous biopsies to come to the correct diagnosis. Diagnosis was significantly aided by immunohistochemical staining for gamma/delta TCR. This patient's disease was refractory to multiagent chemotherapy, a testament to how aggressive this lymphoma can be. Finally, this case serves as a reminder of the challenges face by patients undergoing hematopoietic stem-cell transplantation.

Case 13.2

A 79-year-old woman with a 4-year history of recurrent papules and nodules (<1 cm) on the abdomen presented with a 6-month history of an enlarging 3-cm nodule on her left upper abdomen. The tumor was not responsive to radiation, and it progressed to become a 5-cm crateriform ulcer (Fig. 13.2a). Historically, these nodules resolved with clobetasol ointment and electron beam radiation. Biopsies performed at another institution reported the nodules to be CD4+ small-medium pleomorphic T-cell lymphoma (SMPTCL); TCR clonality was not assessed. The patient denied any constitutional symptoms and had no palpable lymphadenopathy.

Repeat biopsy showed a dermal lichenoid infiltrate of atypical T cells with aggregates of lymphoid cells extending into the subcutis. The atypical cells stained positively for CD3, CD5, CD7, TCR gamma, TCR delta, and perforin without staining for CD4, CD8, CD20, CD30, granzyme B, EBER, and anaplastic lymphoma kinase. Polymerase chain reaction test detected clonal rearrangements of both TCR beta and TCR gamma. The patient was diagnosed with pcGDTCL. Although CT of the chest, abdomen, and pelvis revealed no systemic involvement, peripheral blood flow cytometry showed 1–5 % of peripheral blood cells to be gamma/delta T cells. Review of all prior biopsies revealed changes consistent with pcGDTCL.

Gemcitabine chemotherapy was initiated. Because the patient continued to develop new lesions on the abdomen (Fig. 13.2b), buttocks, and thighs, chemotherapy was discontinued and palliative radiation therapy initiated. Although her cutaneous lesions continue to progress 1 year after presentation, unlike most patients with this disease she shows no evidence of visceral involvement.

Comment As with case 13.1, this patient's lymphoma was only diagnosed after numerous biopsies. Again, her diagnosis was largely dependent on immunohistochemical staining for TCR gamma subunits. This patient's clinical course is less aggressive than that of case 13.1; although she continues to develop new cutaneous lesions, her disease remains skin-limited.

References

1. Gaulard P, Berti E, Willemze R, Jaffe ES. Primary cutaneous peripheral T-cell lymphomas, rare subtypes. In: Swerdlow SH, Campo E, Harris NL, Jaffe ES, Pileri SA, Stein H, et al., editors. WHO classification of tumors of haematopoietic and lymphoid tissues. Lyon: International Agency for Research on Cancer; 2008. p. 302–5.
2. Koch R, Jaffe ES, Mensing C, Zeis M, Schmitz N, Sander CA, et al. Cutaneous gamma/delta T-cell lymphoma. J Dtsch Dermatol Ges. 2009;7:1065–7.
3. Toro JR, Liewehr DJ, Pabby N, Sorbara L, Raffeld M, Steinberg SM, et al. Gamma-delta T-cell phenotype is associated with significantly decreased survival in cutaneous T-cell lymphoma. Blood. 2003;101:3407–12.
4. Tripodo C, Iannitto E, Florena AM, Pucillo CE, Piccaluga PP, Franco V, et al. Gamma-delta T-cell lymphomas. Nat Rev Clin Oncol. 2009;6:707–17.
5. Aguilera P, Mascaró JM, Martinez A, Esteve J, Puig S, Campo E, et al. Cutaneous gamma/delta T-cell lymphoma: a histopathologic mimicker of lupus erythematosus profundus (lupus panniculitis). J Am Acad Dermatol. 2007;56:643–7.
6. Youn SH, Lee YW, Min SK, Park HR, Kim KH, Kim KJ. Fatal cutaneous γ/δ T-cell lymphoma with central nerve system metastasis. Ann Dermatol. 2011;23 Suppl 1:S100–4.
7. Fujii M, Uehara J, Honma M, Ito Y, Takahashi H, Ishida-Yamamoto A, et al. Primary cutaneous γδ-T-cell lymphoma treated with low-dose methotrexate and narrowband ultraviolet B irradiation: report of a case with testicular involvement. J Dermatol. 2011;38:368–72.
8. Chakrapani A, Avery A, Warnke R. Primary cutaneous gamma delta T-cell lymphoma with brain involvement and hemophagocytic syndrome. Am J Dermatopathol. 2013;35:270–2.
9. Willemze R, Jansen PM, Cerroni L, Berti E, Santucci M, Assaf C, et al. Subcutaneous panniculitis-like T-cell lymphoma: definition, classification, and prognostic factors: an EORTC Cutaneous Lymphoma Group Study of 83 cases. Blood. 2008;111:838–45.
10. Kempf W, Kazakov DV, Scheidegger PE, Schlaak M, Tantcheva-Poor I. Two cases of primary cutaneous lymphoma with a γ/δ+phenotype and an indolent course: further evidence of heterogeneity of cutaneous γ/δ+T-cell lymphomas. Am J Dermatopathol. 2014;36:570–7.
11. Ishida M, Iwai M, Yoshida K, Kagotani A, Okabe H. Primary cutaneous B-cell lymphoma with abundant reactive gamma/delta T-cells within the skin lesion and peripheral blood. Int J Clin Exp Pathol. 2014;7:1193–9.
12. Magro CM, Wang X. Indolent primary cutaneous γ/δ T-cell lymphoma localized to the subcutaneous panniculus and its association with atypical lymphocytic lobular panniculitis. Am J Clin Pathol. 2012;138:50–6.
13. Takeshita M, Imayama S, Oshiro Y, Kurihara K, Okamoto S, Matsuki Y, et al. Clinicopathologic analysis of 22 cases of subcutaneous panniculitis-like CD56- or CD56+ lymphoma and review of 44 other reported cases. Am J Clin Pathol. 2004;121:408–16.
14. Nakashima H, Sugaya M, Minatani Y, Ohmatsu H, Asano N, Fujimoto M, et al. Cutaneous gamma/delta T-cell lymphoma treated with retinoid and narrowband ultraviolet B. Clin Exp Dermatol. 2009;34:e345–6.
15. Mehta N, Wayne AS, Kim YH, Hale GA, Alvarao CS, Myskowski P, et al. Bexarotene is active against subcutaneous panniculitis-like T-cell lymphoma in adult and pediatric populations. Clin Lymphoma Myeloma Leuk. 2012;12:20–5.
16. Endly DC, Weenig RH, Peters MS, Viswanatha DS, Comfere NI. Indolent course of cutaneous gamma-delta T-cell lymphoma. J Cutan Pathol. 2013;40:896–902.
17. Garcia-Herrera A, Song JY, Chuang S-S, Villamor N, Colomo L, Pittaluga S, et al. Nonhepatosplenic γδ T-cell lymphomas represent a spectrum of aggressive cytotoxic T-cell lymphomas with a mainly extranodal presentation. Am J Surg Pathol. 2011;35:1214–25.
18. Yamamoto-Sugitani M, Kuroda J, Shimura Y, Nagoshi H, Chinen Y, Ohshiro M, et al. Comprehensive cytogenetic study of primary cutaneous gamma-delta T-cell lymphoma by means of spectral karyotyping and genome-wide single nucleotide polymorphism array. Cancer Genet. 2012;205:459–64.
19. Jaffe ES, Gaulard P, Ralfkiaer E, Cerroni L, Meijer CJLM. Subcutaneous panniculitis-like T-cell lymphoma. In: Swerdlow SH, Campo E, Harris NL, Jaffe ES, Pileri SA, Stein H, et al., editors. WHO classification of tumors of haematopoietic and lymphoid tissues. Lyon: International Agency for Research on Cancer; 2008. p. 294–5.
20. Yu W-W, Hsieh P-P, Chuang S-S. Cutaneous EBV-positive γδ T-cell lymphoma vs. extranodal NK/T-cell lymphoma: a case report and literature review. J Cutan Pathol. 2013;40:310–6.
21. Yi L, Qun S, Wenjie Z, Wen Z, Jian L, Yan Z, et al. The presenting manifestations of subcutaneous panniculitis-like T-cell lymphoma and T-cell lymphoma and cutaneous γδ T-cell lymphoma may mimic those of rheumatic diseases: a report of 11 cases. Clin Rheumatol. 2013;32(8):1169–75.

14 Primary Cutaneous CD4+ Small/Medium Pleomorphic T-Cell Lymphoma

Amrita Goyal, Joi B. Carter, and Lyn McDivitt Duncan

Primary cutaneous CD4+ small/medium pleomorphic T-cell lymphoma (pcSMPTCL) is an extremely rare lymphoma with an overall excellent prognosis. It is a provisional entity in the World Health Organization–European Organization for Research and Treatment of Cancer (WHO/EORTC) guidelines and is considered to have both indolent and aggressive forms. pcSMPTCL typically presents with a persistent, asymptomatic, solitary erythematous nodule or pink plaque on the head, neck, or trunk. Given the generally benign clinical course of this disease, some advocate the use of alternative terms, including T-cell pseudolymphoma, cutaneous nodular proliferation of pleomorphic T lymphocytes of undetermined significance, or clonal T-cell lymphoproliferative disease with indolent behavior [1, 2]. Given the dramatic difference in prognosis between the indolent and aggressive forms, it is possible that this entity, as currently defined, encompasses two distinct diseases. This chapter discusses the clinical presentation, prognosis, treatment, histopathology, immunohistochemistry, molecular characteristics, and differential diagnosis of pcSMPTCL. It closes with a clinical case.

A. Goyal, M.D.
Harvard-MIT Division of Health Sciences and Technology, Harvard Medical School, Boston, MA, USA

J.B. Carter, M.D.
Department of Dermatology, Massachusetts General Hospital, Harvard Medical School, Boston, MA, USA

L.M. Duncan, M.D. (✉)
Dermatopathology Service, Department of Pathology, Massachusetts General Hospital, Harvard Medical School, Boston, MA, USA
e-mail: duncan@helix.mgh.harvard.edu

J.B. Carter et al. (eds.), *Atlas of Cutaneous Lymphomas: Classification and Differential Diagnosis*,
DOI 10.1007/978-3-319-17217-0_14

14.1 Clinical Information

14.1.1 Clinical Presentation

Primary cutaneous CD4+ small/medium pleomorphic T-cell lymphoma (pcSMPTCL) is a provisional entity in the WHO/EORTC listing of cutaneous lymphomas. It constitutes 2–3 % of primary cutaneous lymphomas [3, 4]. While the median age of patients at diagnosis is 53–55 years old, patients aged 3–90 years old have been reported [2, 4]. pcSMPTCL has no gender predilection and patients generally have no history of other cutaneous lymphomas [2].

This T-cell lymphoma manifests as a solitary, erythematous nodule on the head, neck, or trunk, ranging from 1–3 cm in diameter. The nodules of pcSMPTCL develop rapidly over the course of weeks to months, rarely regress spontaneously, and can clinically resemble cysts, furuncles, or dermatofibromas. Patients occasionally demonstrate poikilodermatous or pink plaques (Figs. 14.1 and 14.2) or chronic ulcerations [3–6]. Solitary lesions are seen in 87 % of patients, while 13 % present with multifocal or widespread disease [7]. Patients are otherwise asymptomatic and the plaques/nodules are rarely painful, pruritic, or ulcerated [3, 7].

There are two variants of pcSMPTCL: indolent and aggressive [7, 8]. The vast majority of cases are indolent with small (less than 3 cm) non–progressing solitary lesions, no systemic spread, and a 5-year survival of 90–100 % [2, 4]. However, there are reports of very aggressive cases resulting in systemic spread, central nervous system involvement, and death [8]. Progressive disease and death have been reported in 14 % and 5 % of cases of pcSMPTCL, respectively [7]. Given the marked difference in prognosis between the indolent and aggressive variants, it is possible that the aggressive form of pcSMPTCL is actually a separate entity; at this time the WHO/EORTC classification system does not differentiate between them [2].

14.1.2 Prognosis and Treatment

pcSMPTCL generally has an excellent prognosis, particularly in patients with solitary or localized lesions [1, 3]. Five-year survival rates range from 60 to 100 % overall [2, 3], with rates of over 90 % for patients with solitary lesions [4]. The vast majority of patients experience no spread or dissemination of disease, and excision or radiotherapy is often curative [3, 9]. Patients with aggressive disease have a median survival of 23 months (range, 18–36 months) [8].

Positive prognostic indicators include single lesions, stable or nonprogressing lesions, small size (<3 cm), a low proliferative index, and numerous CD8+ T cells. Patients with aggressive disease tend to have larger lesions (>5 cm), rapid growth or evolution, ulceration, a high proliferative index, and few CD8+ T cells [8].

Given the generally benign nature of this disease, nonaggressive therapy and regular follow-up are recommended [3]. Surgical excision or radiotherapy is often curative in patients with solitary or localized lesions [2, 3]. In aggressive cases of pcSMPTCL with rapid progression and systemic involvement, multiagent chemotherapy may be considered [8].

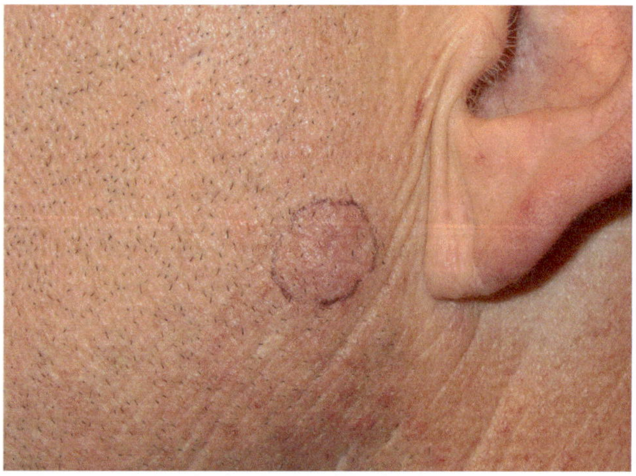

Fig. 14.1 Primary cutaneous CD4+ small/medium pleomorphic T-cell lymphoma. Present on the cheek of a 53-year-old man, just anterior to the ear, is a 5-mm pink indurated plaque (*outlined in pen*)

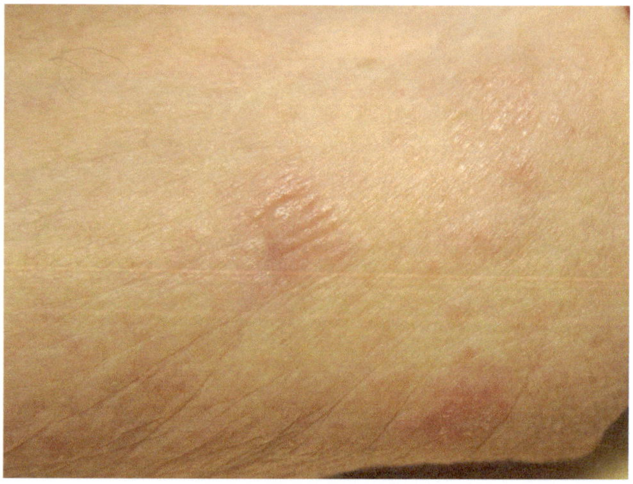

Fig. 14.2 Primary cutaneous CD4+ small/medium pleomorphic T-cell lymphoma, clinical case 14.1. Present on the inner aspect of the patient's right elbow are two dime-sized pink indurated plaques with prominent skin markings and some scale

14.2 Pathology

14.2.1 Histopathology

Skin biopsy demonstrates a dense, nodular or bandlike infiltrate of small to medium pleomorphic mononuclear cells in the dermis and superficial subcutaneous tissue (Fig. 14.3) [2–4, 8]. Focal epidermotropism is occasionally present [6]. Many cases show invasion and destruction of pilosebaceous units [2].

The neoplastic cells of pcSMPTCL are small-to-medium sized lymphocytes with nuclear pleomorphism. Some of the lymphocytes have atypical nuclei with irregular nuclear contours and chromatin clumping [5]. Scattered mitoses are often present [2]. There are often admixed large cells (by definition making up less than 30 % of the infiltrate) [2, 4]. Eosinophils are few to absent [9]. Small granulomas are present near hair follicles or sweat glands in 50 % of cases [2].

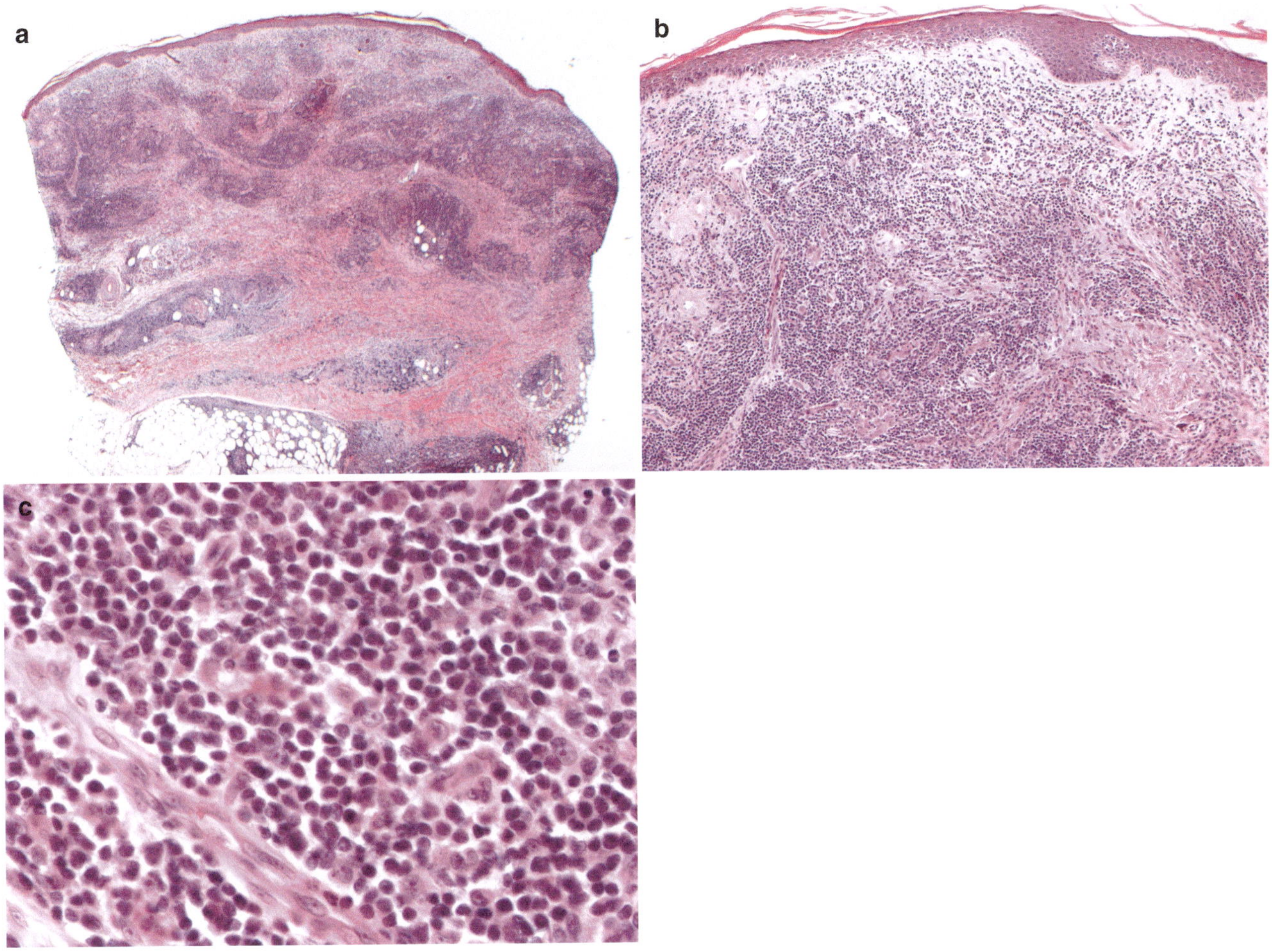

Fig. 14.3 CD4+ small/medium pleomorphic T-cell lymphoma, histopathology, clinical case 14.1. (**a**) Skin biopsy demonstrates a dense nodular infiltrate of atypical cells in the dermis and superficial subcutaneous tissue (H&E, 4×). (**b**) Focal epidermotropism is present. An eccrine duct is surrounded by atypical T cells (H&E, 10×). (**c**) The infiltrate is composed of small-to-medium sized T cells with nuclear pleomorphism and mild cytologic atypia. Nuclei are hyperchromatic and some demonstrate irregular nuclear contours (H&E, 40×)

14.2.2 Immunophenotype and Molecular Findings

The neoplastic cells of pcSMPTCL have recently been described to be CD4+ follicular helper T cells [4, 6]. Consistent with this phenotype, they typically express CD3, CD4, and PD-1 but lack CD8 and CD30 (see Fig. 14.4) [1, 3, 6]. They express alpha and beta T-cell receptor subunits [5].

The neoplastic T cells of pcSMPTCL show variable loss of pan T-cell markers; 13–91 % of cases demonstrate abnormal expression of CD2, CD3, CD5, and/or CD7 [5–8]. The Ki-67 index is often low [8]. Many cases of pcSMPTCL demonstrate rosettes of PD-1+ neoplastic cells [4, 6].

There is often an intense infiltrate of reactive CD8+ T cells and high numbers of CD8+ T cells are associated with a favorable prognosis [2, 8]. B cells are often numerous, making up 10–50 % of the infiltrate [2], and may form nodular aggregates with follicular dendritic cell mesh works. Aggregates of polytypic plasma cells may also be observed [5, 8].

A clonal T-cell receptor is present in 60–100 % of cases [2, 4, 8, 10]. This lymphoma is not associated with Epstein-Barr virus [3, 6]. No consistent genetic abnormalities have been identified [3].

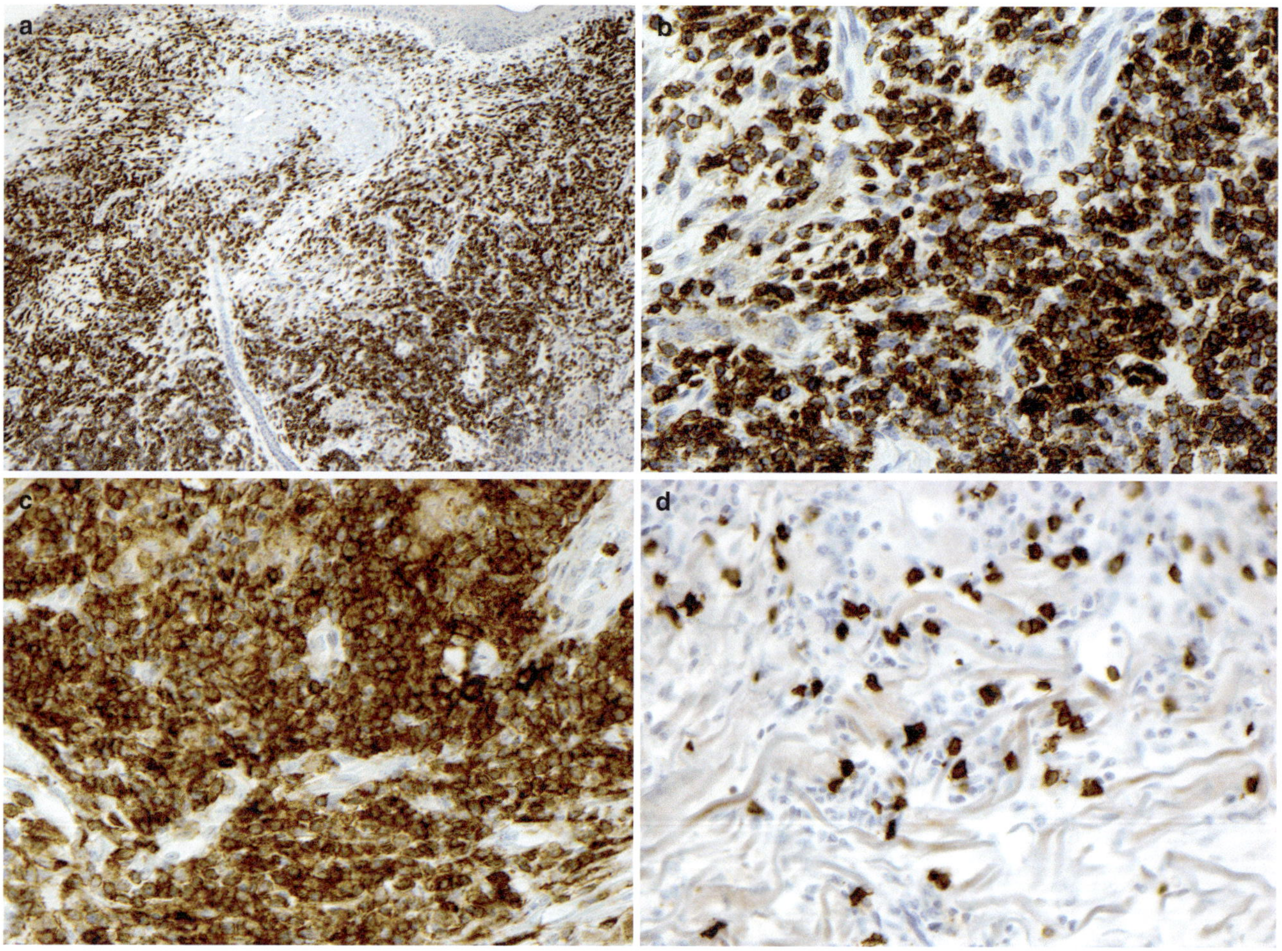

Fig. 14.4 CD4+ small/medium pleomorphic T-cell lymphoma, immunohistochemistry, clinical case 14.1. (**a**) The majority of the dense nodular infiltrate is composed of CD3+ T cells. There is focal involvement of the epidermis. An eccrine duct is spared (CD3, 10×). (**b**) The T cells are small-to-medium sized with nuclear pleomorphism and strong staining for CD3 (CD3, 20×). (**c**) Most of the atypical T cells composing the infiltrate are CD4+ (CD4, 20×). (**d**) There are few scattered CD8+ T cells (CD8, 20×)

14.3 Differential Diagnosis

14.3.1 Diagnostic Considerations

Numerous entities present with similar clinical morphologic appearance resembling that of pcSMPTCL. These include primary cutaneous marginal zone lymphomas (pcMZL), mycosis fungoides (MF, especially plaque and tumor stages), primary cutaneous follicle center lymphoma (pcFCL), and benign cutaneous lymphoid hyperplasia (CLH). Diagnosis of pcSMPTCL can be difficult because of its nonspecific clinical presentation. Diagnosis rests on histopathologic and immunohistochemical analysis.

14.3.2 Cutaneous Lymphoid Hyperplasia (CLH)

CLH, also known as lymphadenosis benigna cutis, lymphocytoma cutis, and pseudolymphoma, is a broad category of non-neoplastic lymphoid proliferations in the skin, commonly presenting as solitary plaques or nodules of the skin. The infiltrates of CLH are a polymorphous mixture of mononuclear cells, histiocytes, plasma cells, and eosinophils. In contrast, pcSMPTCL presents with a relatively monomorphous infiltrate of small-to-medium sized, pleomorphic atypical lymphocytes. The most important factors in differentiating pcSMPTCL and CLH are the lymphocytic atypia and loss of the pan T-cell markers seen in pcSMPTCL. Unlike many cases of CLH, pcSMPTCL is not associated with medications, insect bites, or other immune disorders [7]. However, while PD-1 is commonly present in pcSMPTCL, it may also be seen in reactive dermatoses.

14.3.3 Primary Cutaneous Marginal Zone Lymphoma (pcMZL)

Although the deep-seated, pink to red to violaceous indurated plaques, nodules, or tumors of pcMZL are clinically similar to those of pcSMPTCL, these entities differ significantly histopathologically [11]. pcSMPTCL is a CD4+ T-cell lymphoma, while pcMZL is a B-cell lymphoma characterized by the presence of reactive lymphoid follicles, aggregates of neoplastic marginal zone type B cells, and zones of plasma cells. However, the neoplastic cells of pcMZL can occasionally be difficult to distinguish from the florid B-cell infiltrate of pcSMPTCL [2]. Molecular and immunohistochemical studies can be quite valuable in distinguishing between these entities. Immunohistochemical staining or in situ hybridization studies for kappa and lambda light chains identify light chain restricted plasma cells in approximately 70 % of cases of pcMZL; light chain restriction is absent in pcSMPTCL. Clonality studies may also be helpful in resolving these diagnoses, since pcSMPTCL uniformly lack a clonal immunoglobulin rearrangement [5] while 65–75 % of pcMZLs show clonal immunoglobulin rearrangements [12, 13].

14.3.4 Primary Cutaneous Follicle Center Lymphoma (pcFCL)

This B-cell neoplasm, composed of follicle center B cells, is clinically similar to pcSMPTCL. It too presents with solitary or grouped erythematous, asymptomatic papules or nodules on the head, neck, and trunk [14]. The prominent B-cell infiltrate present in many cases of pcSMPTCL can make these two difficult to distinguish. However, pcSMPTCL does not possess the proliferation of Bcl6+ Bcl2− follicle center cells characteristic of pcFCL [7].

14.3.5 Mycosis Fungoides (MF)

This indolent T-cell lymphoma classically progresses through patch, plaque, and tumor stages, any of which may appear similar to the lesions of pcSMPTCL. However, by definition, pcSMPTCL does not undergo the patch/plaque/tumor progression that is the hallmark of MF. Histopathologically, pcSMPTCL generally lacks the epidermotropism characteristic of MF [2, 3]. Finally, while the cells of pcSMPTCL often express PD-1, this marker is rarely seen in MF [9].

14.4 Clinical Case

Case 14.1

A 79-year-old man presented with a 2-year history of two small asymptomatic papules on his right medial forearm. Two years after their onset, they suddenly swelled and ulcerated, leaving a hemorrhagic crust. He was otherwise well with no constitutional symptoms or major health problems.

Biopsy of a forearm lesion demonstrated surface ulceration and a dense dermal and subcutaneous mononuclear infiltrate of CD3+ CD4+ CD5+ CD43+ T cells, focal aggregates of CD20+ B cells, and a clonal TCR rearrangement (Figs. 14.3 and 14.4). There were no abnormal findings on peripheral blood flow cytometry, and the patient showed no evidence of systemic disease. He was diagnosed with pcSMPTCL.

Although the initial lesions resolved with radiotherapy, the patient experienced local recurrence months later just outside of the radiation field. This recurrence manifested as a pair of dime-sized pink plaques, which were successfully treated with radiation therapy (Fig. 14.2).

Commentary As is expected in pcSMPTCL, this patient had no evidence of extra-cutaneous spread and his disease demonstrated a remarkably indolent clinical course. Although he did experience recurrence after radiation therapy, these recurrent lesions were also amenable to radiation, as characteristic in pcSMPTCL.

References

1. Jaffe ES, Nicolae A, Pittaluga S. Peripheral T-cell and NK-cell lymphomas in the WHO classification: pearls and pitfalls. Mod Pathol. 2013;26 Suppl 1:S71–87.
2. Beltraminelli H, Leinweber B, Kerl H, Cerroni L. Primary cutaneous CD4+ small-/medium-sized pleomorphic T-cell lymphoma: a cutaneous nodular proliferation of pleomorphic T lymphocytes of undetermined significance? A study of 136 cases. Am J Dermatopathol. 2009;31:317–22.
3. Gaulard P, Berti E, Willemze R, Jaffe ES. Primary cutaneous peripheral T-cell lymphomas, rare subtypes. In: Swerdlow SH, Campo E, Harris NL, Jaffe ES, Pileri SA, Stein H, et al., editors. WHO classification of tumors of haematopoietic and lymphoid tissues. Lyon: International Agency for Research on Cancer; 2008. p. 302–5.
4. Ally MS, Prasad Hunasehally RY, Rodriguez-Justo M, Martin B, Verdolini R, Attard N, et al. Evaluation of follicular T-helper cells in primary cutaneous CD4+ small/medium pleomorphic T-cell lymphoma and dermatitis. J Cutan Pathol. 2013;40:1006–13.
5. Grogg KL, Jung S, Erickson LA, McClure RF, Dogan A. Primary cutaneous CD4-positive small/medium-sized pleomorphic T-cell lymphoma: a clonal T-cell lymphoproliferative disorder with indolent behavior. Mod Pathol. 2008;21:708–15.
6. Rodríguez Pinilla SM, Roncador G, Rodríguez-Peralto JL, Mollejo M, García JF, Montes-Moreno S, et al. Primary cutaneous CD4+ small/medium-sized pleomorphic T-cell lymphoma expresses follicular T-cell markers. Am J Surg Pathol. 2009;33:81–90.
7. Williams VL, Torres-cabala CA, Duvic M. Primary cutaneous small- to medium-sized CD4+ pleomorphic T-cell lymphoma. Am J Clin Dermatol. 2011;12:389–401.
8. Garcia-Herrera A, Colomo L, Camós M, Carreras J, Balague O, Martinez A, et al. Primary cutaneous small/medium CD4+ T-cell lymphomas: a heterogeneous group of tumors with different clinicopathologic features and outcome. J Clin Oncol. 2008;26:3364–71.
9. Cetinozman F, Jansen PM, Willemze R. Expression of programmed death-1 in primary cutaneous CD4-positive small/medium-sized pleomorphic T-cell lymphoma, cutaneous pseudo-T-cell lymphoma, and other types of cutaneous T-cell lymphoma. Am J Surg Pathol. 2012;36:109–16.
10. Baum CL, Link BK, Neppalli VT, Swick BL, Liu V. Reappraisal of the provisional entity primary cutaneous CD4+ small/medium pleomorphic T-cell lymphoma: a series of 10 adult and pediatric patients and review of the literature. J Am Acad Dermatol. 2011;65:739–48.
11. Isaacson P, Chott A, Nakamura S, Muller-Hermelink HK, Harris NL, Swerdlow SH. Extranodal marginal zone lymphoma of mucosa-associated lymphoid tissue (MALT lymphoma). In: Swerdlow SH, Campo E, Harris NL, Jaffe ES, Pileri SA, Stein H, et al., editors. WHO classification of tumors of haematopoietic and lymphoid tissues. 4th ed. Lyon: International Agency for Research on Cancer; 2008. p. 214–7.
12. Servitje O, Gallardo F, Estrach T, Pujol RM, Blanco A. Clinical and laboratory investigations primary cutaneous marginal zone B-cell lymphoma: a clinical, histopathological, immunophenotypic and molecular genetic study of 22 cases. Br J Dermatol. 2002;147:1147–58.
13. Geyer JT, Ferry JA, Longtine JA, Flotte TJ, Harris NL, Zukerberg LR. Characteristics of cutaneous marginal zone lymphomas with marked plasmacytic differentiation and a T cell-rich background. Am J Clin Pathol. 2010;133(1):59–69.
14. Senff NJ, Hoefnagel JJ, Jansen PM, Vermeer MH, van Baarlen J, Blokx WA, et al. Reclassification of 300 primary cutaneous B-cell lymphomas according to the new WHO-EORTC classification for cutaneous lymphomas: comparison with previous classifications and identification of prognostic markers. J Clin Oncol. 2007;25:1581–7.

Introduction to the B-Cell Lymphomas

15

Amrita Goyal, Aliyah R. Sohani, Alexandra E. Kovach, Joi B. Carter, Jeffrey A. Barnes, and Lyn McDivitt Duncan

The human body contains a vast array of B cells, with phenotypes ranging from the naïve B cell to the centrocyte, centroblast, immunoblast, plasmablast, and plasma cell. Each of these B-cell subsets has different functional, proliferative, and migratory capacities, and the diversity of cutaneous B-cell lymphoma (CBCL) reflects the variety of non-neoplastic B-cell counterparts. The WHO-EORTC classification [1] recognizes four cutaneous B-cell lymphomas: primary cutaneous marginal zone lymphoma (pcMZL or MALT lymphoma), primary cutaneous follicle-center lymphoma (pcFCL), primary cutaneous diffuse large B-cell lymphoma, leg-type (pcDLBCL), and intravascular large B-cell lymphoma (ivLBCL). Here we offer a schema for understanding and distinguishing these lymphomas. Each lymphoma is addressed individually in subsequent chapters.

A. Goyal, M.D.
Harvard-MIT Division of Health Sciences and Technology, Harvard Medical School, Boston, MA, USA

A.R. Sohani, M.D.
Hematopathology Service, Department of Pathology, Massachusetts General Hospital, Harvard Medical School, Boston, MA, USA

A.E. Kovach, M.D.
Department of Pathology, Boston Children's Hospital, Boston, MA, USA

J.B. Carter, M.D.
Department of Dermatology, Massachusetts General Hospital, Harvard Medical School, Boston, MA, USA

J.A. Barnes, M.D., Ph.D.
Comprehensive Cutaneous Lymphoma Program, Department of Medicine, Massachusetts General Hospital Cancer Center, Boston, MA, USA

L.M. Duncan, M.D. (✉)
Dermatopathology Service, Department of Pathology, Massachusetts General Hospital, Harvard Medical School, Boston, MA, USA
e-mail: duncan@helix.mgh.harvard.edu

J.B. Carter et al. (eds.), *Atlas of Cutaneous Lymphomas: Classification and Differential Diagnosis*, DOI 10.1007/978-3-319-17217-0_15

15.1 Classification and Frequency of Cutaneous B-Cell Lymphomas

Although the majority of *systemic* lymphomas are of B-cell origin, only 25 % of cutaneous lymphomas are derived from B cells. The current edition of the WHO/EORTC classification guidelines includes four CBCLs: primary cutaneous marginal zone lymphoma of mucosa-associated lymphoid tissue (pcMZL also known as MALT lymphoma), primary cutaneous follicle center lymphoma (pcFCL), primary cutaneous diffuse large B-cell lymphoma, leg-type (pcDLBCL), and intravascular large B-cell lymphoma (ivLBCL). While the first three are primary cutaneous lymphomas, ivLBCL is a rare systemic lymphoma that may present with prominent cutaneous findings and is thus included in the classification. The relative frequencies of these lymphomas are listed in Table 15.1.

Table 15.1 Frequency of cutaneous B-cell lymphomas

Lymphoma	Frequency (%) (among B-cell lymphomas)[a]
pcMZL	30
pcFCL	48
pcDLBCL, leg type	20
ivLBCL	1

Data from Willemze et al. [1]

ivLBCL intravascular large B-cell lymphoma, *pcDLBCL* primary cutaneous diffuse large B-cell lymphoma, *pcFCL* primary cutaneous follicle center lymphoma, *pcMZL* primary cutaneous marginal zone lymphoma

[a]Does not add up to 100 % because the study also included cases of pcDLBCL, other (1 %)

15.2 Clinical Presentation and Prognosis of Cutaneous B-Cell Lymphomas

The majority of CBCLs are clinically similar, presenting as dome-shaped, smooth, asymptomatic, erythematous to violaceous plaques, nodules, or tumors. ivLBCL is the exception and may demonstrate a wide variety of cutaneous manifestations (or none at all) (*see* Chap. 19). The clinical characteristics of the B-cell lymphomas are listed in Table 15.2. Cutaneous lymphoid hyperplasia (CLH) is included in this table because it is the primary differential diagnostic entity for the low-grade CLBLs (pcMZL and pcFCL).

CBCL can roughly be broken down by prognosis (Table 15.2). While pcFCL and pcMZL have excellent prognoses marked by repeated recurrences but minimal mortality, diagnoses of pcDLBCL or ivLBCL portend a much poorer outcome. This division is depicted in Fig. 15.1.

Table 15.2 Clinical characteristics of cutaneous B-cell lymphomas and cutaneous lymphoid hyperplasia

	pcMZL	pcFCL	pcDLBCL, leg type	ivLBCL	CLH
Clinical presentation	Solitary or multiple erythematous-to-violaceous plaques, nodules, or tumors	Solitary or grouped erythematous-to-violaceous plaques, nodules, or tumors	Solitary or multiple red or blue-red tumors on lower leg (unilateral or bilateral)	*Western*—cutaneous and CNS manifestations *Eastern*—hemophagocytic syndrome	Firm skin-colored to erythematous to violaceous nodule/tumor or infiltrated plaques
Location	Trunk, extremities	Head, trunk	Lower leg, often in areas of venous stasis; rare cases meeting diagnostic criteria may occur at other sites	Systemic	Face (70 %), chest (36 %), upper extremities (25 %)
Associated symptoms	None	None	Often none	B symptoms, neurologic abnormalities, hemophagocytic syndrome	Often at sites of bites, trauma, vaccinations, tattoos
Median age	60s	50s	70s	60s	30s
Gender predilection	Male	None	Female	None	Female
Common treatment	Radiotherapy, excision, intralesional steroids	Radiotherapy, excision, intralesional steroids	Radiotherapy, multiagent chemotherapy with rituximab	Chemotherapy	Excision, intralesional steroids
Likelihood of extracutaneous spread	5 %	5–10 %	50 %	Systemic at diagnosis	None
5-year survival	100 %	95 %	50 %	<30 %	100 %

Data from Bergman [2], Senff et al. [3, 4], Swerdlow et al. [5]
CLH cutaneous lymphoid hyperplasia, *CNS* central nervous system, *ivLBCL* intravascular large B-cell lymphoma, *pcDLBCL* primary cutaneous diffuse large B-cell lymphoma, *pcFCL* primary cutaneous follicle center lymphoma, *pcMZL* primary cutaneous marginal zone lymphoma, leg type

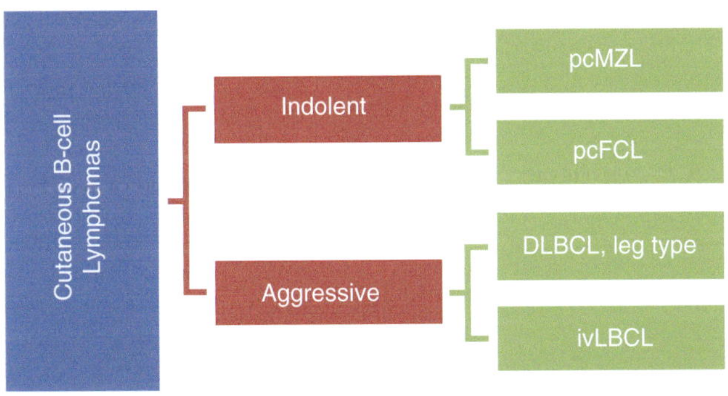

Fig. 15.1 CBCL categorized by prognosis. *ivLBCL* intravascular large B-cell lymphoma, *pcDLBCL* primary cutaneous diffuse large B-cell lymphoma, *pcFCL* primary cutaneous follicle center lymphoma, *pcMZL* primary cutaneous marginal zone lymphoma

15.3 Pathologic Algorithms for Understanding Cutaneous B-Cell Lymphomas

Although CBCLs occur less frequently than cutaneous T-cell lymphomas, there are many nuances involved in making a diagnosis of CBCL. Because of their clinical homogeneity, differentiating B-cell lymphomas is largely dependent on pathology, which in turn requires a synthesis of cytology, histology, and immunohistochemistry analysis. This section elaborates on the role of histopathology and immunohistochemistry in diagnosing cutaneous B-cell lymphomas. Table 15.3 outlines major characteristics that may help differentiate the cutaneous B-cell lymphomas.

Table 15.3 Histopathologic and molecular characteristics of cutaneous B-cell lymphomas (CBCLs) and cutaneous lymphoid hyperplasia (CLH)

	pcFCL	pcMZL	pcDLBCL	ivLBCL	CLH
Cellular morphology	Medium to large centrocytes and centroblasts	Centrocyte-like marginal zone B cells, variable lymphoplasmacytoid and plasma cells, rare immunoblasts	Confluent sheets of large cells resembling immunoblasts or centroblasts	Large atypical B cells in vascular lumina	Polymorphous lymphocytes with admixed histiocytes, eosinophils, and plasma cells
Distribution of lymphoid infiltrate	Follicular, diffuse, or follicular and diffuse patterns; normal reactive follicles usually absent	Dense, nodular, dermal, and subcutaneous; intact and colonized reactive lymphoid follicles may be present	Diffuse infiltrates or confluent sheets; no follicle formation	Intravascular	Nodular or diffuse infiltrate with reactive follicles
Distinctive features	Ill-defined follicles with absent mantle zones	Sheets of marginal zone B cells and aggregates of lymphoplasmacytoid cells; occasional mature plasma cells; rare immunoblasts; occasionally frequent non-neoplastic T cells	Monomorphous sheets of large cells	Intravascular	No abnormal follicle architecture, no light-chain restriction
Immunohistochemical markers	CD20+	CD20+	CD20+	CD20+	Admixed infiltrate of CD3+ T cells that often predominates. CD20+ B cells, occasionally with well-formed reactive lymphoid follicles
	PAX5+	PAX5+	PAX5+	PAX5+	
	CD79a+	CD79a+	CD79a+	CD79a+	
	Bcl6+	Bcl6–	Bcl6–/+	Bcl6+/–	
	CD10+/–	CD10–	CD10–	CD10– (80 % of cases)	
	Bcl2–/+	Bcl2+	Bcl2+	Bcl2+	
	MUM1–	MUM1+	MUM1+	MUM1+	
	FoxP1–	CyclinD1–	FoxP1+		
	IgM-	CD5–	IgM+		
		IgM –/+			
Molecular genetic features	Amplification of *REL* gene	*IGH, MALT1, API2*, and *FOXP1* translocations [6]	*IGH, BCL6* and/or *MYC* translocation(s)	Unknown; reports of chromosome number abnormalities	No clonally rearranged *IGH*
	Loss of *CDKN2A* and *CDKN2A* rare		9p21.3 deletion (loss of *CDKN2A* and *CDKN2B*)		May see rearranged TCR in reactive/oligoclonal responses in the skin
	t(14;18) absent		*BCL2* amplification		
			t(14;18) absent		
Immunoglobulin (Ig) clonality	Monoclonal surface Ig	Monoclonal cytoplasmic Ig	Monoclonal surface or cytoplasmic Ig	Often monoclonal surface Ig	Polyclonal Ig
Light-chain restriction	Absent in plasma cells	Often present in plasma cells (can be demonstrated in up to 70 % cases)	Present, but absent in plasma cells	Present, but absent in plasma cells	Absent

CLH data from Ploysangam et al. [7]

CLH cutaneous lymphoid hyperplasia, *ivLBCL* intravascular large B-cell lymphoma, *pcDLBCL* primary cutaneous diffuse large B-cell lymphoma, leg type, *pcFCL* primary cutaneous follicle center lymphoma, *pcMZL* primary cutaneous marginal zone lymphoma

15.3.1 Histopathology in Diagnosis of CBCL

There are three main histopathologic patterns of cutaneous involvement commonly seen in CBCL: nodular or follicular, diffuse, and intravascular. Neoplasms with a nodular/follicular pattern have aggregates of lymphoid cells in the dermis; the structure of the lymphoid follicles can be critical in diagnosis and is discussed later in this chapter. Diffuse patterns of infiltration are characterized by sheets of neoplastic cells occupying the dermis. Finally, neoplasms with intravascular involvement manifest as tumor cells within the lumina of vessels.

The distribution of the lymphoid infiltrate can be quite informative. For example, although ivLBCL and pcDLBCL may share similar cytology, ivLBCL is readily distinguished by the presence of the atypical cells within the vasculature. This is in contrast to pcDLBCL, in which the dermis is overrun by sheets of large neoplastic cells. The nodular or follicular and diffuse patterns are slightly less informative. A nodular or follicular lymphoid infiltrate may be consistent with either pcFCL or pcMZL; likewise, a diffuse pattern may be seen in either pcDLBCL or pcFCL (Fig. 15.2). Thus, histopathology alone is helpful but insufficient for diagnosis; additional information from immunohistochemistry and molecular testing is often necessary.

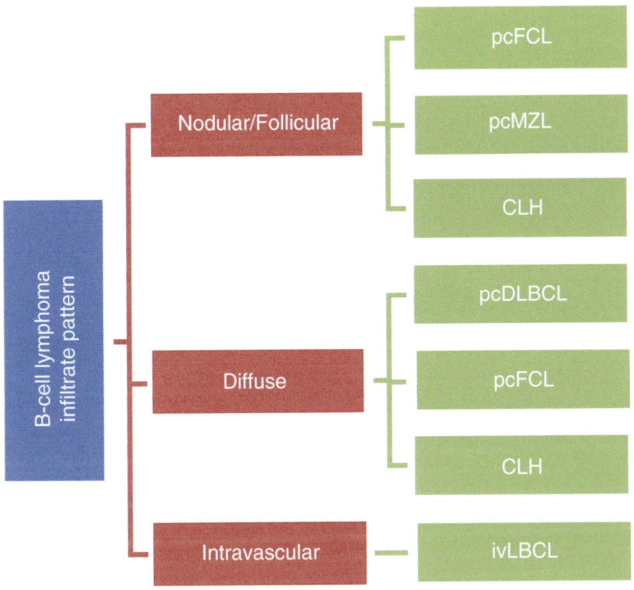

Fig. 15.2 CBCLs categorized by histopathologic characteristics. The cutaneous B-cell lymphomas can be organized based on the pattern of infiltration. Three major patterns considered in cutaneous B-cell lymphomas are nodular/follicular, diffuse, and intravascular. Although some lymphomas have unique histology (e.g., ivLBCL), others have more heterogeneous presentations, e.g., pcFCL is present twice in this flow chart because it can present with follicular, diffuse, or follicular and diffuse patterns

15.3.2 Immunohistochemistry in the Diagnosis of CBCL

Immunophenotypic analysis is critical for accurate diagnosis of cutaneous B-cell lymphomas. The most commonly used B-cell markers include CD20, CD79a, and PAX5. Of note, PAX5, a nuclear marker, may be easier to interpret and less susceptible to overestimation of the B-cell burden. It is also important to note whether a patient has received rituximab or other anti-CD20 therapy before relying on CD20 to define a B-cell population. Additionally, immunohistochemical stains for germinal center markers (CD10, Bcl6) or postgerminal center origin, including plasma cells (MUM1), the anti-apoptotic marker Bcl2, follicular dendritic cells (CD21, CD23), a pan-T-cell marker (most commonly CD3), and evaluation of kappa and lambda immunoglobulin light chains by immunohistochemistry or in situ hybridization are usually part of the diagnostic testing panel.

The immunohistochemical staining patterns for the cutaneous B-cell lymphomas are complex. Here we present a possible schema for categorizing immunohistochemical patterns of neoplastic B-cells (Fig. 15.3; *see* Table 15.3); it is possible to generate numerous others. This schema is meant to serve as a simplified starting point for learning how to consider these lymphomas in a diagnostic context. It is important to note that there are always numerous reactive T cells present in the skin, even in the setting of a B-cell lymphoma.

Because the majority of cutaneous and systemic B-cell lymphomas are derived from germinal center B cells, the immunophenotypes of the B-cell lymphomas can be more easily understood in the setting of B-cell development within the germinal center; this is further discussed later on in the chapter.

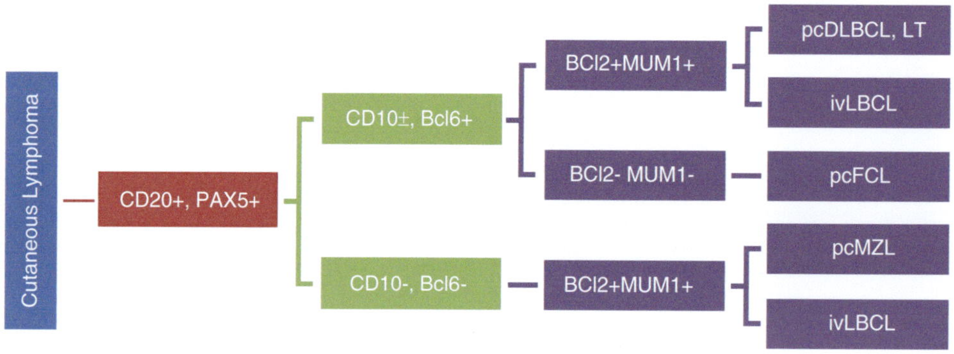

Fig. 15.3 CBCLs based on immunophenotype of the neoplastic B cells. Because these cutaneous tumors always have an admixed infiltrate of reactive lymphocytes, the distribution of the infiltrate, the architecture of lymphoid follicles (if present), and the presence or absence of light-chain restriction are also necessary to define a neoplastic population. The immunophenotypes shown here correspond to those most commonly reported for each entity, but exceptions do exist

15.4 Understanding the Cutaneous B-Cell Lymphomas

Diagnosing cutaneous B-cell lymphomas can be very difficult, and accurate identification requires a solid understanding of cytology, immunohistochemistry, and lymphoid follicle architecture and development. In this section, we will review B-cell cytology, immunohistochemical staining patterns of B cells throughout their development, and the structure of normal and abnormal lymphoid follicles.

15.4.1 B-Cell Cytology

A significant component of the diagnosis of B-cell lymphomas rests in identifying cells on the basis of their cytology. Thus, recognition of the cytologic characteristics of the various types of non-neoplastic B-cell counterparts is helpful.

Naïve B cells have a small, round nucleus with a thin rim of cytoplasm (Fig. 15.4a). Centroblasts, the next stage in B-cell activation, have medium-sized to large nuclei, open or vesicular chromatin, several basophilic peripherally placed nucleoli that often "cling" to the nuclear membrane, and a small-to-moderate amount of eosinophilic cytoplasm. Centroblast nuclei are usually round but may demonstrate indentations, notches, or grooves (Fig. 15.4b). Centrocytes are the progeny of centroblasts and have small- to medium-sized cleaved or folded nuclei, moderately dispersed chromatin, inconspicuous nucleoli, and a thin rim of cytoplasm. Particularly in reference to cytologic preparations or in peripheral smears with circulating centrocytes in systemic follicular lymphoma, centrocytes have been referred to as "buttock cells" because of their characteristically cleaved nuclei (Fig. 15.4c). Of note, lymphocytes of the marginal zone of the follicle are commonly described as showing centrocyte-like features.

Immunoblasts and plasmablasts are derived from centrocytes and are precursors of the plasma cell. Immunoblasts have large nuclei with a moderate amount of cytoplasm, dispersed or open nuclear chromatin, and a prominent centrally placed eosinophilic macronucleolus (Fig. 15.4d). Plasmablasts are more similar to plasma cells but somewhat larger, with an eccentrically placed nucleus and a paranuclear clearing or "hof," an area of cytoplasm where immunoglobulin has begun to accumulate (Fig. 15.4e). Unlike plasma cells, plasmablasts usually have a single nucleolus. Mature plasma cells have round nuclei, eccentrically placed abundant eosinophilic cytoplasm, and a usually well-defined hof. The nuclei of plasma cells have a characteristic "clock face" nuclear chromatin pattern with peripherally located regions of condensed chromatin (Fig. 15.4f). Some plasma cells have prominent pink cytoplasmic immunoglobulin inclusions (Russell bodies); a plasma cell stuffed with multiple Russell bodies is termed a Mott cell. Immunoglobulin pseudoinclusions in the nucleus, termed Dutcher bodies, are said to occur exclusively in neoplastic proliferations with plasmacytic differentiation; for example, their presence may favor cutaneous marginal zone lymphoma over a differential diagnosis of cutaneous lymphoid hyperplasia with plasmacytic differentiation.

15.4.2 Using B-Cell Development and Germinal Center Architecture to Understand the B-Cell Lymphomas

The majority of B-cell lymphomas originate from germinal center B cells, probably the result of high levels of cellular proliferation and somatic hypermutation (SHM) [8]. One of the keys to understanding the B-cell lymphomas is an appreciation of the structure of a normal germinal follicle and the events that occur within it. Germinal follicles are found in secondary lymphoid organs, including lymph nodes, Peyer patches, and tonsils, among others.

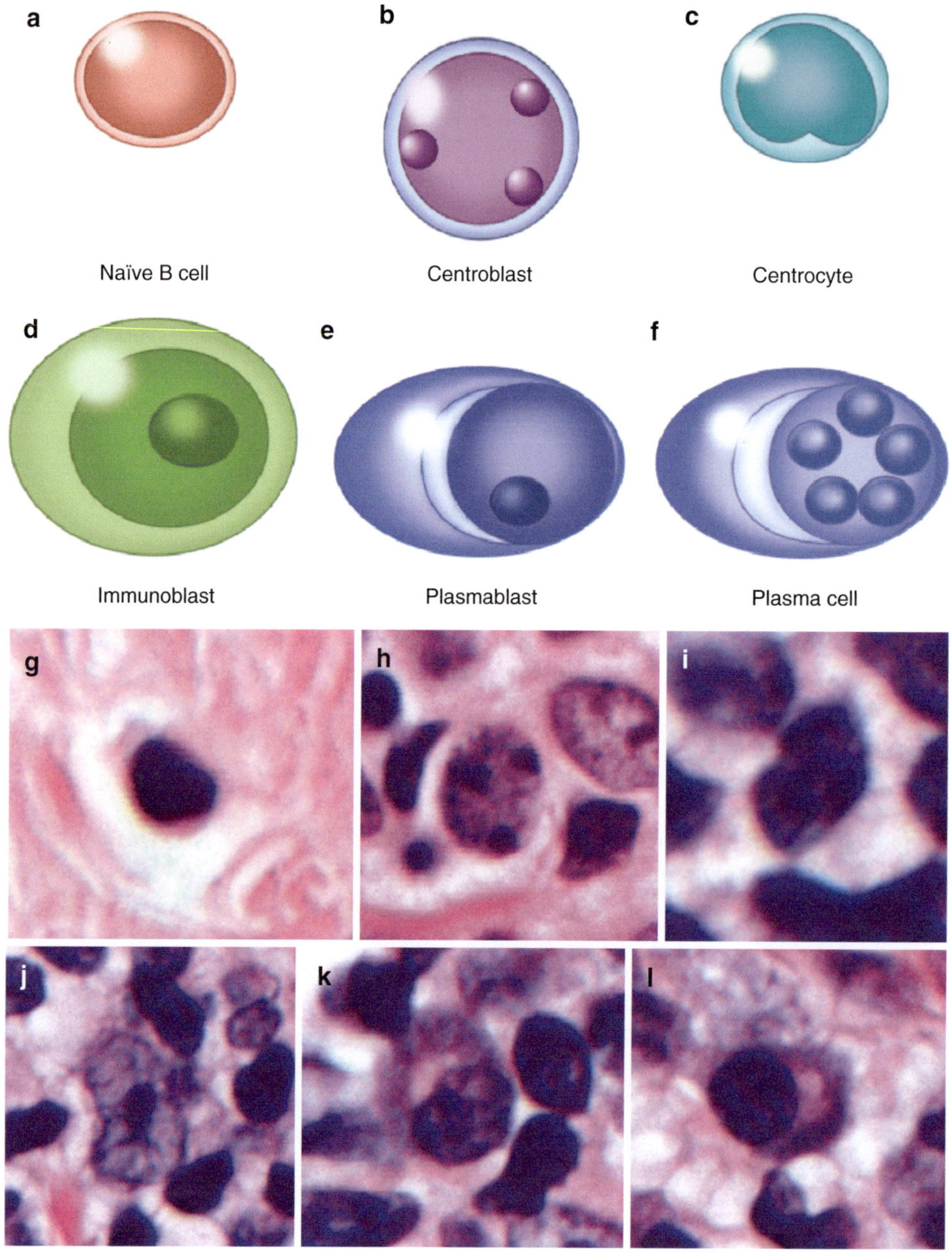

Fig. 15.4 Morphology of B-cell subtypes. These illustrations and histological images depict the major cytologic features characteristic of the cell types commonly seen in B-cell lymphomas. **a**, **g**) Naïve B cells have a small, round nucleus with a thin rim of cytoplasm. **b**, **h**) Centroblasts have medium-sized to large nuclei, open or vesicular chromatin, several basophilic peripherally placed nucleoli which often "cling" to the nuclear membrane, and a small-to-moderate amount of eosinophilic cytoplasm. **c**, **i**) Centrocytes have small to medium-sized cleaved or folded nuclei, moderately dispersed chromatin, inconspicuous nucleoli, and a thin rim of cytoplasm. **d**, **j**) Immunoblasts have large nuclei with a moderate amount of cytoplasm, dispersed or open nuclear chromatin, and a prominent centrally placed eosinophilic macronucleolus. **e**, **k**) Plasmablasts have an eccentrically placed nucleus and a paranuclear clearing, or "hof," an area of cytoplasm where immunoglobulin has begun to accumulate. **f**, **l**) Mature plasma cells have round nuclei, eccentrically placed abundant eosinophilic cytoplasm, and a usually well-defined hof. The nuclei of plasma cells have a characteristic "clock face" nuclear chromatin pattern with peripherally located regions of condensed chromatin

15.4.2.1 Development of the Germinal Follicle

The lymphoid follicle of a secondary lymphoid organ is composed of three variably prominent zones: a germinal center, a surrounding mantle zone, and an outer marginal zone [9]. B cells arrive in the germinal center from the mantle zone as mature naïve cells, possessing a unique immunoglobulin heavy chain but not yet having been exposed to their cognate antigen. These naïve, mature B cells migrate to T-cell rich "dark" zones of the germinal center, where they become activated secondary to interaction with the CD4+ T cells, follicular dendritic cells (FDCs), or other antigen presenting cells [10, 11].

Activation results in the transformation of the B cells into centroblasts, the proliferating germinal center B cells [10, 12]. For reasons that are poorly understood, these cells have a high rate of mutation at the immunoglobulin heavy- and light-chain loci. Hence, during SHM, the germinal center B cells accumulate numerous point mutations, leading to further diversification of the immunoglobulin repertoire. Once SHM is complete, the B cells are exposed to FDCs. The B cells with a high affinity for antigens presented by FDCs are permitted to live, while their co-cells of lesser affinity perish. These cells then undergo clonal expansion through rapid division. This population growth results in expansion of the germinal center, with a germinal center "light zone" composed of matured centrocytes, FDCs, T cells, and macrophages and a remaining dark zone concentrated in centroblasts [10]; since SHM, the newly diversified B cells have become smaller, nondividing centrocytes, capable of further differentiation and migration to the light zone.

The light zone of the germinal center is the site of class-switch recombination (CSR), high-affinity antibody production, and B-cell differentiation [10]. Once in the light zone, centrocytes undergo selection [10]. They may then have one of three outcomes: differentiation into memory B cells or plasma cells, apoptosis, or regression into centroblasts [10, 13]. There are additional recognized intermediate cell types in each of these pathways. For example, as previously described, the centrocyte becomes an immunoblast and then a plasmablast en route to becoming a plasma cell [10].

The cells experience dramatic changes in gene expression patterns and cell surface markers as part of this activation process, resulting in differences in germinal B-cell and activated/postgerminal B-cell phenotypes [14, 15]. These alterations in gene and cell surface marker expression can be valuable in attempting to trace the origin or non-neoplastic counterpart of a neoplastic cell for accurate classification (Fig. 15.5).

15.4.2.2 Application to the Cutaneous B-Cell Lymphomas

An understanding of the structure of the lymphoid follicle and the patterns of gene expression through B-cell development is indispensable to conceptualizing the phenotypes of the cutaneous B-cell lymphomas. For example, pcFCL is a lymphoma composed of centrocytes and centroblasts, cells derived from the follicle center (hence the name *follicle center* lymphoma). These cells have a germinal B-cell phenotype, as do normal follicle center cells. Because pcFCL is derived from mature B cells, the cells of pcFCL have a clonal immunoglobulin heavy chain (*IGH*) gene rearrangement. The immunohistochemical phenotype of the neoplastic cells of most cases of pcFCL is similar to that of normal follicle center cells: CD20+, CD79a+, CD10+, Bcl6+, Bcl2−, and MUM1−.

MALT lymphomas, on the other hand, are lymphomas of marginal zone B cells (often described as centrocyte-like or monocytoid in appearance) with some centroblasts and immunoblasts and variable plasmacytic differentiation, manifesting morphologically with lymphoplasmacytoid cells and mature plasma cells. These cells have an activated or postgerminal center phenotype and have undergone SHM. As with pcFCL, pcMZL is derived from mature B cells and thus both have a clonal *IGH* rearrangement. The immunophenotype of MALT lymphoma cells in most cases is similar to that of normal marginal zone cells: CD20+, CD79+, CD10−, Bcl6−, Bcl2+, and MUM1+. Most cases have detectable light-chain restriction in plasma cells and at least a subset of lymphocytes with plasmacytic differentiation. As previously described, the presence of Dutcher bodies (immunoglobulin nuclear pseudoinclusions) can be a helpful clue that a proliferation is neoplastic in nature. Diagnosis can be challenging, as plasmacytic differentiation can be minimal, and the numerous admixed small non-neoplastic T cells can occasionally outnumber the neoplastic B cells.

pcDLBCL and ivLBCL are lymphomas of large B cells. The cells of these lymphomas appear malignant. They usually have an activated or postgerminal center B cell phenotype and thus demonstrate clonal *IGH* rearrangements. Their morphology and immunophenotype are similar to those of large transformed cells such as centroblasts, immunoblasts, or, more rarely, plasmablasts: CD20+, CD79+, CD10−, Bcl6−/+, Bcl2+, and MUM1+. Of note, Bcl6 has been directly implicated in lymphomagenesis [18].

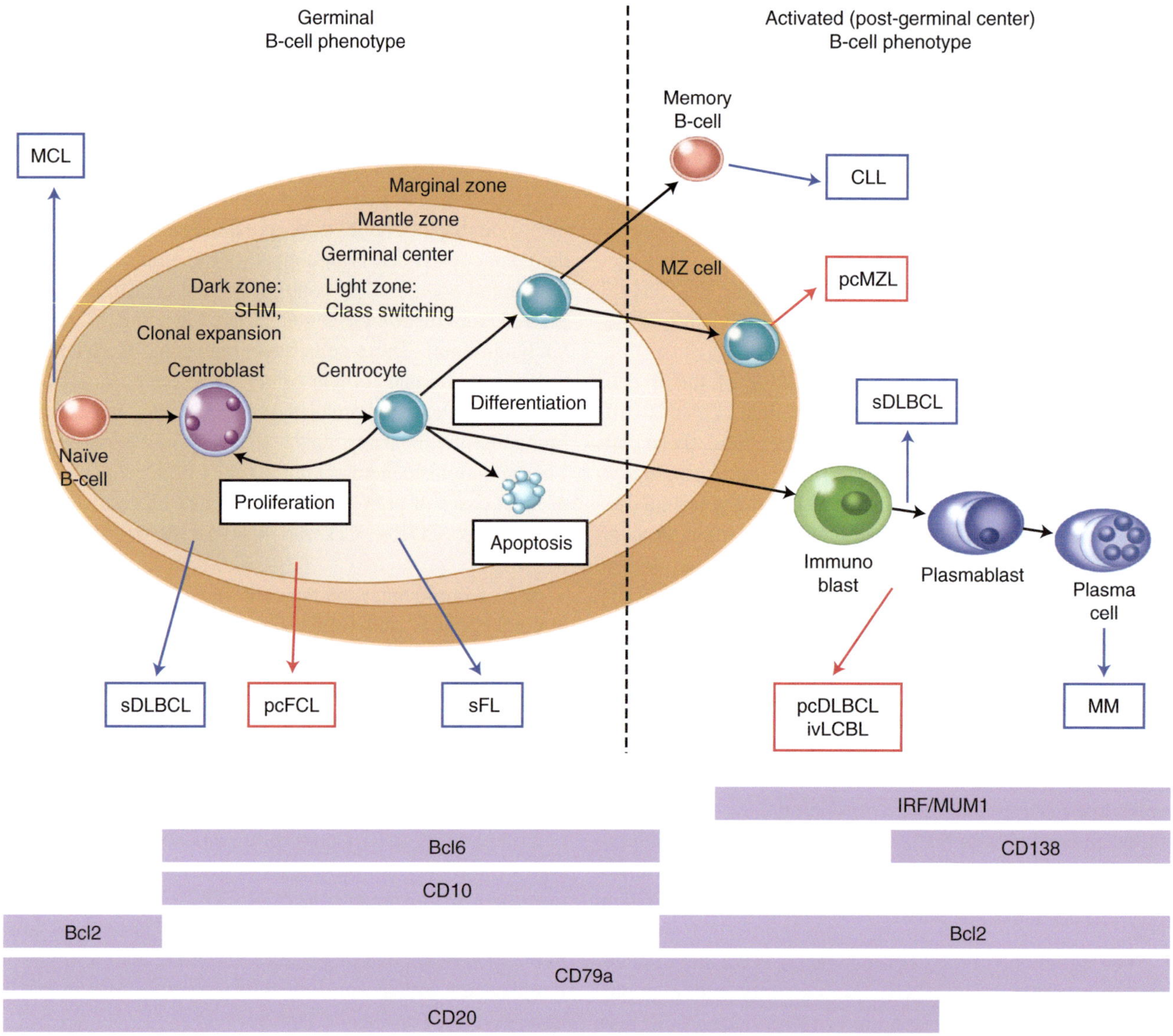

Fig. 15.5 The relationship between the normal germinal center and B-cell lymphomas**.** The germinal follicle is composed of three variably prominent zones: germinal center, mantle zone, and marginal zone. B cells arrive as naïve mature cells. Upon exposure to antigen, the B cells become centroblasts and undergo somatic hypermutation (*SHM*) and clonal expansion, creating the dark zone of the germinal center. The centroblasts then differentiate into centrocytes, which travel to the light zone of the germinal cell to undergo selection. Selection may result in apoptosis, with regression to centroblasts and cycling back to the dark zone, or differentiation into plasma cells or memory cells. In order to differentiate into plasma cells, the centrocytes must transition into immunoblasts, then plasmablasts, and finally plasma cells. Over the course of B-cell development and differentiation, there are many dramatic changes in gene expression. The timing of expression of several key proteins is depicted at the *bottom* of the figure; the bars approximate the portion of development over which the gene is expressed. Note that during their transition through the germinal center, the B cells have a germinal center B-cell phenotype with cells that are CD10+, BCL6+, and MUM1−. Following this stage of differentiation, there are many changes in gene expression, resulting in an activated or postgerminal center B-cell phenotype (typically defined by expression of MUM1). Many B-cell lymphomas can be traced to a germinal center B-cell origin, particularly systemic follicular lymphomas and some systemic DLBCLs; on the other hand, up to one third of cases of DLBCL are of the activated B-cell phenotype (ABC). This distinction, which has prognostic and evolving therapeutic implications, was originally described through gene expression profile work [16], with an immunohistochemical algorithm using CD10, BCL6, and MUM1 serving as a common surrogate in individual clinical cases [17]. In the figure above, lymphomas included in the WHO-EORTC classification of cutaneous lymphomas are in red boxes; other common systemic B-cell malignancies are in blue. In accordance with its normal counterpart, pcFCL has a germinal B-cell phenotype, while pcMZL, pcDLBCL, and ivLBCL have an activated/postgerminal center B-cell phenotype. *CLL* chronic lymphocytic leukemia, *MCL* mantle cell lymphoma, *pcFCL* primary cutaneous follicle center lymphoma, *pcDLBCL* primary cutaneous diffuse large B-cell lymphoma, leg type, *ivLBCL* intravascular large B-cell lymphoma, *sDLBCL* systemic diffuse large B-cell lymphoma, *sFL* systemic follicular lymphoma, *MM* multiple myeloma (plasma cell myeloma), *pcMZL* primary cutaneous marginal zone lymphoma, *SHM* somatic hypermutation, *MZ* marginal zone

15.4.3 Reactive and Neoplastic Lymphoid Follicle Structure

Lymphoid follicles are not normally present in the skin. When they are, an explanation should be sought, either reactive or neoplastic. Differences in lymphoid follicle structure can help to distinguish between neoplastic and non-neoplastic follicles as well as help to differentiate the various types of neoplasms, particularly pcFCL and MALT lymphoma.

A normal reactive lymphoid follicle has a well-defined germinal center composed of a light zone containing centrocytes, a dark zone of centroblasts and an associated encompassing follicular dendritic cell (FDC) meshwork. The germinal center is surrounded by a marginal zone and an often inconspicuous inner mantle zone (Fig. 15.6a). This normal follicular architecture is disrupted in both pcMZL and pcFCL, where the follicles are composed of neoplastic cells (as in pcFCL) or overrun by them (as in pcMZL). Typically, the term "germinal center" is used to describe reactive follicles, while "follicle center" is used to describe neoplastic follicles.

pcMZL is a neoplastic proliferation of cells along the spectrum of marginal zone cells and cells with plasmacytic differentiation. Occasional large transformed cells with the appearance of immunoblasts may be present, but these do not predominate. Accordingly, there is an expansion of the marginal zone, with marginal zone cells, lymphoplasmacytoid cells, and rare immunoblasts spilling out of the marginal zone into the surrounding dermis and, in some cases, invading or colonizing the residual reactive germinal centers. These colonized reactive follicles show disruption of their normal architecture, with scattered clusters of germinal center cells and disruption or splaying of the FDC meshwork (Fig. 15.6b) [19].

The neoplastic follicles of pcFCL can be conceptually thought of as "opposite" to those of pcMZL. pcFCL is a neoplasm of follicle center cells; hence, there is expansion of the follicle center with associated expansion rather than disruption of the FDC meshwork. The neoplastic cells may compress the marginal zone to a thin rim around the follicle center, or the cells may spill out of the follicle into the surrounding dermis. One feature of pcFCL characteristic of cutaneous but not nodal-based follicular lymphoma is the "naked" or "inside-out" follicle, with outer centrocyte and centroblast B cells and centrally located marginal zone cells or even small T cells (see Chap. 17; Fig. 15.6c) [19].

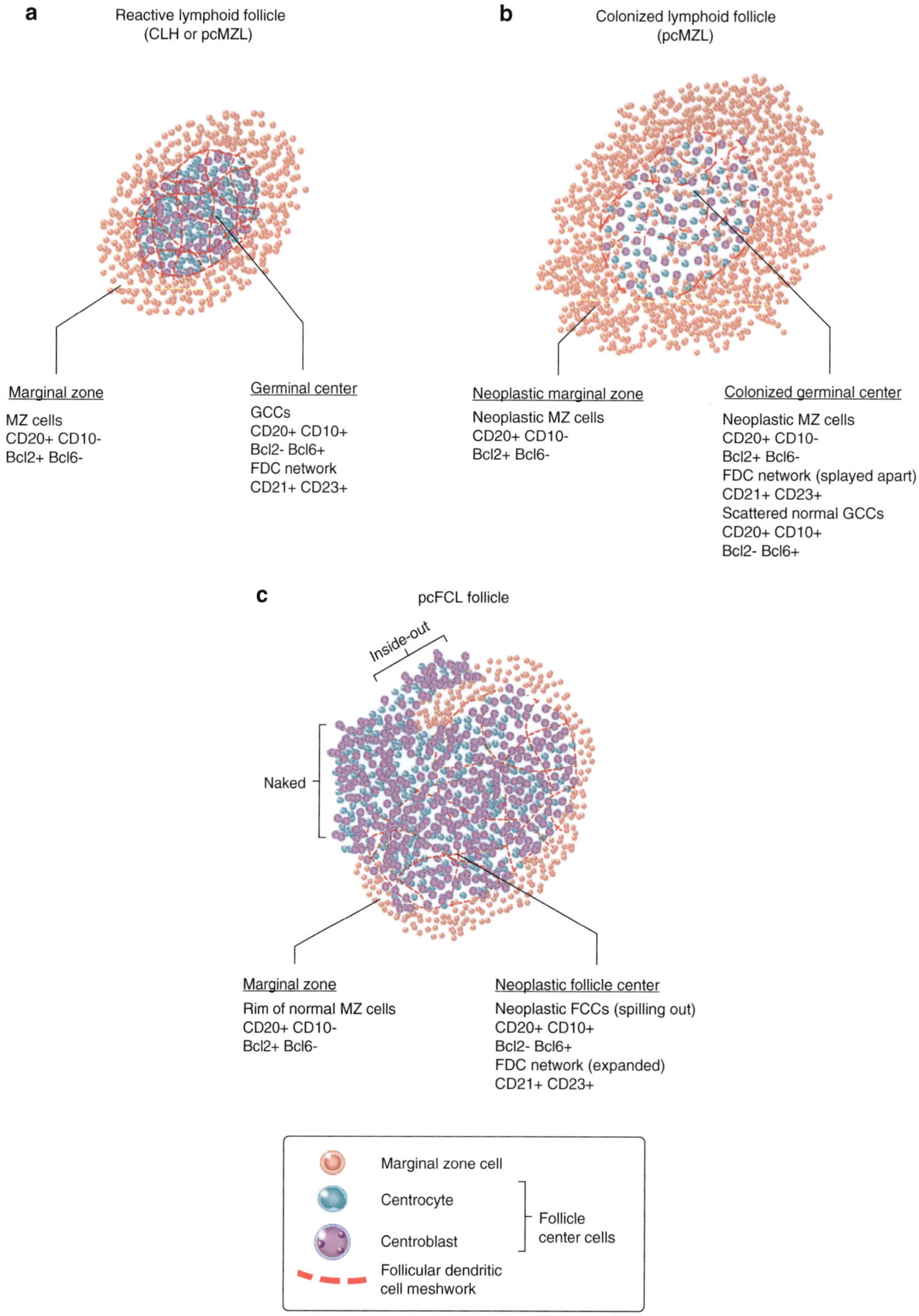

Fig. 15.6 Reactive and neoplastic cutaneous lymphoid follicles. (**a**) Reactive lymphoid follicles are well-defined, with a regularly shaped germinal center (composed of centrocytes, centroblasts, and follicular dendritic cells) and a surrounding marginal zone. (**b**) The lymphoid follicles of pcMZL may be similar to those of reactive lymphoid follicles or may be irregularly shaped and overrun by neoplastic marginal zone cells (termed "colonization" of the germinal center), which manifests as disruption or splaying of the follicular dendritic cell network. (**c**) In pcFCL, on the other hand, the follicle center is expanded. The neoplastic follicle center cells may spill out into the dermis; direct juxtaposition of the medium-large follicle center cells against dermal collagen may result in the appearance of a "naked" follicle. When the follicle center cells surround aggregates of small marginal zone cells, an "inside-out" appearing lymphoid follicle may form, with the small cells in the center and larger cells at the periphery. Immunophenotypes are as indicated in the diagram [19]. *CLH* cutaneous lymphoid hyperplasia, *MZ* marginal zone, *GCC* germinal center cells, *FCC* follicle center cells, *pcMZL* primary cutaneous marginal zone lymphoma, *pcFCL* primary cutaneous follicle center lymphoma

References

1. Willemze R, Jaffe ES, Burg G, Cerroni L, Berti E, Swerdlow SH, et al. WHO-EORTC classification for cutaneous lymphomas. Blood. 2005;105:3768–85.
2. Bergman R. Pseudolymphoma and cutaneous lymphoma: facts and controversies. Clin Dermatol. 2010;28:568–74.
3. Senff NJ, Hoefnagel JJ, Jansen PM, Vermeer MH, van Baarlen J, Blokx WA, et al. Reclassification of 300 primary cutaneous B-cell lymphomas according to the new WHO-EORTC classification for cutaneous lymphomas: comparison with previous classifications and identification of prognostic markers. J Clin Oncol. 2007;25:1581–7.
4. Senff NJ, Noordijk EM, Kim YH, Bagot M, Berti E, Cerroni L, et al. European Organization for Research and Treatment of Cancer and International Society for Cutaneous Lymphoma consensus recommendations for the management of cutaneous B-cell lymphomas. Blood. 2008;112:1600–9.
5. Swerdlow SH, Campo E, Harris NL, Jaffe ES, Pileri SA, Stein H, et al., editors. WHO classification of tumors of haematopoietic and lymphoid tissues. 4th ed. Lyon: International Agency for Research on Cancer; 2008.
6. Fernandez-Flores A. Current concepts on cutaneous MALT lymphomas. Am J Dermatopathol. 2013;35:477–84.
7. Ploysangam T, Breneman DL, Mutasim DF. Cutaneous pseudolymphomas. J Am Acad Dermatol. 1998;38:877–98.
8. Küppers R. Mechanisms of B-cell lymphoma pathogenesis. Nat Rev Cancer. 2005;5:251–62.
9. Hauser A, Kerfoot S, Haberman A. Cellular choreography in the germinal center: new visions from in vivo imaging. Semin Immunopathol. 2010;32:239–55.
10. Klein U, Dalla-Favera R. Germinal centres: role in B-cell physiology and malignancy. Nat Rev Immunol. 2008;8:22–33.
11. Gatto D, Brink R. The germinal center reaction. J Allergy Clin Immunol. 2010;126:898–907; quiz 908–9.
12. Victora GD, Schwickert TA, Fooksman DR, Kamphorst AO, Meyer-Hermann M, Dustin ML, et al. Germinal center dynamics revealed by multiphoton microscopy with a photoactivatable fluorescent reporter. Cell. 2010;143:592–605.
13. Bannard O, Horton RM, Allen CDC, An J, Nagasawa T, Cyster JG. Germinal center centroblasts transition to a centrocyte phenotype according to a timed program and depend on the dark zone for effective selection. Immunity. 2013;39:912–24.
14. Nakayama Y, Stabach P, Maher SE, Mahajan MC, Masiar P, Liao C, et al. A limited number of genes are involved in the differentiation of germinal center B cells. J Cell Biochem. 2006;99:1308–25.
15. Klein U, Tu Y, Stolovitzky GA, Keller JL, Haddad J, Miljkovic V, et al. Transcriptional analysis of the B cell germinal center reaction. Proc Natl Acad Sci U S A. 2003;100:2639–44.
16. Alizadeh AA, Eisen MB, Davis RE, Ma C, Lossos IS, Rosenwald A, et al. Distinct types of diffuse large B-cell lymphoma identified by gene expression profiling. Nature. 2000;403:503–11.
17. Hans CP, Weisenburger DD, Greiner TC, Gascoyne RD, Delabie J, Ott G, et al. Confirmation of the molecular classification of diffuse large B-cell lymphoma by immunohistochemistry using a tissue microarray. Blood. 2004;103:275–82.
18. Ranuncolo SM, Polo JM, Dierov J, Singer M, Kuo T, Greally J, et al. Bcl-6 mediates the germinal center B cell phenotype and lymphomagenesis through transcriptional repression of the DNA-damage sensor ATR. Nat Immunol. 2007;8:705–14.
19. de Leval L, Harris NL, Longtine J, Ferry JA, Duncan LM. Cutaneous B-cell lymphomas of follicular and marginal zone types: use of Bcl-6, CD10, Bcl-2, and CD21 in diagnosis and classification. Am J Surg Pathol. 2001;25:732–41.

Primary Cutaneous Marginal Zone Lymphoma

16

Amrita Goyal, Joi B. Carter, Jeffrey A. Barnes, and Lyn McDivitt Duncan

Primary cutaneous marginal zone lymphoma (pcMZL) is an indolent B-cell lymphoma that commonly presents with red to violaceous plaques, nodules, or tumors. It has an excellent prognosis. This entity has also been known as cutaneous marginal zone lymphoma (CMZL), extranodal marginal zone lymphoma of mucosa associated lymphoid tissue (MZL or MALT lymphoma), primary cutaneous immunocytoma, primary cutaneous plasmacytoma, and lymphoma cutis [1, 2]. This chapter will discuss the clinical presentation, prognosis, treatment, histopathology, immunophenotype, and differential diagnosis of pcMZL. It closes with a clinical case, including clinical images and histopathology.

A. Goyal, M.D.
Harvard-MIT Division of Health Sciences and Technology, Harvard Medical School, Boston, MA, USA

J.B. Carter, M.D.
Department of Dermatology, Massachusetts General Hospital, Harvard Medical School, Boston, MA, USA

J.A. Barnes, M.D., Ph.D.
Comprehensive Cutaneous Lymphoma Program, Department of Medicine, Massachusetts General Hospital Cancer Center, Boston, MA, USA

L.M. Duncan, M.D. (✉)
Dermatopathology Service, Department of Pathology, Massachusetts General Hospital, Harvard Medical School, Boston, MA, USA
e-mail: duncan@helix.mgh.harvard.edu

J.B. Carter et al. (eds.), *Atlas of Cutaneous Lymphomas: Classification and Differential Diagnosis*, DOI 10.1007/978-3-319-17217-0_16

16.1 Clinical

16.1.1 Clinical Presentation

pcMZL is the second most common cutaneous B-cell lymphoma, accounting for nearly 25 % of cutaneous B-cell lymphomas [3]. The skin is the second most common site for extranodal marginal zone lymphomas overall, after the gastrointestinal tract [4]. Although the median age of patients with this lymphoma is 50–53 years old, cases have been reported over a range of 21–93 years. This lymphoma is found in men nearly twice as often as women [2, 5, 6].

pcMZL typically presents with a solitary or regional grouping of deep-seated, red to violaceous indurated plaques, nodules, or tumors that may be surrounded by diffuse or annular erythema (Fig. 16.1) [2, 4, 7]. The lesions have a predilection for the trunk (46–60 %), upper extremities (17 %), and face and scalp (13 %) [2, 5, 8]. Twenty-eight to fifty-eight percent of patients present with a single lesion, 24–72 % with multifocal regional lesions, and 0–17 % with disseminated disease; these values range widely among studies because of the small number of patients [2, 5]. Patients are otherwise asymptomatic. Although nodal dissemination and large cell transformation are possible, the vast majority of patients never experience extracutaneous spread of their disease [2, 5, 9].

Studies have offered some evidence of an association between pcMZL and *Borrelia burgdorferi* in European populations, analogous to the role of *Helicobacter pylori* in the pathogenesis of gastric marginal zone lymphoma (MZL or MALT lymphoma). However, this has not been substantiated in North American or Asian studies [5]. Although many gastric MZLs demonstrate complete resolution with antibiotic therapy against *H. pylori*, a handful of case reports from Europe describe minimal to partial improvement of cutaneous pcMZLs with antibiotic treatment for *B. burgdorferi* infection [10, 11].

16.1.2 Prognosis and Treatment

This lymphoma is markedly indolent, with a very low incidence of extracutaneous spread and minimal risk of death [2, 12]. The overall 5-year survival rate is estimated at nearly 97 % [9]. The lesions of pcMZL are very responsive to treatment: 93 % of patients with solitary lesions and 75 % of those with multifocal lesions attain a complete response to therapy [2]. However, 39 and 77 % of those patients, respectively, experience relapses within 5 years [2].

The only factor with prognostic value is the number of lesions—patients with a single lesion have a higher survival rate than those with regional or disseminated disease [5, 9]. Poor prognosis has been reported in rare cases of large cell transformation or pcMZL with head and neck involvement [7].

Although there is no standardized treatment protocol, single or localized lesions are typically treated with intralesional steroids, surgical excision, and/or radiotherapy [2]. Recurrent lesions tend to be outside of the irradiated area. Retrospective studies have demonstrated a response rate to systemic rituximab approaching 90 % [13].

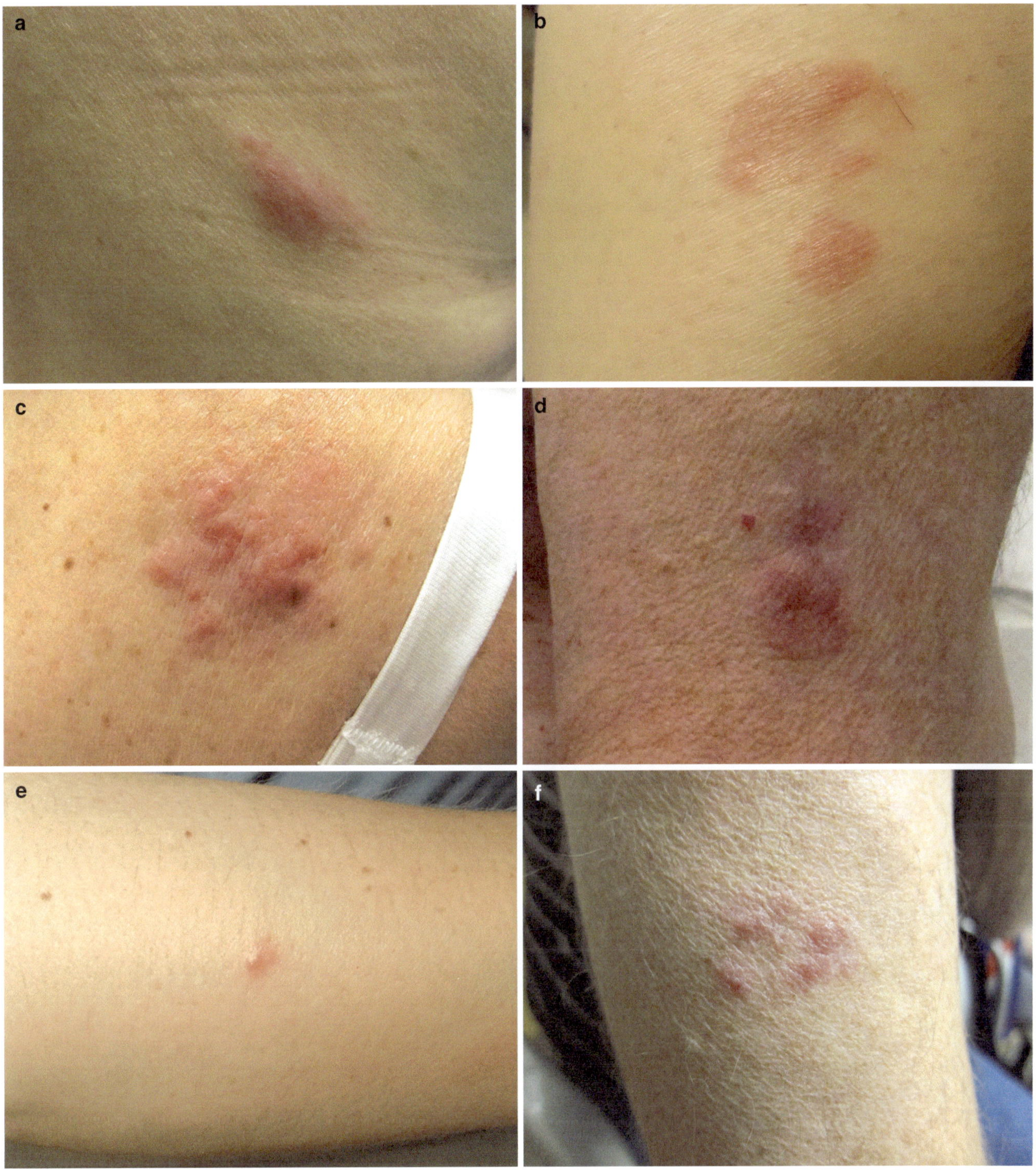

Fig. 16.1 Primary cutaneous marginal zone lymphoma (pcMZL), varied clinical morphologies. (**a**) Bright pink, 2- × 3-cm tumor on the upper back of the patient (Case 16.1). (**b**) Thin, pink to erythematous, irregularly shaped, 1- to 3-cm plaques on the calf of a 61-year-old woman. (**c**) Multiple erythematous 0.5- to 1-cm nodules coalescing into a 5-cm plaque on the upper back of an 80-year-old woman. (**d**) Two erythematous, indurated, annular, 0.5- to 1.5-cm plaques on the upper arm of a 70-year-old man. (**e**) Pink papule (3 mm) on the forearm of a 41-year-old woman. (**f**) 2.5 cm plaque of indurated pink smooth coalescing papules on the right upper arm of a 63 year old man

16.2 Pathology

16.2.1 Histopathology

This lymphoma is characterized by a dense, nodular, non-epidermotropic, dermal, and subcutaneous lymphocytic B-cell infiltrate composed of centrocyte-like marginal zone cells, lymphoplasmacytoid cells, and plasma cells (Fig. 16.2) [2, 4, 5, 7]. The cellular composition can range from prominent plasma cell infiltrates to a predominance of monocytoid B cells with few plasma cells. Zones of neoplastic plasma cells occur in more than two thirds of cases [6, 14]. Reactive germinal centers are present in most cases (Fig. 16.3) and are occasionally colonized by neoplastic cells (Fig. 16.4) [15].

The centrocyte-like marginal zone cells have cleaved nuclei with dispersed chromatin and pale amphophilic cytoplasm [4, 7]; the large amount of cytoplasm can give a monocytoid appearance [4]. The reniform (bean-shaped) nuclei usually have inconspicuous nucleoli (*see* Fig. 16.1c) [4, 12]. Dutcher bodies (intranuclear PAS+ immunoglobulin pseudo-inclusions found in plasma cells) may also be present.

Findings that may confound the identification of the neoplastic B cells include a typically dense infiltrate of benign reactive CD3+ CD45RO+ T-cells [4, 7]. Scattered centroblasts and immunoblasts (from disrupted follicle centers) may be seen, particularly in the setting of follicular colonization. Variable numbers of CD30+ large cells may also be present [7].

Adnexal involvement may be seen; both eccrine and follicular involvement has been reported [14]. Formation of lymphoepithelial lesions (groups of three or more marginal zone cells with destruction of epithelium) involving adnexal structures is diagnostically helpful but often absent [4, 7].

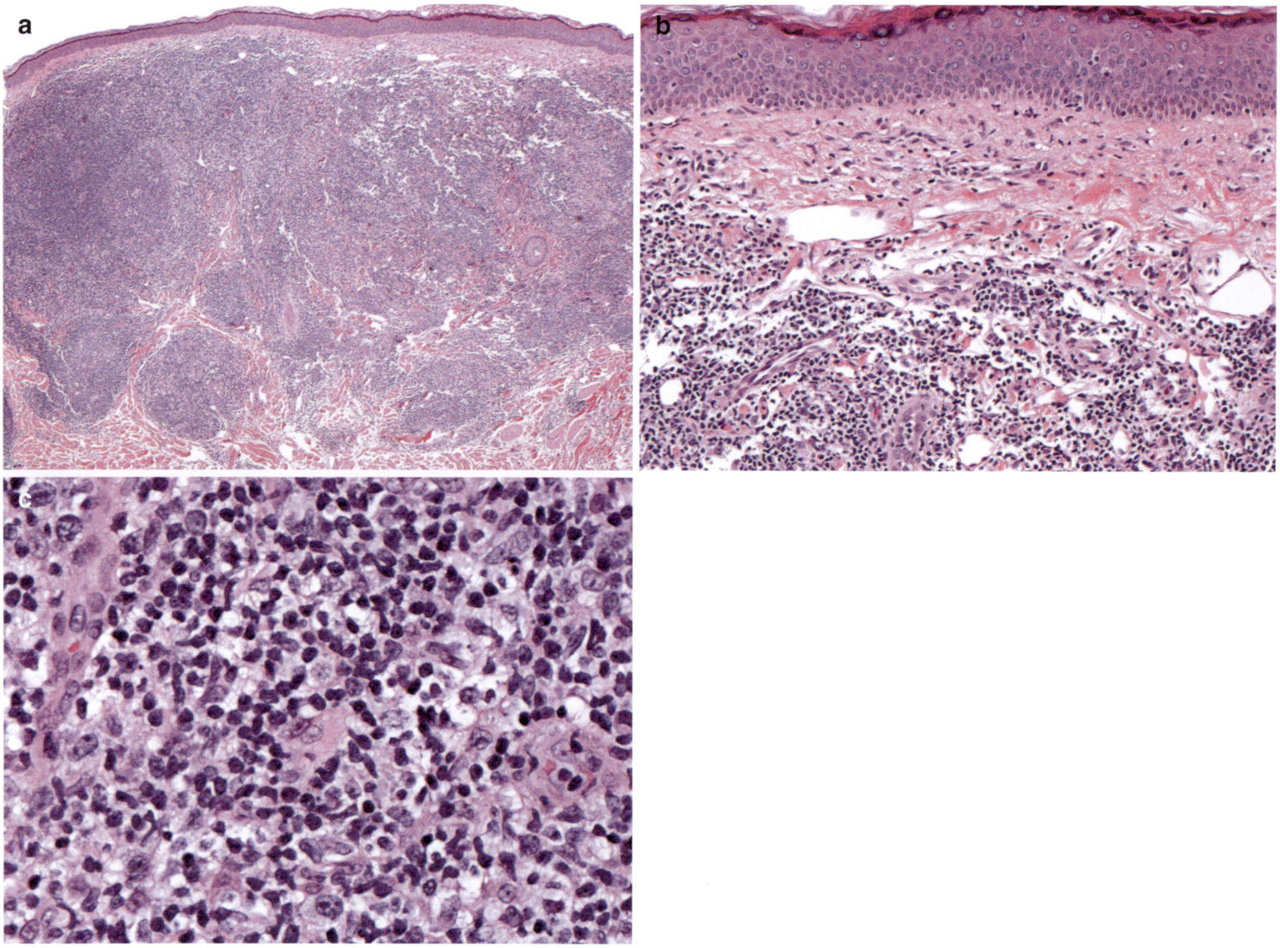

Fig. 16.2 Primary cutaneous marginal zone lymphoma (pcMZL), histopathology (Case 16.1). (**a**) Superficial and deep dermal nodular and diffuse lymphoid infiltrate (H&E, 4×). (**b**) A grenz zone is present, and the epidermis is uninvolved (H&E, 1×). (**c**) The infiltrate is composed of numerous centrocytes with small-to-medium sized cleaved nuclei and many centroblasts with round nuclei, open chromatin, and basophilic nucleoli at the nuclear margins. There are scattered plasma cells (H&E, 40×)

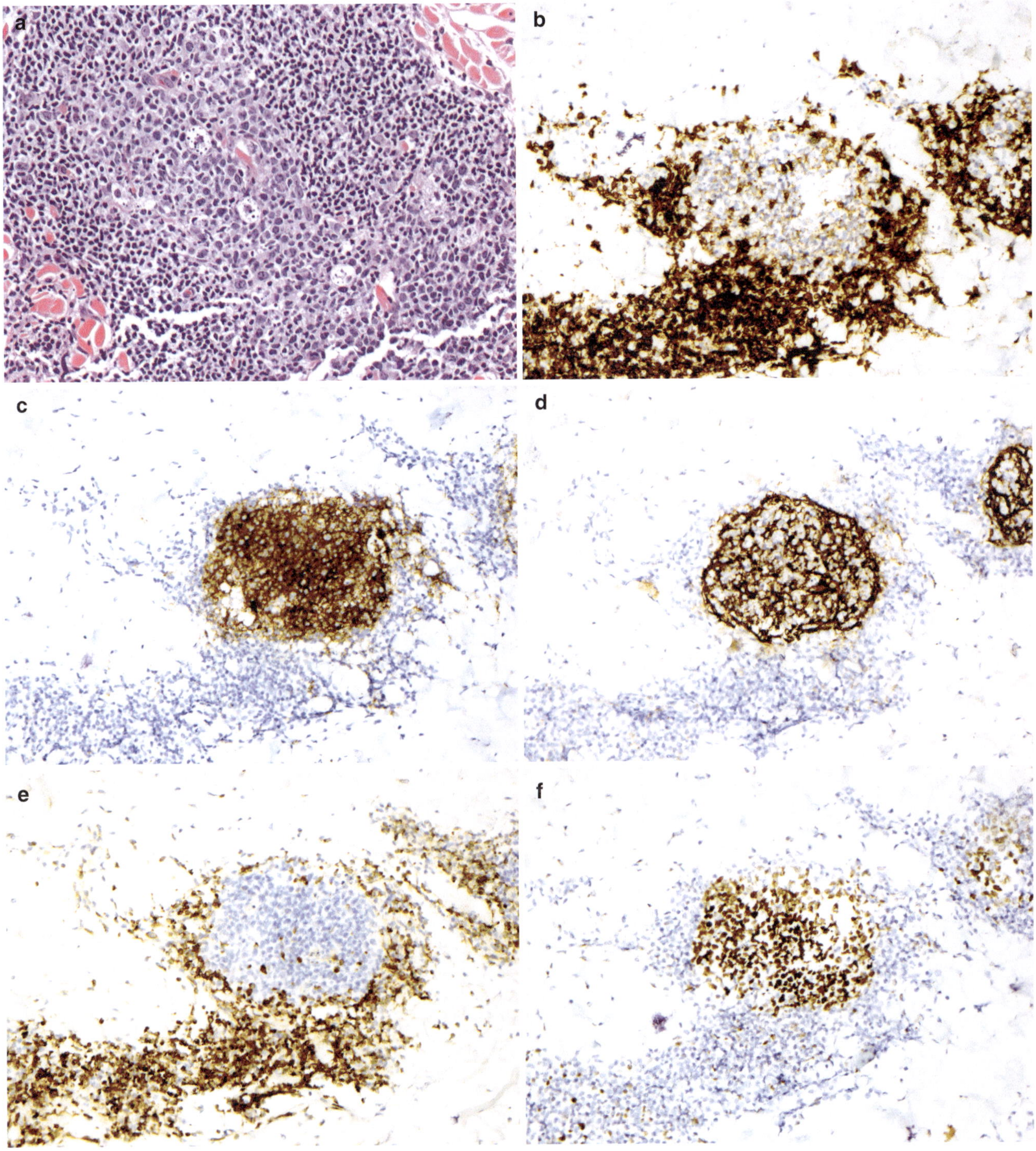

Fig. 16.3 Primary cutaneous marginal zone lymphoma (pcMZL), reactive follicle (Case 16.1). (**a**) A reactive lymphoid follicle in the dermis is composed of a central aggregate of follicle center cells surrounded by a mantle zone of small lymphocytes with scant cytoplasm (H&E, 20×). (**b**) Numerous CD3+ T cells in and around the reactive follicle (CD3, 20×) (**c**) The majority of cells in the reactive follicle are CD20+ B cells (CD20, 20×) (**d**) CD21+ follicular dendritic cell meshwork of the follicle is intact (CD21, 20×). (**e**) The B cells within the reactive follicle are negative for Bcl2 (in contrast to those in the obliterated follicle in Fig. 16.4e). The surrounding T and B cells express Bcl2 (Bcl2, 20×). (**f**) The cells within the follicle express Bcl6 (unlike many of the B cells in Fig. 16.4f) (Bcl6, 20×)

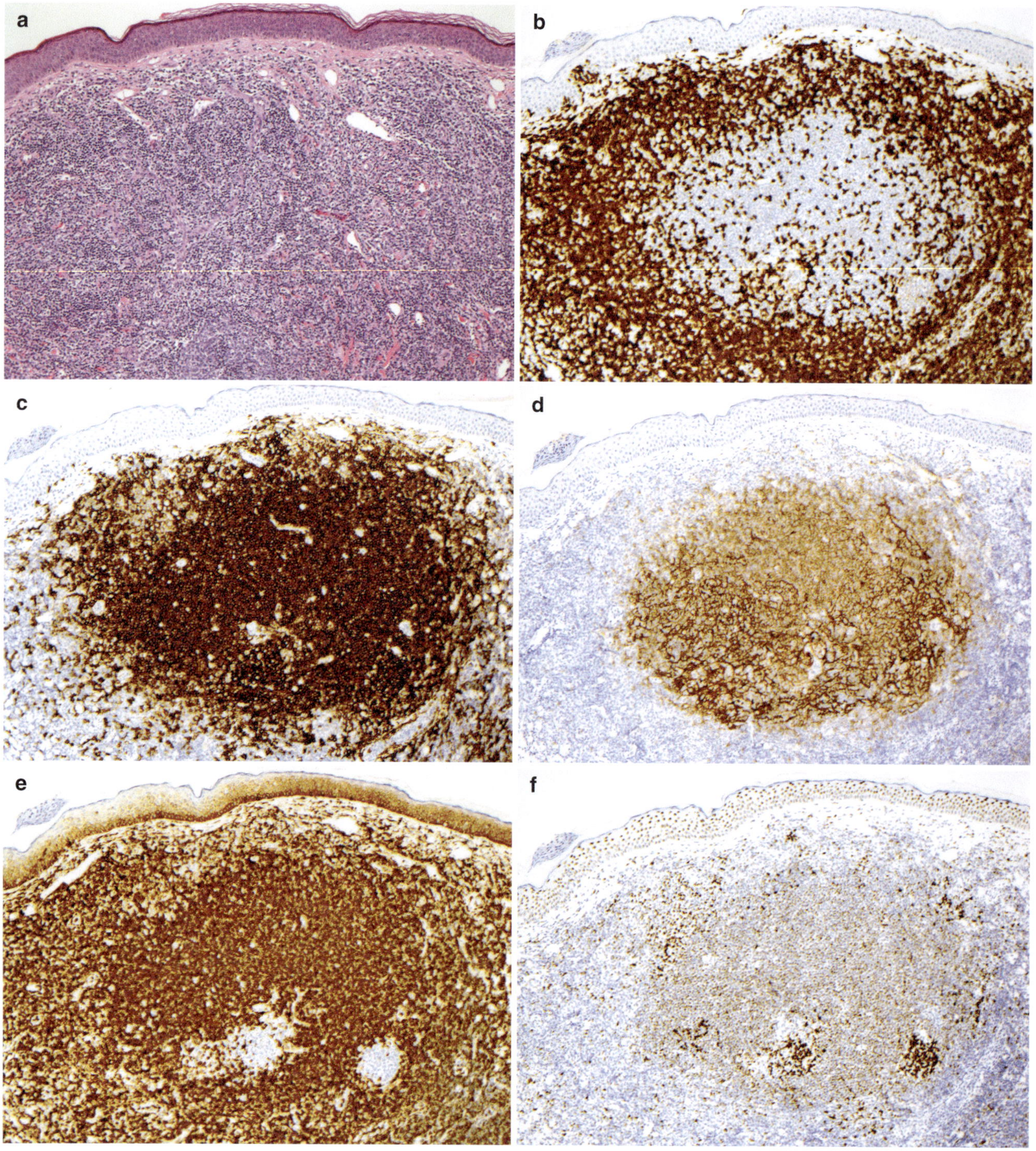

Fig. 16.4 pcMZL, colonized follicle (Case 16.1). (**a**) One of many follicles that has been colonized by neoplastic B cells (H&E, 10×). (**b**) Numerous CD3+ T cells surround the colonized follicle (CD3, 10×). (**c**) The majority of the cells in the follicle are CD20+ atypical B cells (CD20, 10×). (**d**) Staining for CD21 shows a preserved follicular dendritic cell meshwork. (CD21, 10×) (**e**) The neoplastic B cells in the follicle and T cells surrounding it stain strongly for Bcl2. (Bcl2, 10×) (**f**) Only scattered residual follicle center cells stain positively for Bcl6; the neoplastic cells colonizing the follicle do not express Bcl6. The Bcl2+ Bcl6− immunophenotype indicates that this follicle has been colonized by neoplastic B cells (Bcl6, 10×)

16.2.2 Immunophenotype and Molecular Findings

The neoplastic B cells have an immunohistochemical phenotype similar to that of marginal zone cells: the neoplastic cells typically express CD20, Bcl2, and CD79a but lack Bcl6. The plasma cells demonstrate monotypic light-chain expression in 70 % of cases (Fig. 16.5) [6]. Cells express IgG more commonly than IgM, IgA, or IgD; this is in contrast to MZLs at other extranodal sites, which typically express IgM [4].

Other features distinguishing pcMZL from extracutaneous disease include the absence of CXCR3 expression and the presence of a Th2 type cytokine milieu (with higher levels of IL-4) in pcMZL compared with extracutaneous MZL [16]. In addition, the t(14;18)(q32;q21) IgH gene translocation is observed in fewer than 20 % of cases [2].

Abnormalities in the MALT1 gene and trisomy 18 have been described in 25 % of cases [2]. The neoplastic cells have a postgerminal center phenotype, and many cases demonstrate aberrant somatic hypermutation of PAX5, RhoH/TTF, cMYC, and PIM1 [4, 17].

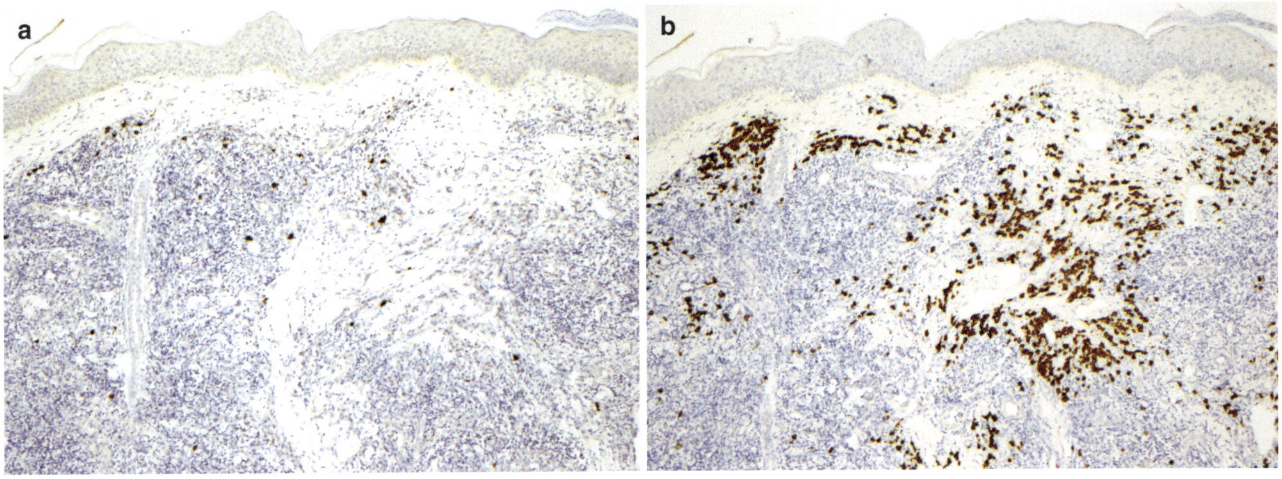

Fig. 16.5 pcMZL, plasma cells demonstrate light-chain restriction. (**a**) *In situ* hybridization for the kappa light chain shows few positively staining plasma cells (ISH for kappa light chain, 20×). (**b**) *In situ* hybridization for the lambda light chain demonstrates plasma cells expressing lambda light chains around the superficial vasculature (ISH for lambda light chain, 10×)

16.3 Differential Diagnosis

16.3.1 Diagnostic Considerations

The keys to diagnosis lie in the patient demographics, physical examination (including assessment of lesion location, characteristic, and number), and biopsy results.

16.3.2 Differential Diagnosis

16.3.2.1 Cutaneous Lymphoid Hyperplasia (CLH)

The cutaneous lesions of CLH may demonstrate similar clinical morphology to those of pcMZL, given that they both often present as solitary nodules, plaques, or tumors [2, 8]. On biopsy, both conditions show a dense lymphocytic infiltrate and a grenz zone. However, Dutcher bodies, aggregates of marginal zone cells, and sheets of plasma cells strongly support a diagnosis of pcMZL over CLH [8, 18]. CLH more often displays epidermal changes, including spongiosis, dyskeratosis, and parakeratosis, whereas pcMZLs usually are separated from the overlying epidermis by a grenz zone of uninvolved papillary dermis. While CLH is polytypic, pcMZLs typically show light-chain restriction of plasma cells [8].

16.3.2.2 Primary Cutaneous Follicle Center Lymphoma (pcFCL)

pcFCL also often presents with solitary firm erythematous papules or plaques on the head, neck, or upper extremities without systemic involvement [2, 7, 19]. Both pcMZL and pcFCL are characterized by the presence of lymphoid follicles, which are defined as aggregates of CD21+ follicular dendritic cells associated with BCL-6+ and BCL-2− follicle center cells.

The architecture of these follicles is often helpful in distinguishing these two most common forms of cutaneous B-cell lymphoma. In pcMZL the reactive follicles may be infiltrated by Bcl2+ Bcl6− marginal zone B-cells, leading to dispersion of the Bcl6+ follicle center cells. This is not a characteristic of pcFCL. In pcFCL the neoplastic follicle center cells may form irregularly shaped nodules and surround aggregates of small lymphocytes, forming "inside-out" follicles. The proliferation of follicle center cells in pcFCL may also be directly apposed to reticular dermal collagen fibers without a mantle zone of small lymphocytes, so-called "naked" follicles. "Inside-out" and "naked" lymphoid follicles are characteristic of pcFCL and not a feature of pcMZL.

Immunohistochemical stains for Bcl6, Bcl2, CD21, CD10, and kappa and lambda light chains are indispensable in this differential diagnosis [19]. While neoplastic cells in pcMZL are Bcl2+ Bcl6− small cleaved cells, monocytoid B cells or lymphoplasmacytoid cells, the neoplastic cells of pcFCL are Bcl2− Bcl6+ follicle center cells (i.e., centrocytes, centroblasts, and immunoblasts) [4, 20]. Immunohistochemical or in situ hybridization analysis of kappa and lambda light chains demonstrates light-chain restricted plasma cells in greater than 70 % of pcMZL of the skin [6], a finding absent in pcFCL [21].

16.3.2.3 Primary Cutaneous Diffuse Large B-Cell Lymphoma, Leg Type (pcDLBCL)

Although pcDLBCL and pcMZLs have very different prognoses, the lesions of these two lymphomas may be impossible to distinguish in the absence of histopathology and immunohistochemical studies, particularly when pcDLBCL manifests on locations other than the leg. Fortunately, these tumors are usually easy to distinguish based on the cytologic and histomorphologic features. On biopsy, pcDLBCL appears with a diffuse monomorphic infiltrate of large B cells [22]. pcMZLs, on the other hand, present with a dense, nodular, nonepidermotropic, dermal, and subcutaneous infiltrate of small to medium-sized B cells [4]. Immunohistochemistry is often helpful: while the neoplastic cells of pcDLBCL may express Bcl6, those of pcMZL do not [4, 22]. Note that tumor cells in both pcDLBCL and MZL are Bcl2+.

16.3.2.4 Secondary Cutaneous Marginal Zone Lymphoma

MZLs and secondary cutaneous involvement by systemic lymphomas can be very difficult to distinguish clinically and pathologically. While there are some molecular and immunophenotypic trends that differ between extracutaneous and cutaneous pcMZL, patients must be staged for systemic disease in order to rule out extracutaneous lymphoma.

16.4 Clinical Case

Case 16.1

A 73-year-old woman presented with numerous persistent pink papules, nodules, and tumors on her back that had been present for 3 months and that she thought were bug bites (*see* Fig. 16.1a). She had no constitutional symptoms. Biopsy of one of the tumors demonstrated an atypical B-cell infiltrate of Bcl6– Bcl2+ cells (*see* Figs. 16.2 and 16.4). Lambda light-chain restriction was present (*see* Fig. 16.5). A PET-CT scan showed no marked lymphadenopathy, and blood tests showed no peripheral blood involvement. The patient was diagnosed with pcMZL and treated with radiation therapy. While the initial lesions cleared with radiation, 2 years after diagnosis she continues to develop new nodules, which respond well to repeat low-dose radiation. She is otherwise well.

Commentary This patient's lesions—asymptomatic, persistent pink papules without overlying epidermal change on the trunk—are characteristic of primary cutaneous pcMZL. In addition, this patient's atypical cells were Bcl6– Bcl2+, as is expected in pcMZL. In order to definitively diagnose her disease as primarily cutaneous, systemic MZL lymphoma must be ruled out by means of bloodwork and CT scans. Low-dose radiation treatment can be highly effective in treating pcMZL lymphoma.

References

1. Geyer JT, Ferry JA, Longtine JA, Flotte TJ, Harris NL, Zukerberg LR. Characteristics of cutaneous marginal zone lymphomas with marked plasmacytic differentiation and a T cell–rich background. Am J Clin Pathol. 2010;133:59–69.
2. Hoefnagel J, Vermeer MH, Jansen PM, Heule F, van Voorst Vader PC, Sanders CJG, et al. Primary cutaneous marginal zone B-cell lymphoma: clinical and therapeutic features in 50 cases. Arch Dermatol. 2005;141:1139–45.
3. Bradford PT, Devesa SS, Anderson WF, Toro JR. Cutaneous lymphoma incidence patterns in the United States: a population-based study of 3884 cases. Blood. 2009;113:5064–73.
4. Isaacson P, Chott A, Nakamura S, Muller-Hermelink HK, Harris NL, Swerdlow SH. Extranodal marginal zone lymphoma of mucosa-associated lymphoid tissue (MALT lymphoma). In: Swerdlow SH, Campo E, Harris NL, Jaffe ES, Pileri SA, Stein H, et al., editors. WHO classification of tumors of hematopoietic and lymphoid tissues. 4th ed. Lyon: International Agency for Research on Cancer; 2008. p. 214–7.
5. Dalle S, Thomas L, Balme B, Dumontet C, Thieblemont C. Primary cutaneous marginal zone lymphoma. Crit Rev Oncol Hematol. 2010;74:156–62.
6. Cerroni L, Signoretti S, Höfler G, Annessi G, Pütz B, Lackinger E, et al. Primary cutaneous marginal zone B-cell lymphoma: a recently described entity of low-grade malignant cutaneous B-cell lymphoma. Am J Surg Pathol. 1997;21:1307–15.
7. Servitje O, Gallardo F, Estrach T, Pujol RM, Blanco A. Clinical and laboratory investigations. Primary cutaneous marginal zone B-cell lymphoma: a clinical, histopathological, immunophenotypic and molecular genetic study of 22 cases. Br J Dermatol. 2002;147:1147–58.
8. Baldassano MF, Bailey EM, Ferry JA, Harris NL, Duncan LM. Cutaneous lymphoid hyperplasia and cutaneous marginal zone lymphoma: comparison of morphologic and immunophenotypic features. Am J Surg Pathol. 1999;23:88–96.
9. Zinzani PL, Quaglino P, Pimpinelli N, Berti E, Baliva G, Rupoli S, et al. Prognostic factors in primary cutaneous B-cell lymphoma: the Italian Study Group for Cutaneous Lymphomas. J Clin Oncol. 2006;24:1376–82.
10. Kütting B, Bonsmann G, Metze D, Luger TA, Cerroni L. *Borrelia burgdorferi*—associated primary cutaneous B cell lymphoma: complete clearing of skin lesions after antibiotic pulse therapy or intralesional injection of interferon alfa-2a. J Am Acad Dermatol. 1997;36:311–4.
11. Roggero E, Zucca E, Mainetti C, Bertoni F, Valsangiacomo C, Pedrinis E, et al. Eradication of *Borrelia burgdorferi* infection in primary marginal zone B-cell lymphoma of the skin. Hum Pathol. 2000;31:263–8.
12. Gerami P, Wickless SC, Rosen S, Kuzel TM, Ciurea A, Havey J, et al. Applying the new TNM classification system for primary cutaneous lymphomas other than mycosis fungoides and Sézary syndrome in primary cutaneous marginal zone lymphoma. J Am Acad Dermatol. 2008;59:245–54.
13. Morales AV, Advani R, Horwitz SM, Riaz N, Reddy S, Hoppe RT, et al. Indolent primary cutaneous B-cell lymphoma: experience using systemic rituximab. J Am Acad Dermatol. 2008;59:953–7.
14. Bailey EM, Ferry JA, Harris NL, Mihm MC, Jacobson JO, Duncan LM. Marginal zone lymphoma (low-grade B-cell lymphoma of mucosa-associated lymphoid tissue type) of skin and subcutaneous tissue: a study of 15 patients. Am J Surg Pathol. 1996;20:1011–23.
15. Cho-Vega JH, Vega F, Rassidakis G, Medeiros LJ. Primary cutaneous marginal zone B-cell lymphoma. Am J Clin Pathol. 2006;125:S38–49.
16. Duncan LM, Baran JL, Ferry JA. Cutaneous lymphomas. In: Ferry JA, editor. Extranodal lymphomas. Philadelphia: Elsevier Saunders; 2011.
17. Deutsch AJA, Fru M, Aigelsreiter A, Cerroni L, Neumeister P. Primary cutaneous marginal zone B-cell lymphomas are targeted by aberrant somatic hypermutation. J Invest Dermatol. 2009;129:476–9.
18. Bain BJ. Dutcher bodies. Am J Hematol. 2009;84:589.
19. de Leval L, Harris NL, Longtine J, Ferry JA, Duncan LM. Cutaneous B-cell lymphomas of follicular and marginal zone types: use of Bcl-6, CD10, Bcl-2, and CD21 in differential diagnosis and classification. Am J Surg Pathol. 2001;25:732–41.
20. Willemze R, Swerdlow SH, Harris NL, Vergier B. Primary cutaneous follicle centre lymphoma. In: Swerdlow SH, Campo E, Harris NL, Jaffe ES, Pileri SA, Stein H, et al., editors. WHO classification of tumors of hematopoietic and lymphoid tissues. 4th ed. Lyon: International Agency for Research on Cancer; 2008. p. 227–8.
21. Cerroni L, Arzberger E, Pütz B, Höfler G, Metze D, Sander CA, et al. Primary cutaneous follicle center cell lymphoma with follicular growth pattern. Blood. 2000;95:3922–8.
22. Meijer CJLM, Vergier B, Duncan LM, Willemze R. Primary cutaneous DLBCL, leg type. In: Swerdlow SH, Campo E, Harris NL, Jaffe ES, Pileri SA, Stein H, et al., editors. WHO classification of tumors of hematopoietic and lymphoid tissues. 4th ed. Lyon: International Agency for Research on Cancer; 2008. p. 242.

17 Primary Cutaneous Follicle Center Lymphoma

Amrita Goyal, Joi B. Carter, Jeffrey A. Barnes, and Lyn McDivitt Duncan

Primary cutaneous follicle center lymphoma (pcFCL) is an indolent B-cell lymphoma with a remarkably good prognosis. This neoplasm of mature germinal center B cells constitutes 60 % of all primary cutaneous B-cell lymphomas and 9–11 % of all cutaneous lymphomas [1, 2]. It also comprises 5 % of all follicular lymphomas, nodal and extranodal [3]. It typically presents with firm, erythematous to violaceous papules, plaques, and tumors on the scalp, trunk, and upper extremities. When it occurs on the back, it has been referred to in the past as Crosti lymphoma or reticulohistiocytoma of the dorsum [1, 4]. Differentiation of pcFCL from systemic follicular lymphomas is critical, given the substantially worse prognosis of systemic follicular lymphomas. This chapter addresses the clinical presentation, prognosis, treatment, histopathology, immunophenotype, and differential diagnosis of pcFCL. It closes with two clinical cases, including clinical images and histopathology.

A. Goyal, M.D.
Harvard-MIT Division of Health Sciences and Technology, Harvard Medical School, Boston, MA, USA

J.B. Carter, M.D.
Department of Dermatology, Massachusetts General Hospital, Harvard Medical School, Boston, MA, USA

J.A. Barnes, M.D., Ph.D.
Comprehensive Cutaneous Lymphoma Program, Department of Medicine, Massachusetts General Hospital Cancer Center, Boston, MA, USA

L.M. Duncan, M.D. (✉)
Dermatopathology Service, Department of Pathology, Massachusetts General Hospital, Harvard Medical School, Boston, MA, USA
e-mail: duncan@helix.mgh.harvard.edu

J.B. Carter et al. (eds.), *Atlas of Cutaneous Lymphomas: Classification and Differential Diagnosis*, DOI 10.1007/978-3-319-17217-0_17

17.1 Clinical Information

17.1.1 Clinical Presentation

Primary cutaneous follicle center lymphoma (pcFCL) accounts for 60 % of primary cutaneous B-cell lymphomas and has an excellent prognosis. Patients with pcFCL have a median age of 51 years, and this lymphoma impacts men 1.5 times more often than women [1].

Typical lesions of pcFCL are slow growing 2- to 5-cm firm, smooth, rarely ulcerated, erythematous to violaceous plaques, nodules, or tumors, often with telangiectasias (see Figs. 17.1, 17.2, and 17.3) [1, 5, 6]. These tumors primarily occur on the head and neck (61 %), upper extremities (23 %), and trunk (16 %) [1, 5]. More than 80 % of patients present with a single lesion; of the 20 % of patients with multiple lesions, the vast majority have localized or regional disease [1, 5, 6]. While untreated lesions continue to grow, extracutaneous involvement of pcFCL occurs in less than 10 % of patients [1].

Several patterns of cutaneous involvement have been described. The majority of patients present with solitary plaques or nodules on the scalp, forehead, and trunk, as described above [1]. Patients may also manifest with what was formerly referred to as Crosti lymphoma (see Fig. 17.4): large erythematous infiltrated plaques on the back with surrounding erythematous macules and papules; the surrounding papules may be located up to 10–15 cm from the main lesion [2, 4]. Finally, a small group of patients may show multiple, miliary, agminated papules [2, 7]. In spite of these morphologic differences, these variants all share the same excellent prognosis, and there is no evidence that they should be further subdivided [2].

17.1.2 Prognosis and Treatment

pcFCL has a 95 % disease-specific 5-year survival rate [1]. With treatment, nearly 99 % of patients have complete remission, and while 30 % of patients will experience recurrence, only 10 % of patients develop extracutaneous progression. Interestingly, cutaneous relapses do not indicate progression of disease [6]. There is no prognostic significance in the histologic growth pattern, the number of blastic cells, the expression of Bcl2, or multifocal disease [1, 6]. However, location on the leg has been associated with a worse prognosis: patients with pcFCL on the legs have a higher relapse rate (63 %) and lower disease-specific survival (44 %) than those with disease at other locations (25 % relapse rate; 99 % disease-specific survival) [8].

The first-line treatments for solitary lesions is intralesional steroids, local radiation, or excision; lesions have also been successfully managed with intralesional interferon alpha or intralesional rituximab [4, 6, 9]. Radiation therapy can also be used successfully for late relapses [10]. Systemic rituximab and chemotherapy are only recommended for very extensive, thick lesions or extracutaneous involvement [1, 11, 12]. Radiotherapy may be as effective as multiagent chemotherapy even in the case of multifocal disease [9, 11, 13].

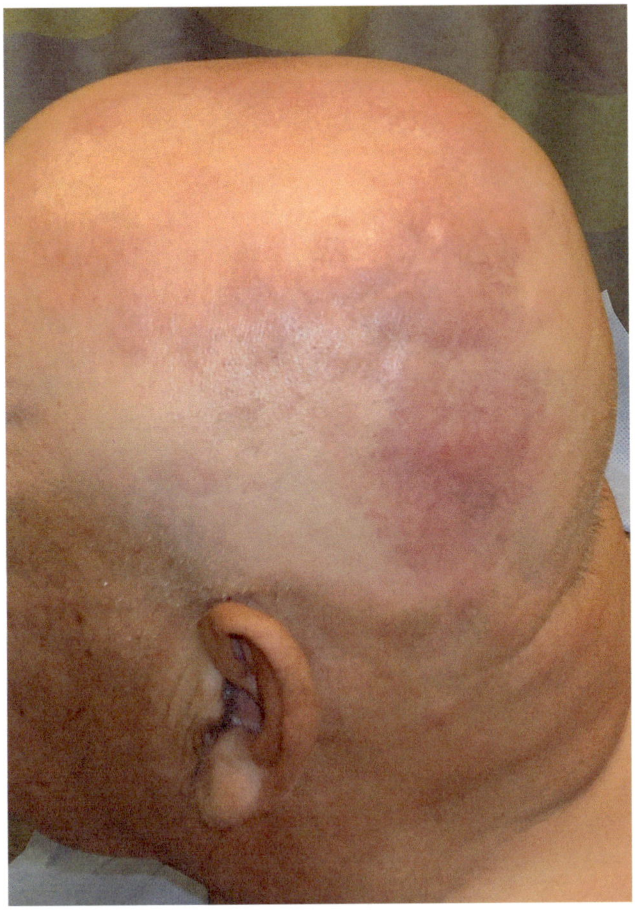

Fig. 17.1 Primary cutaneous follicle center lymphoma (pcFCL), clinical image. Numerous 1- to 5- cm well-demarcated, erythematous, indurated plaques are seen on the scalp of a 71-year-old man

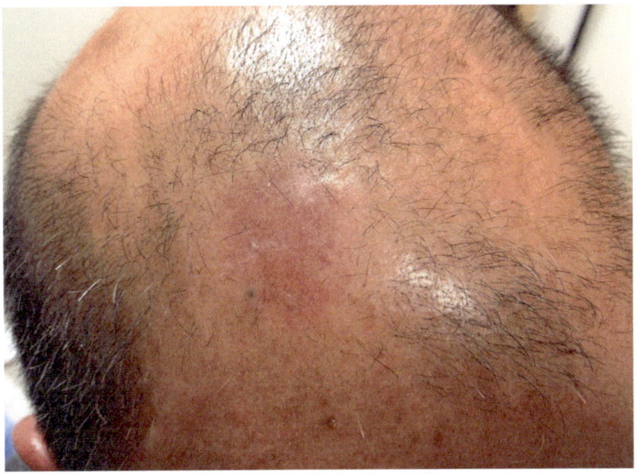

Fig. 17.2 Primary cutaneous follicle center lymphoma (pcFCL), clinical image. A solitary, pink, 2-cm dermal plaque on the anterior scalp of a 51-year-old man

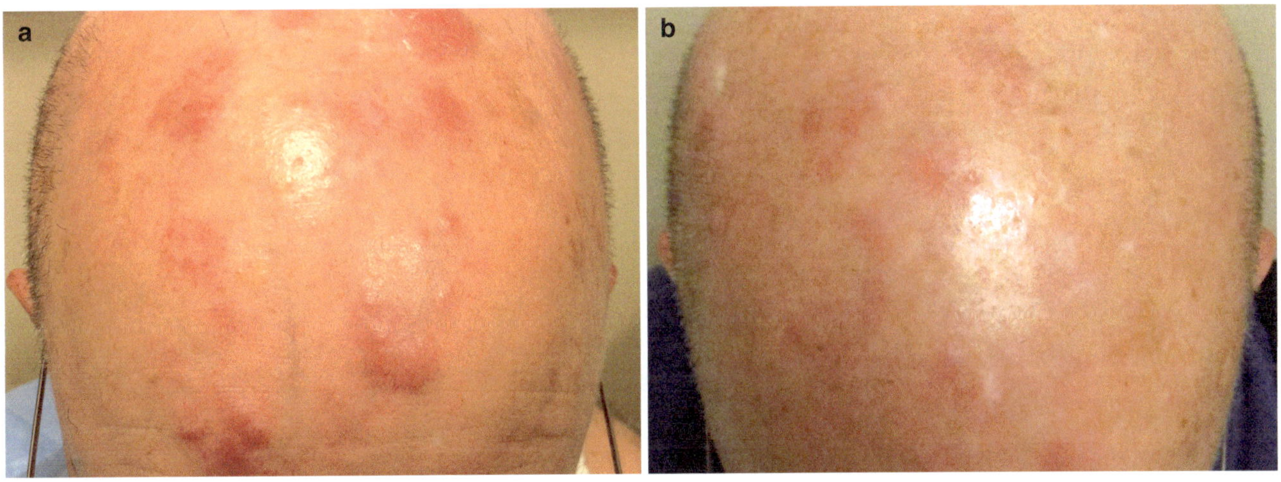

Fig. 17.3 Primary cutaneous follicle center lymphoma (pcFCL), diffuse type, clinical images from Case 17.1. (**a**) This patient with diffuse type pcFCL has multiple firm, shiny, pink to violaceous dermal nodules and plaques of varying thickness on his forehead and scalp. (**b**) Recurrence of nodules and plaques after radiation therapy. Although some of these lesions are at the same site as prior nodules or plaques, several are in previously unaffected areas

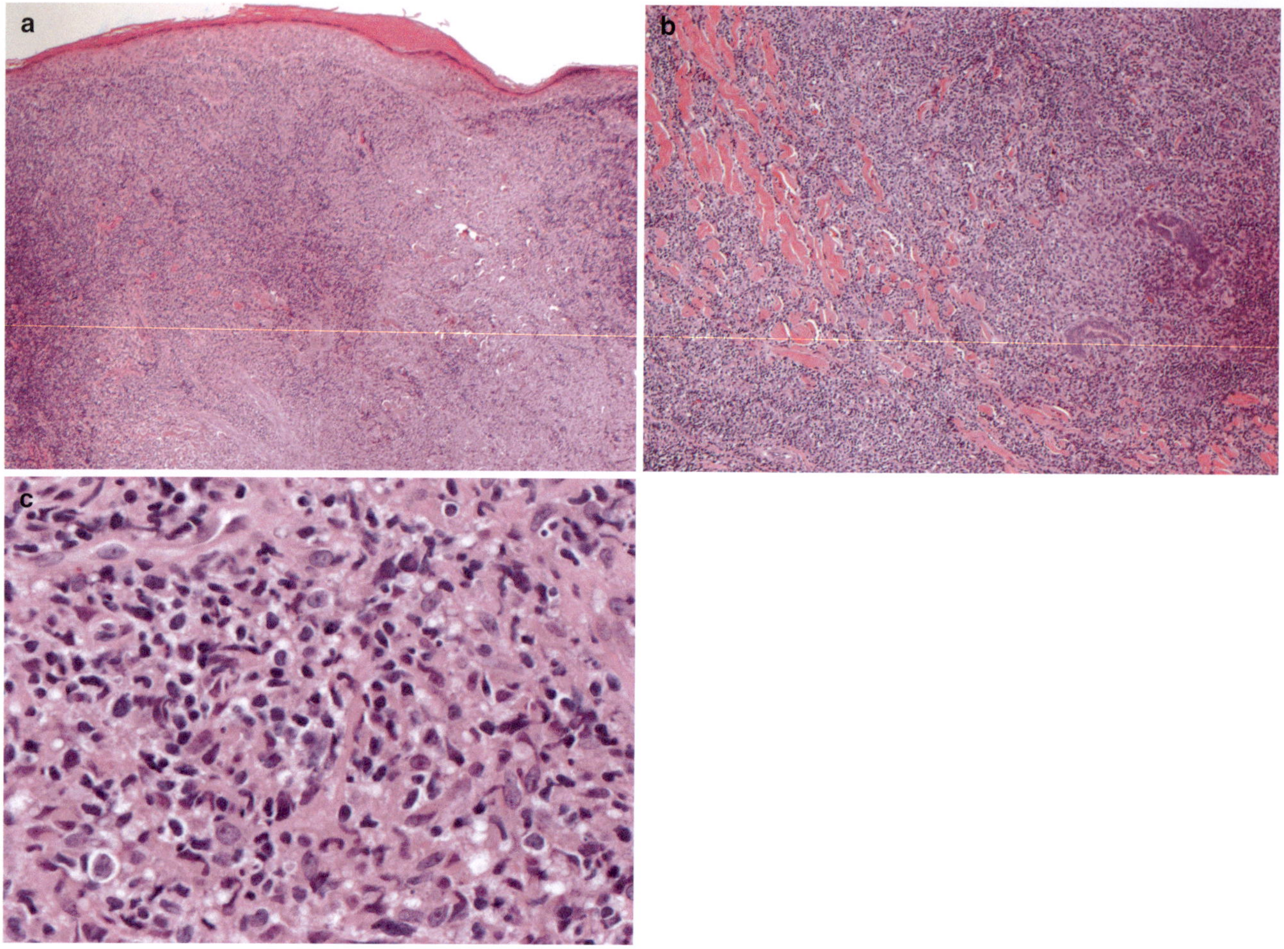

Fig. 17.4 Primary cutaneous follicle center lymphoma (pcFCL), diffuse type, histopathology, from Case 17.1. (**a**) The papillary and deep dermis are occupied by a dense, diffuse infiltrate of neoplastic B cells. The epidermis is uninvolved. No follicles are present, a finding confirmed on immunohistochemical staining for follicular dendritic cell meshwork (not pictured) (H&E, 4×). (**b**) Disruption of the collagen fibers of the dermis is visible. The eccrine ducts on the right side of the image are surrounded by but not invaded by neoplastic cells (H&E, 20×). (**c**) The neoplastic B cells are remarkably atypical with hyperchromatic, angulated, irregularly shaped nuclei. Several large centroblasts are present (H&E, 63×)

17.2 Pathology

17.2.1 Histopathology

The neoplastic infiltrate of pcFCL is characterized by a dermal infiltrate of atypical B cells that may extend into the subcutaneous fat [1, 4, 14]. The epidermis is nearly always spared [1]. Skin biopsy may demonstrate one of three patterns of infiltration by neoplastic cells: follicular, follicular and diffuse, or diffuse [1, 6]. These occur in 2, 34, and 64 % of cases, respectively [6].

The lymphoid follicles of pcFCL are often poorly defined, with a proliferation of neoplastic follicle center cells supported by an expanded follicular dendritic cell meshwork [14]. Alternatively, these tumors may present with a diffuse infiltrate characterized by a proliferation of large centrocytes and variable numbers of centroblasts [1, 2]. The neoplastic follicle center cells may surround aggregates of small T cells and B cells, forming so-called "inside-out follicles" (*see* Fig. 17.5a). The presence of "naked follicles," collections of follicle center cells apposed to the reticular dermal collagen without an intervening mantle zone of small lymphocytes (*see* Fig. 17.5b), is also supportive of this diagnosis [14]. Large numbers of reactive T cells are usually present, and stromal proliferation is common [1].

17.2.2 Immunophenotype and Molecular Findings

The neoplastic cells of pcFCL are follicle center B cells with a germinal center phenotype [1, 15, 16]. These cells typically express CD20, CD79a, and Bcl6 [1, 14, 17] and lack Bcl2, MUM1, FoxP1, CD5, and CD43 (*see* Fig. 17.6) [1, 14]. While CD10 is typically absent in cases with a diffuse histopathologic growth pattern, the neoplastic B cells of lymphomas with a follicular growth pattern may express CD10 [1].

A monoclonal Ig rearrangement is typically present [1], and the same clone is often seen in multiple lesions of the same patient [18]. However, the presence of two distinct clones should not prevent a diagnosis of pcFCL if other clinical and pathologic features are consistent with the diagnosis [18]. These studies are performed by means of polymerase chain reaction, as described in Chap. 3. Of note, light-chain restriction is characteristically not detected in plasma cells.

Half of cases do show point mutations in *BCL6*, *MYC*, *RhoH/TTF*, and P*ax*5 secondary to aberrant somatic hypermutation [17, 19]. Unlike in DLBCL, deletions of 9p21.3 (carrying the *CDKN2A* and *CDNK2B* genes) are uncommon [1]. The *BCL2* rearrangement is typically absent [1].

Complex karyotypes are common [2]. Although the t(14;18) translocation is absent in the majority of cases, it has been reported [20–22].

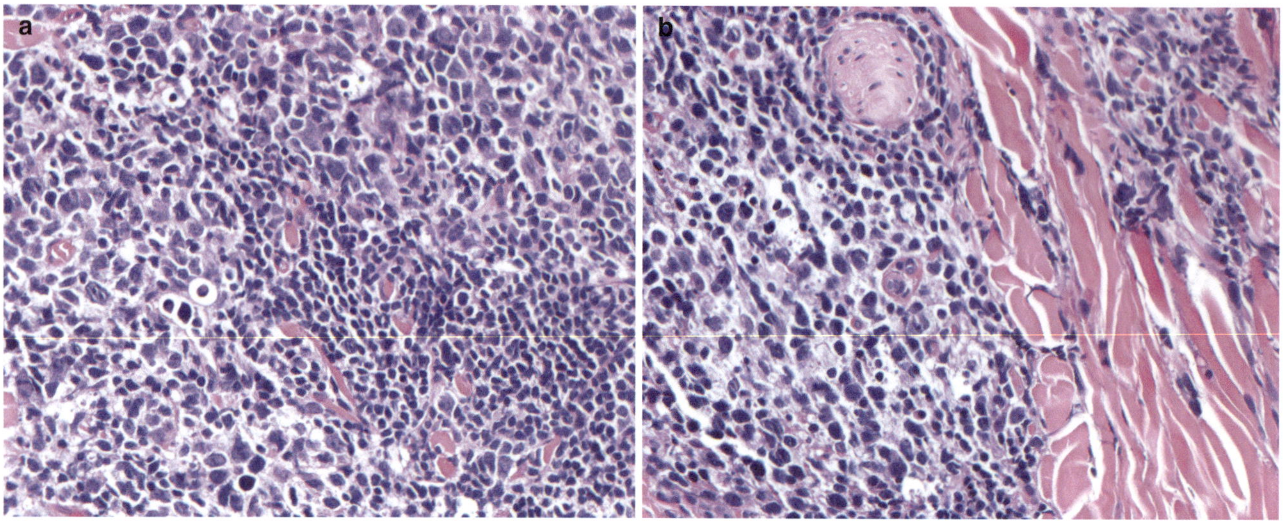

Fig. 17.5 Primary cutaneous follicle center lymphoma (pcFCL), naked and inside out follicles Case 17.2. (**a**) An inside out follicle displays the large neoplastic follicle center cells surrounding an aggregate of small reactive lymphocytes (H&E, 40×). (**b**) A naked follicle is seen with the neoplastic follicle center cells directly apposed to the reticular dermal collagen without an intervening mantle zone of small lymphocytes (H&E, 40×)

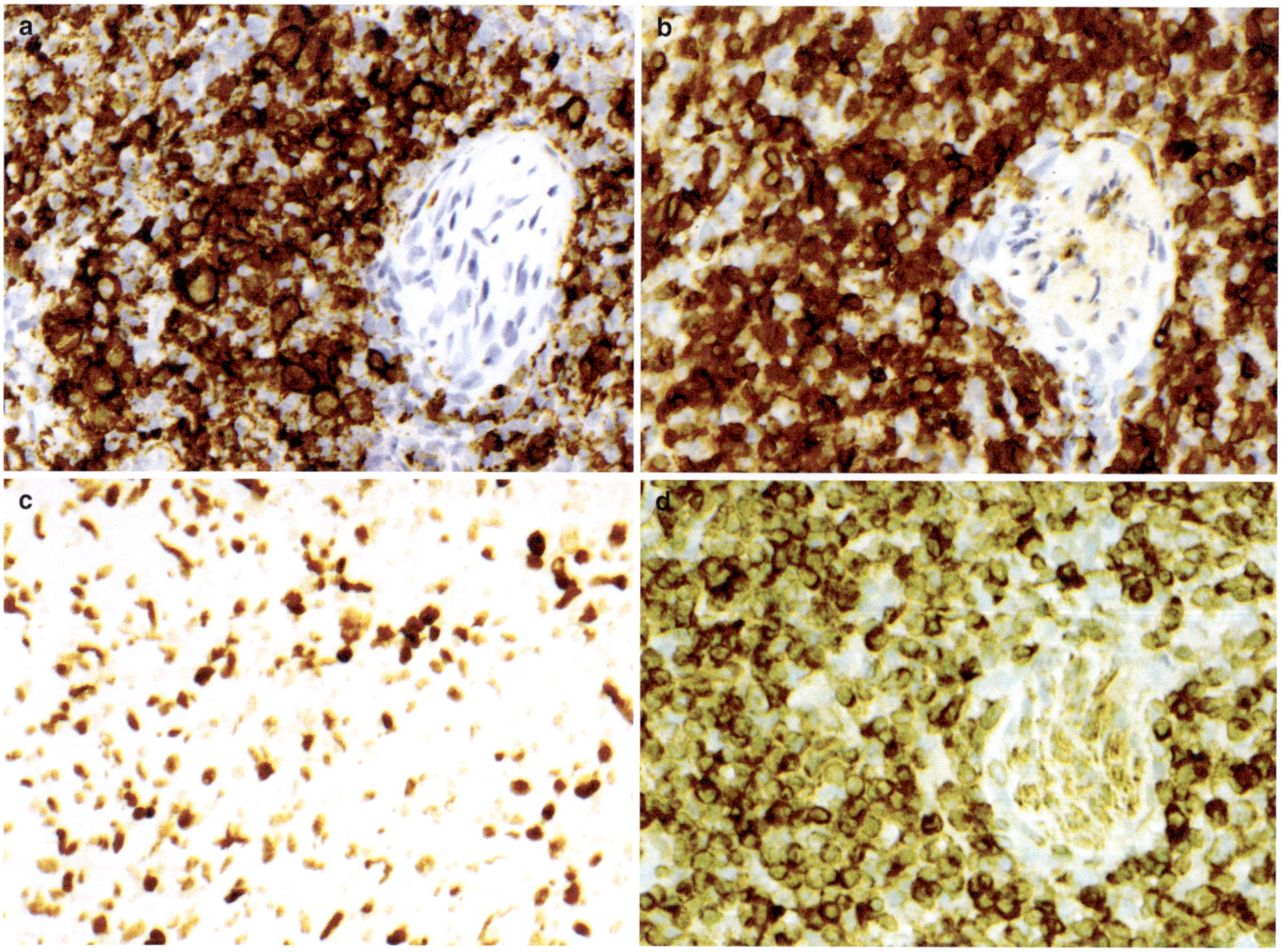

Fig. 17.6 Primary cutaneous follicle center lymphoma (pcFCL), diffuse type, immunohistochemistry, from Case 17.1. (**a**) Numerous very large, highly atypical CD20+ neoplastic B cells (CD20, 10×). (**b**) Large numbers of small round CD3+ reactive T cells are also present (CD3, 10×). (**c**) The neoplastic cells are negative for Bcl2, although some smaller cells stain positively (Bcl2, 40×). (**d**) The large neoplastic B cells (around a nerve) stain positively for Bcl6 (Bcl6, 40×)

17.3 Differential Diagnosis

17.3.1 Diagnostic Considerations

As with all other cutaneous lymphomas, diagnosis rests on a synthesis of clinical, histopathologic, and immunohistochemical findings. Although pcFCL has a remarkably good prognosis with and without treatment, it must be distinguished from other more life-threatening lymphomas such as diffuse large B-cell lymphoma, leg type, and systemic follicular lymphoma. Other more common conditions may mimic pcFCL, including pcMZL and cutaneous lymphoid hyperplasias.

17.3.2 Differential Diagnosis

17.3.2.1 Cutaneous Lymphoid Hyperplasia (CLH)

Cutaneous lymphoid hyperplasia (CLH)—also known as "pseudolymphoma" or cutaneous follicular hyperplasia — shows benign proliferations of lymphocytes that can be clinically and histologically similar to pcFCL. Histopathologic findings that help in differentiating these conditions include round or oval lymphoid follicle centers with maintained mantle zone architecture. In contrast, the follicles of pcFCL are more irregularly shaped. The neoplastic follicle center cells may surround aggregates of small reactive lymphocytes, forming inside-out follicles with the small cells in the center and large cells at the periphery. Aggregates or nodules of follicle center cells without surrounding small lymphocytes are termed naked follicles and are characteristic of pcFCL. Immunohistochemical stains for Bcl6, Bcl2, and CD21 help to reveal the architecture of lymphoid follicles: follicle center cells have a Bcl6+ Bcl2- immunophenotype and are supported by a CD21+ follicular dendritic cell meshwork. Irregularly expanded follicular dendritic cell meshwork is also commonly seen in pcFCL [1]. Clonal Ig rearrangements are present in 95 % of B-cell lymphomas but in only 17 % of benign cutaneous lymphoid infiltrates [18].

17.3.2.2 Systemic Follicular Lymphoma (sFL) with Secondary Cutaneous Involvement

Systemic follicular lymphoma (sFL) with secondary cutaneous involvement, although nearly identical in terms of clinical morphology to pcFCL has distinct genetic underpinnings and treatment [23]. Differentiation of sFL and pcFCL requires a thorough staging evaluation to assess for extracutaneous disease [3, 23]. Expression of Bcl2 and/or the presence of the t(14;18) translocation or other *Bcl2* rearrangement should increase concern for nodal follicular lymphoma with secondary cutaneous involvement [20, 23].

17.3.2.3 Primary Cutaneous Marginal Zone Lymphoma (pcMZL)

Primary cutaneous marginal zone lymphoma (pcMZL) also often presents with solitary, firm, erythematous papules or plaques on the head, neck, and upper extremities and thus can be difficult to distinguish from pcFCL clinically. To further complicate this differential diagnosis, both tumors are characterized by the presence of lymphoid follicles on skin biopsy. The architecture of these follicles is often helpful in distinguishing these two most common forms of cutaneous B-cell lymphoma. In pcFCL the neoplastic follicle center cells may form irregularly shaped nodules and surround aggregates of small lymphocytes, forming inside-out follicles. The proliferation of follicle center cells in pcFCL may also be directly apposed to reticular dermal collagen fibers without a mantle zone of small lymphocytes, so-called naked follicles. Inside-out and naked lymphoid follicles are characteristic of pcFCL and not a feature of pcMZL. Immunohistochemical stains for Bcl6, Bcl2, CD21, CD10, and kappa and lambda light chains are indispensable in this differential diagnosis [14]. In pcMZL the reactive follicles may be infiltrated by Bcl2+ Bcl6- marginal zone B cells, leading to dispersion of the BCL6+ follicle center cells. This is not a characteristic of pcFCL.

While the neoplastic cells of both lymphomas are CD20+ and CD79+ B cells, the neoplastic cells in pcMZL are Bcl2+ Bcl6- small cleaved cells, monocytoid B cells, or lymphoplasmacytoid cells, while the neoplastic cells of pcFCL are Bcl2-Bcl6+ follicle center cells (centrocytes and centro-

Table 17.1 Immunohistochemical markers for differentiation of pcDLBCL, pcFCL, and MALT lymphoma

	CD20	CD79	CD10	Bcl6	MUM1	Bcl2	FoxP1	IgM [26]
pcMZL	+	+	–	–	+	+		–/+
pcFCL	+	+	±[a]	+	–	–	–	–
pcDLBCL	+	+	–	±	+	+	+	+

Adapted from Jaffe et al. [27]

pcDLBCL primary cutaneous diffuse large B-cell lymphoma, *pcFCL* primary cutaneous follicle center lymphomas, *pcMZL* primary cutaneous marginal zone lymphoma

[a]CD10 positive in follicular pattern, negative in diffuse pattern of FCL

blasts) (Table 17.1) [1, 24]. Follicle structure may also be helpful in differentiating these entities: pcFCL is characterized by a proliferation of neoplastic follicle center cells supported by an expanded follicular dendritic cell meshwork. CD21 staining of follicular dendritic cells is helpful in identifying the sites of lymphoid follicles.

Immunohistochemical or in situ hybridization analysis of kappa and lambda light chains demonstrates light-chain restricted plasma cells in more than 70 % of pcMZLs of the skin [25], a finding absent in pcFCL [23].

17.3.2.4 Diffuse Large B-Cell Lymphoma, Leg Type (DLBCL, LT)

Diffuse large B-cell lymphoma, leg type (DLBCL, LT), particularly in cases presenting on the lower leg, can be very difficult to distinguish from pcFCL. These tumors may also mimic one another histopathologically when pcFCL manifests with a diffuse pattern. The presence of many admixed T cells, stromal reaction, and remnants of networks of follicular dendritic cells supports a diagnosis of pcFCL [6]. The tumor cells of DLBCL usually have large round non-cleaved nuclei of centroblasts in contrast to the mixed proliferation of centrocytes, centroblasts and immunoblasts observed in pcFCL. Immunohistochemistry is often indispensable in elucidating the correct diagnosis. While pcFCL is typically Bcl2− Bcl6+, FoxP1−, IgM−, and MUM1−, pcDLBCL is typically Bcl2+ Bcl6± FoxP1+ IgM+, and MUM1+ (*see* Table 17.1).

17.4 Clinical Case

17.4.1 Primary Cutaneous Follicle Center Lymphoma, Diffuse Type

Case 17.1

A 66-year-old man presented with a 15-year history of multiple 1- to 3-cm, pink to violaceous smooth papules, plaques, and nodules on his scalp and forehead (see Fig. 17.3a). He had no systemic symptoms or palpable lymphadenopathy.

A biopsy of one of the plaques demonstrated a dense CD20+ B-cell infiltrate throughout the superficial and deep dermis with numerous admixed CD3+ T cells. The epidermis was spared (see Fig. 17.4). The atypical B cells were positive for Bcl6 but negative for Bcl2, and there was no evidence of follicular dendritic cell meshwork with CD21 (Fig. 17.6). A clonal IgH gene rearrangement was detected by polymerase chain reaction. On CT scan, there was no evidence of systemic malignancy. The patient was diagnosed with primary cutaneous follicle center lymphoma, diffuse type.

The cutaneous lesions largely resolved with local radiation therapy. However, 4 months after treatment the patient developed new lesions within the radiation field (*see* Fig 17.3b). Otherwise he continues to be well.

Commentary This case serves to illustrate three points. First, as in this patient, pcFCL most commonly occurs on the head and neck, with a particular predilection for the scalp. The nodules are asymptomatic, and extracutaneous manifestations are exceedingly rare. Second, pcFCL is exquisitely responsive to radiation therapy but has a tendency to recur. The final point is histopathologic. There are three histopathologic variants of pcFCL: diffuse, follicular, and follicular and diffuse. This patient's biopsies demonstrated diffuse architecture, which in some cases can be difficult to distinguish from pcDLBCL.

17.4.2 Primary Cutaneous Follicle Center Lymphoma, Follicular Type

Case 17.2

An 85-year-old woman presented with a 1-year history of a pruritic, poorly demarcated, indurated pink plaque on her forehead (no clinical photographs available). She had no systemic complaints, and her physical examination was otherwise unremarkable.

A biopsy of this plaque revealed a dense dermal lymphoid infiltrate with expansile nodules of follicle center cells within irregularly shaped meshwork of CD21+ follicular dendritic cells (Fig. 17.7); naked and inside out follicles were present. The follicle center cells stained positively for CD20 and Bcl6 but did not express Bcl2 (Fig. 17.8). There were numerous admixed CD3+ T cells. A clonal IgH gene rearrangement was present. The patient was diagnosed with primary cutaneous follicle center lymphoma, follicular type.

The patient was treated with localized radiation therapy, resulting in complete resolution of the plaque. One year after treatment she is well, with no evidence of recurrence.

Commentary The clinical findings in this case are typical of pcFCL: a plaque located on the head. The histology offers an example of follicular-type pcFCL, with discrete follicles. The staining patterns seen both cases are classic for pcFCL.

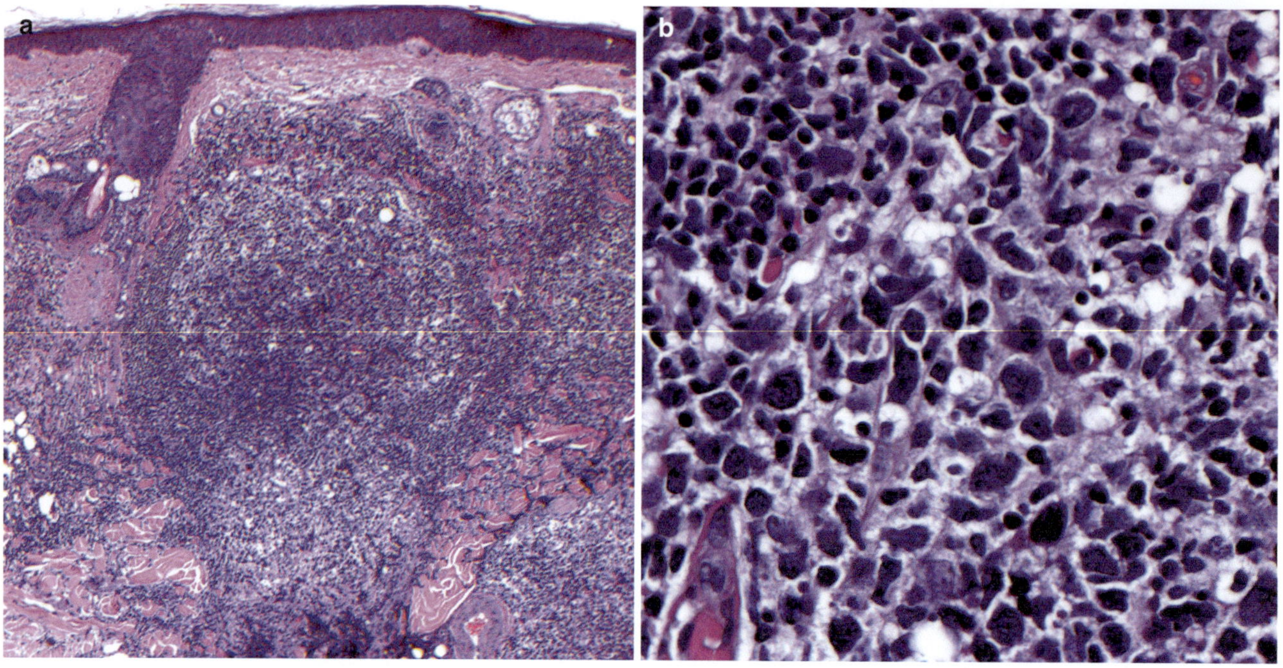

Fig. 17.7 Primary cutaneous follicle center lymphoma (pcFCL), follicular pattern Case 17.2. (**a**) The dermis is occupied by several dense follicular aggregates of neoplastic B cells. The follicles are poorly defined and composed of neoplastic follicle center B cells (H&E, 4×). (**b**) The neoplastic cells are centrocytes with medium-sized densely chromatic cleaved nuclei and centroblasts with large round nuclei and basophilic nucleoli at the nuclear margin. The atypical cytologic findings include increased nuclear to cytoplasmic ratio and irregularly shaped hyperchromatic nuclei (H&E, 63×)

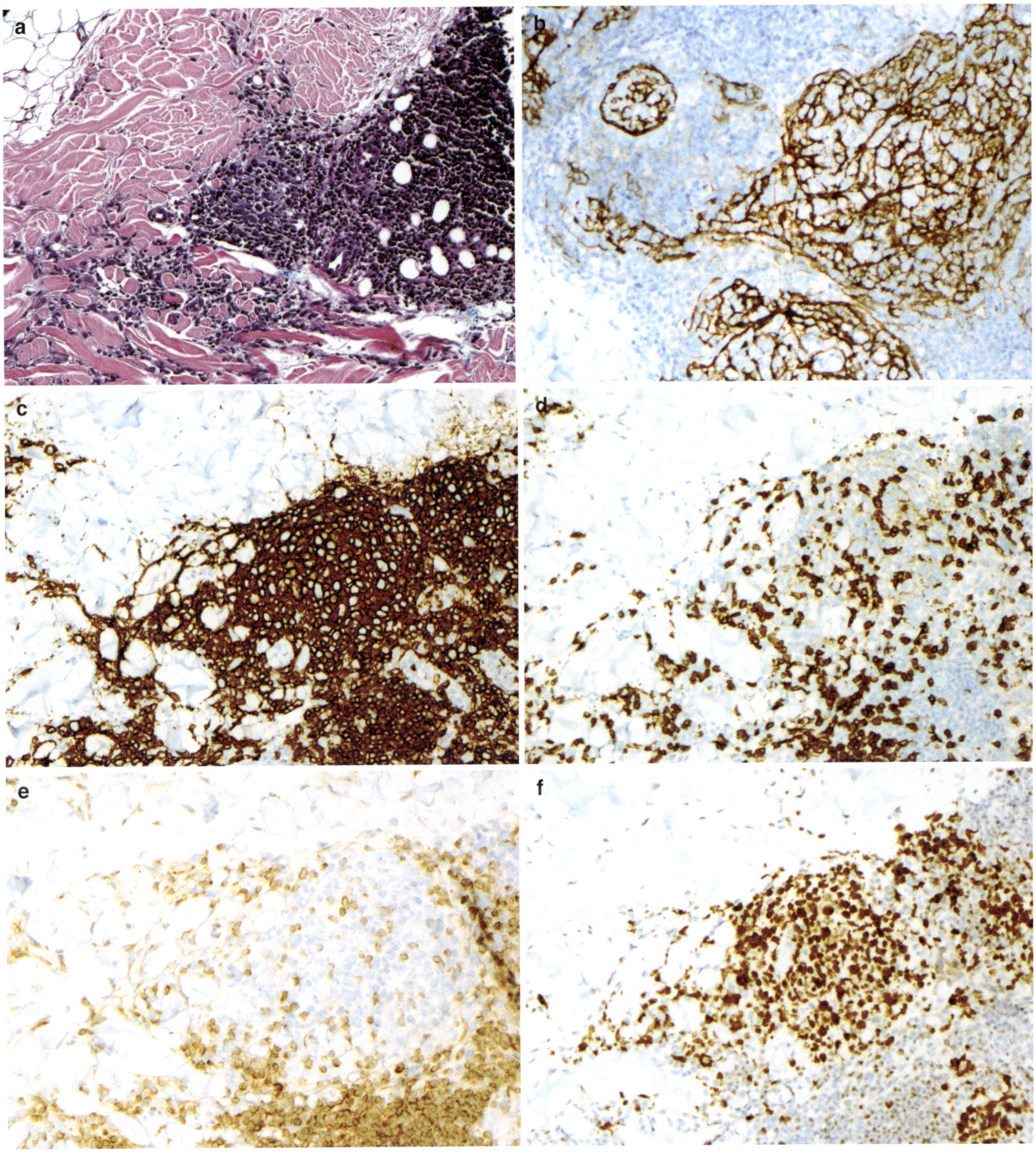

Fig. 17.8 Primary cutaneous follicle center lymphoma (pcFCL), follicular type, immunohistochemistry, Case 17.2. (**a**) A dense aggregate of neoplastic follicle center B cells, reactive T cells, and follicular dendritic cells forms an expansile lymphoid follicle deep in the dermis (H&E, 20×). (**b**) Immunohistochemistry for CD21 reveals an intact irregularly shaped follicular dendritic cell meshwork (CD21, 20×). (**c**) The follicle center cells are CD20+ B cells (CD20, 20×). (**d**) Scattered CD3+ T cells are admixed within and around the follicle (CD3, 20×). (**e**) The CD20+ B cells within the follicle do not express Bcl2 (Bcl2, 20×). (**f**) The neoplastic B cells stain positively for Bcl6 (Bcl6, 20×)

References

1. Willemze R, Swerdlow SH, Harris NL, Vergier B. Primary cutaneous follicle centre lymphoma. In: Swerdlow SH, Campo E, Harris NL, Jaffe ES, Pileri SA, Stein H, et al., editors. WHO classification of tumors haematopathol lymphoid tissues. 4th ed. Lyon: International Agency for Research on Cancer; 2008. p. 227–8.
2. Swerdlow SH, Quintanilla-Martinez L, Willemze R, Kinney MC. Cutaneous B-cell lymphoproliferative disorders: report of the 2011 Society for Hematopathology/European Association for Haematopathology workshop. Am J Clin Pathol. 2013;139:515–35.
3. Fernán de zdeLarrea C, Martínez-Pozo A, Mercadal S, García A, Gutierrez-García G, Valera A, et al. Initial features and outcome of cutaneous and non-cutaneous primary extranodal follicular lymphoma. Br J Haematol. 2011;153:334–40.
4. Gulia A, Saggini A, Wiesner T, Fink-Puches R, Argenyi Z, Ferrara G, et al. Clinicopathologic features of early lesions of primary cutaneous follicle center lymphoma, diffuse type: implications for early diagnosis and treatment. J Am Acad Dermatol. 2011;65:991–1000.
5. Hamilton SN, Wai ES, Tan K, Alexander C, Gascoyne RD, Connors JM. Treatment and outcomes in patients with primary cutaneous B-cell lymphoma: the BC Cancer Agency experience. Int J Radiat Oncol. 2013;87:719–25.
6. Senff NJ, Hoefnagel JJ, Jansen PM, Vermeer MH, van Baarlen J, Blokx WA, et al. Reclassification of 300 primary cutaneous B-Cell lymphomas according to the new WHO-EORTC classification for cutaneous lymphomas: comparison with previous classifications and identification of prognostic markers. J Clin Oncol. 2007;25:1581–7.
7. Massone C, Chott A, Metze D, Kerl K, Citarella L, Vale E. Subcutaneous, blastic natural killer (NK), NK/T-cell, and other cytotoxic lymphomas of the skin: a morphologic, immunophenotypic, and molecular study of 50 patients. Am J Surg Pathol. 2004;28:719–35.
8. Senff NJ, Hoefnagel JJ, Neelis KJ, Vermeer MH, Noordijk EM, Willemze R. Results of radiotherapy in 153 primary cutaneous B-Cell lymphomas classified according to the WHO-EORTC classification. Arch Dermatol. 2007;143:1520–6.
9. Senff NJ, Noordijk EM, Kim YH, Bagot M, Berti E, Cerroni L, et al. European Organization for Research and Treatment of Cancer and International Society for Cutaneous Lymphoma consensus recommendations for the management of cutaneous B-cell lymphomas. Blood. 2008;112:1600–9.
10. Fernandez-Flores A, Smucler-Simonovich A, Escalante F, Manjon JA. The differential diagnosis between primary cutaneous large B-cell lymphoma and cutaneous follicular lymphoma: prognostic and therapeutic implications. Am J Dermatopathol. 2011;33:819–26.
11. Bekkenk MW, Vermeer MH, Geerts ML, Noordijk EM, Heule F, van Voorst Vader PC, et al. Treatment of multifocal primary cutaneous B-cell lymphoma: a clinical follow-up study of 29 patients. J Clin Oncol. 1999;17:2471–8.
12. Quéreux G, Brocard A, Peuvrel L, Nguyen JM, Knol A-C, Dréno B. Systemic rituximab in multifocal primary cutaneous follicle centre lymphoma. Acta Derm Venereol. 2011;91:562–7.
13. Ceovic R, Jovanovic I, Kostovic K, Rados J, Dotlic S, Radman I, et al. Radiotherapy of primary cutaneous follicle center lymphoma: case report and review of literature. Radiat Oncol. 2013;8:147.
14. De Leval L, Harris NL, Longtine J, Ferry JA, Duncan LM. Cutaneous B-cell lymphomas of follicular and marginal zone types: use of Bcl-6, CD10, Bcl-2, and CD21 in diagnosis and classification. Am J Surg Pathol. 2001;25:732–41.
15. Gellrich S, Rutz S, Golembowski S, Jacobs C, von Zimmermann M, Lorenz P, et al. Primary cutaneous follicle center cell lymphomas and large B cell lymphomas of the leg descend from germinal center cells. A single cell polymerase chain reaction analysis. J Invest Dermatol. 2001;117:1512–20.
16. Hoefnagel JJ, Dijkman R, Basso K, Jansen PM, Hallermann C, Willemze R, et al. Distinct types of primary cutaneous large B-cell lymphoma identified by gene expression profiling. Blood. 2005;105:3671–8.
17. Hoefnagel JJ, Vermeer MH, Jansen PM, Fleuren GJ, Meijer CJLM, Willemze R. Bcl-2, Bcl-6 and CD10 expression in cutaneous B-cell lymphoma: further support for a follicle centre cell origin and differential diagnostic significance. Br J Dermatol. 2003;149:1183–91.
18. Fujiwara M, Morales AV, Seo K, Kim YH, Arber DA. Sundram UN Clonal identity and differences in primary cutaneous B-cell lymphoma occurring at different sites or time points in the same patient. Am J Dermatopathol. 2013;35:11–8.
19. Dijkman R, Tensen CP, Jordanova ES, Knijnenburg J, Hoefnagel JJ, Mulder AA, et al. Array-based comparative genomic hybridization analysis reveals recurrent chromosomal alterations and prognostic parameters in primary cutaneous large B-cell lymphoma. J Clin Oncol. 2006;24:296–305.
20. Child FJ, Russell-Jones R, Woolford AJ, Calonje E, Photiou A, Orchard G, et al. Absence of the t(14;18) chromosomal translocation in primary cutaneous B-cell lymphoma. Br J Dermatol. 2001;144:735–44.
21. Hallermann C, Kaune KM, Gesk S, Martin-Subero JI, Gunawan B, Griesinger F, et al. Molecular cytogenetic analysis of chromosomal breakpoints in the IGH, MYC, BCL6, and MALT1 gene loci in primary cutaneous B-cell lymphomas. J Invest Dermatol. 2004;123:213–9.
22. Mirza I, Macpherson N. Primary cutaneous follicular lymphoma: an assessment of clinical, histopathologic, immunophenotypic, and molecular features. J Clin Oncol. 2002;20:647–55.
23. Cerroni L, Arzberger E, Pütz B, Höfler G, Metze D, Sander CA, et al. Primary cutaneous follicle center cell lymphoma with follicular growth pattern. Blood. 2000;95:3922–8.
24. Isaacson P, Chott A, Nakamura S, Muller-Hermelink HK, Harris NL, Swerdlow SH. Extranodal marginal zone lymphoma of mucosa-associated lymphoid tissue (MALT lymphoma). In: Swerdlow SH, Campo E, Harris NL, Jaffe ES, Pileri SA, Stein H, et al., editors. WHO classification of tumors haematopathol lymphoid tissues. 4th ed. Lyon: International Agency for Research on Cancer; 2008. p. 214–7.
25. Cerroni L, Signoretti S, Höfler G, Annessi G, Pütz B, Lackinger E, et al. Primary cutaneous marginal zone B-cell lymphoma: a recently described entity of low-grade malignant cutaneous B-cell lymphoma. Am J Surg Pathol. 1997;21:1307–15.
26. Demirkesen C, Tüzüner N, Esen T, Lebe B, Ozkal S. The expression of IgM is helpful in the differentiation of primary cutaneous diffuse large B cell lymphoma and follicle center lymphoma. Leuk Res. 2011;35:1269–72.
27. Jaffe ES, Harris NL, Stein H, Campo E, Pileri SA, Swerdlow SH. Introduction and overview of the classification of the lymphoid neoplasms. In: Swerdlow SH, Campo E, Harris NL, Jaffe ES, Pileri SA, Stein H, et al., editors. WHO classification of tumors haematopathol lymphoid tissues. 4th ed. Lyon: International Agency for Research on Cancer; 2008. p. 158–66.

18 Primary Cutaneous Diffuse Large B-Cell Lymphoma, Leg Type

Amrita Goyal, Joi B. Carter, Jeffrey A. Barnes, and Lyn McDivitt Duncan

Primary cutaneous diffuse large B-cell lymphoma (pcDLBCL), leg type, is a rare B-cell lymphoma of post-germinal B cells. Although this lymphoma classically presents on the leg with erythematous or violaceous tumors or nodules, it can also present elsewhere on the body. Patients with pcDLBCL have a moderately poor prognosis and experience frequent systemic dissemination. Though small case series have reported dramatic improvements in survival with combination chemotherapy and rituximab, treatment is largely limited by patient age and functional status. This chapter discusses the clinical presentation, prognosis, treatment, histopathology, immunohistochemistry, molecular characteristics, and differential diagnosis of pcDLBCL. The chapter closes with two clinical cases: one case of pcDLBCL occurring on the leg and one occurring on the scalp.

A. Goyal, M.D.
Harvard-MIT Division of Health Sciences and Technology, Harvard Medical School, Boston, MA, USA

J.B. Carter, M.D.
Department of Dermatology, Massachusetts General Hospital, Harvard Medical School, Boston, MA, USA

J.A. Barnes, M.D., Ph.D.
Comprehensive Cutaneous Lymphoma Program, Department of Medicine, Massachusetts General Hospital Cancer Center, Boston, MA, USA

L.M. Duncan, M.D. (✉)
Dermatopathology Service, Department of Pathology, Massachusetts General Hospital, Harvard Medical School, Boston, MA, USA
e-mail: duncan@helix.mgh.harvard.edu

J.B. Carter et al. (eds.), *Atlas of Cutaneous Lymphomas: Classification and Differential Diagnosis*, DOI 10.1007/978-3-319-17217-0_18

18.1 Clinical

18.1.1 Clinical Presentation

Primary cutaneous diffuse large B-cell lymphoma (pcDLBCL), leg type, is a subtype of diffuse large B-cell lymphoma that accounts for 10–20 % of cutaneous B-cell lymphomas and 2.6 % of all cutaneous lymphomas [1–3]. This lymphoma primarily impacts the elderly, with a median age of onset in the seventh decade [1, 2, 4]. As with many other B-cell lymphomas, Asians and Pacific Islanders have a higher rate of pcDLBCL than other ethnic groups [2]. In contrast to most other primary cutaneous B-cell lymphomas, pcDLBCL is two to four times more common in women than in men [1, 5–7].

pcDLBCL typically presents with 2- to 5-cm erythematous to violaceous tumors or coalescing nodules on the lower legs (see Figs. 18.1 and 18.2) [1, 7, 8]. Although the lymphoma is termed "leg type," 10–15 % of patients present with this lymphoma at other sites, including the head, trunk, and upper limbs (see Fig. 18.3). Most patients have a single lesion at diagnosis [8]. Patients with leg involvement have higher rates of extracutaneous dissemination (33 %) than those who do not (18 %) [9].

18.1.2 Prognosis and Treatment

Patients with a diagnosis of pcDLBCL have a 5-year disease-specific survival rate of 50–70 % [1, 2, 4]. Most deaths occur in the first year after diagnosis [4]. Negative clinical prognostic factors include presentation on the leg, multiple lesions on the skin at diagnosis, and age older than 75 years [1, 9].

Tumor location is a key negative prognostic indicator: patients with tumors on the leg have a mean 5-year survival rate of 43 %, compared with 77 % for patients with a non-leg location [9]. Patients with multiple lesions have a 5-year survival rate of 39 %, compared with over 70 % for those with a single lesion [9]. Clinical factors that do not change patient outcome include gender, patient baseline performance status, serum lactate dehydrogenase (LDH), and the duration of the lesions prior to diagnosis [9, 10]. Molecular markers of prognostic significance are discussed below.

Patients diagnosed with pcDLBCL are often elderly and frail, with a poor performance status at baseline; they are poor candidates for chemotherapy [4]. Intravenous rituximab and combination chemotherapy are the standards of care for pcDLBCL [9, 11–13]; limited-stage non-Hodgkin's lymphoma patients (a category including those with pcDLBCL) who are treated with a combination of chemotherapy and radiation may have a better outcome than those treated with chemotherapy alone [14, 15]. There is a trend towards improved survival with the combination of multiagent chemotherapy and rituximab; small, retrospective studies have shown a 60–90 % response rate and a 3-year survival rate of up to 80–90 % with this treatment regimen [8, 12, 16]. Even with the combination of radiation, chemotherapy, and rituximab, however, patients commonly experience relapses and systemic dissemination [1, 9].

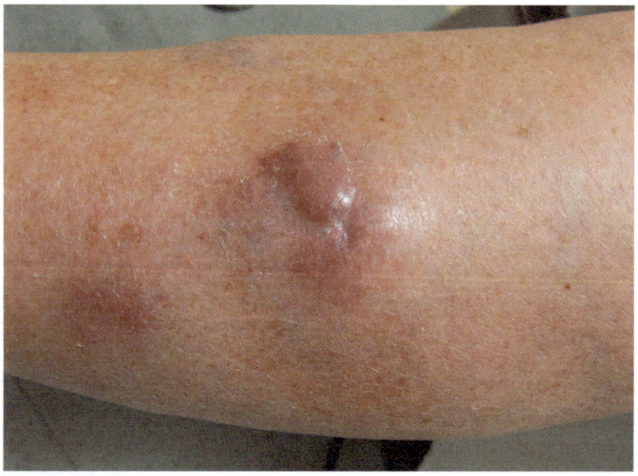

Fig. 18.1 Primary cutaneous diffuse large B-cell lymphoma, leg type (pcDLBCL, LT), presenting with pink, indurated plaques and nodules on the anterior shin of an 84-year-old woman

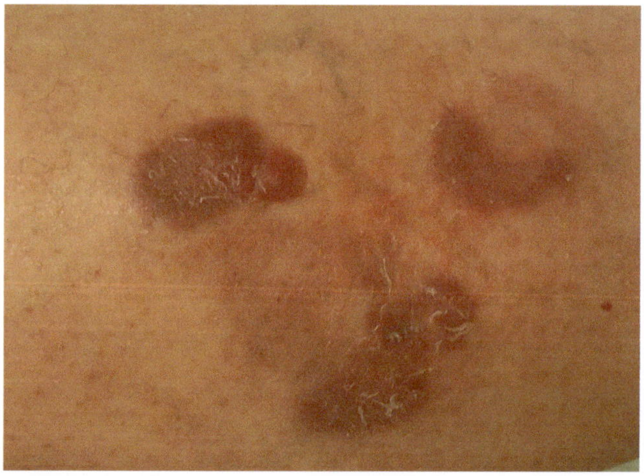

Fig. 18.2 This clinical photo of pcDLBCL, LT shows three indurated, dark pink to erythematous plaques on the calf of Case 18.1. The plaques range from 1 to 3 cm in size. There is some overlying scale and surrounding areas of dyspigmentation

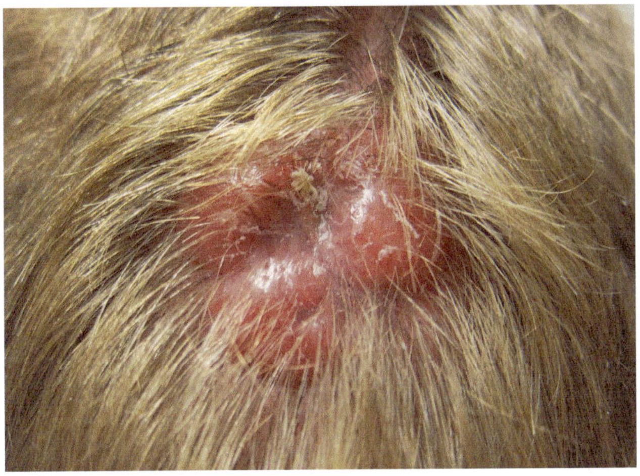

Fig. 18.3 This clinical photo (Case 18.2) shows pcDLBCL, LT on the crown of the head, appearing as a 3.5 × 3 cm firm, multilobulated tumor on a pink, edematous background. Central erosion and crust are present at the site of a prior biopsy

18.2 Pathology

18.2.1 Histopathology

Cutaneous biopsy specimens of pcDLBCL are characterized by a monotonous, dense, diffuse, superficial, and deep dermal infiltrate of large, atypical B cells forming confluent sheets [1, 17, 18]. Epidermal involvement is absent (see Figs. 18.4 and 18.5) [1].

The atypical B cells of pcDLBCL are large, round, and noncleaved, often resembling centroblasts. Mitoses are common [1].

There are few perivascular reactive T cells, and the reactive infiltrate is sparse compared with that of other cutaneous B-cell lymphomas [1, 18].

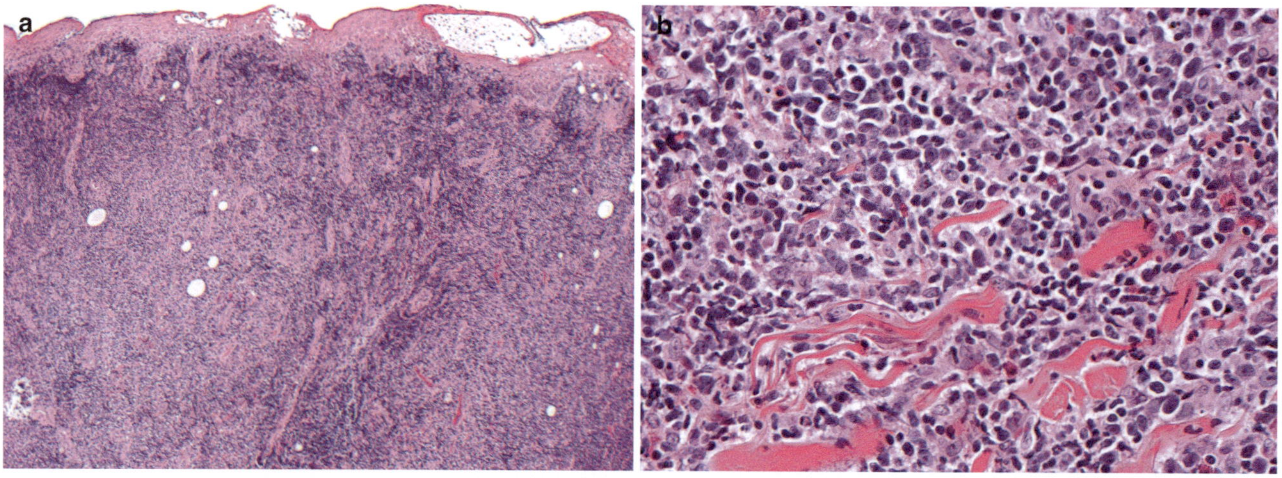

Fig. 18.4 Histology of pcDLBCL, LT from Case 18.1. (**a**) A diffuse, dense, monotonous sheet-like infiltrate of atypical B cells occupies the papillary and reticular dermis. The epidermis is spared (HE, 10×). (**b**) Sheets of large, atypical B cells disrupt the collagen of the dermis. The neoplastic cells have large, round, and noncleaved nuclei (H&E, 40×)

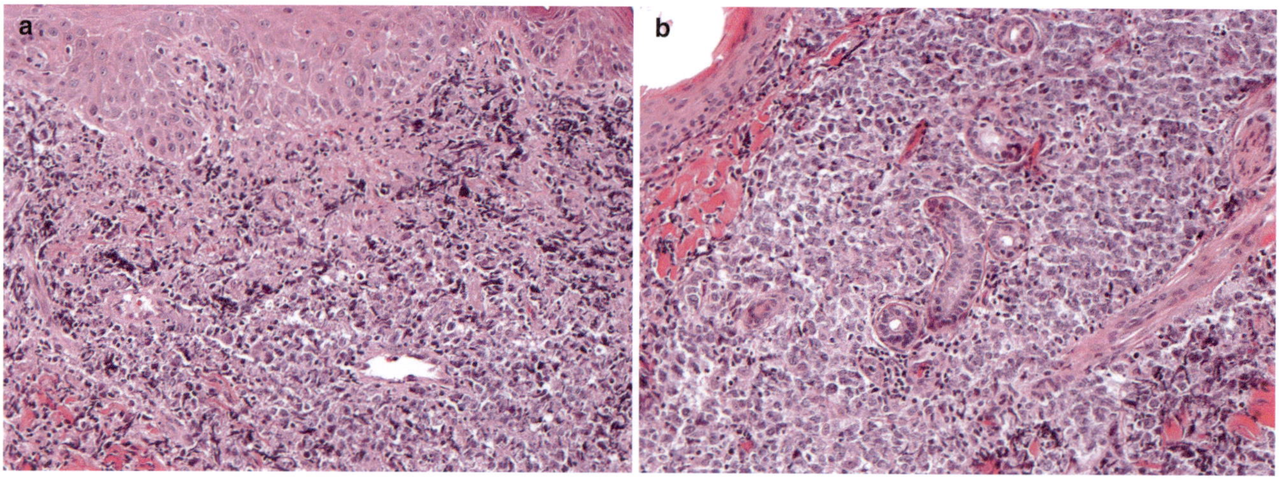

Fig. 18.5 Histopathology of pcDLBCL, LT from Case 18.2. Although this biopsy specimen is from a lesion occurring on the patient's scalp, the histopathology is identical to that seen in lesions located on the leg (see Fig. 18.4). (**a**) Sheets of large, atypical B cells occupy the dermis with minimal epidermal involvement (H&E, 10×). (**b**) The eccrine unit in the middle of the field, although surrounded by large neoplastic B cells, is uninvolved (H&E, 20×)

18.2.2 Immunophenotype and Molecular Findings

The neoplastic B cells of pcDLBCL express CD20, CD79a, monotypic Ig, MUM1/IRF4, Bcl2, Bcl6, and FoxP1. Approximately 10 % of cases lack Bcl2 and/or MUM1 expression. Bcl6 staining is often dim, and CD10 staining is usually absent (see Figs. 18.6 and 18.7) [1]. As in all B-cell neoplasms, the neoplastic cells of pcDLBCL express the transcription factor Pax5 [19].

Nearly all cases of pcDLBCL demonstrate chromosomal imbalances [20]. Deletions of 18q and 6q occur much more frequently in pcDLBCL than in primary cutaneous marginal zone lymphoma (pcMZL) or primary cutaneous follicle center lymphoma (pcFCL) [20]. Deletion of 9p21.3 (containing the *CDKN2A* and *CDKN2B* genes) is present in 67 % of tumors, and patients with decreased expression of the *CDKN2A* and *CDKN2B* genes secondary to deletion or hypermethylation have a worse prognosis [1, 21, 22]. Two thirds of tumors have amplification of 18q21.31–q21.33, a region that includes the genes *BCL2* and *MALT1* [1]. Of note, the t(14;18) translocation is typically absent [1].

Molecular markers with negative prognostic significance include expression of MUM1, expression of transcription factors OCT2 [1, 20] or FoxP1 [23], and inactivation of the *CDKN2A* gene [1, 21]. The prognostic significance of Bcl2 expression is unclear [10, 17, 21, 24]. High expression of FoxP3 by tumor cells and regulatory T cells in the tumor is associated with a better prognosis [25].

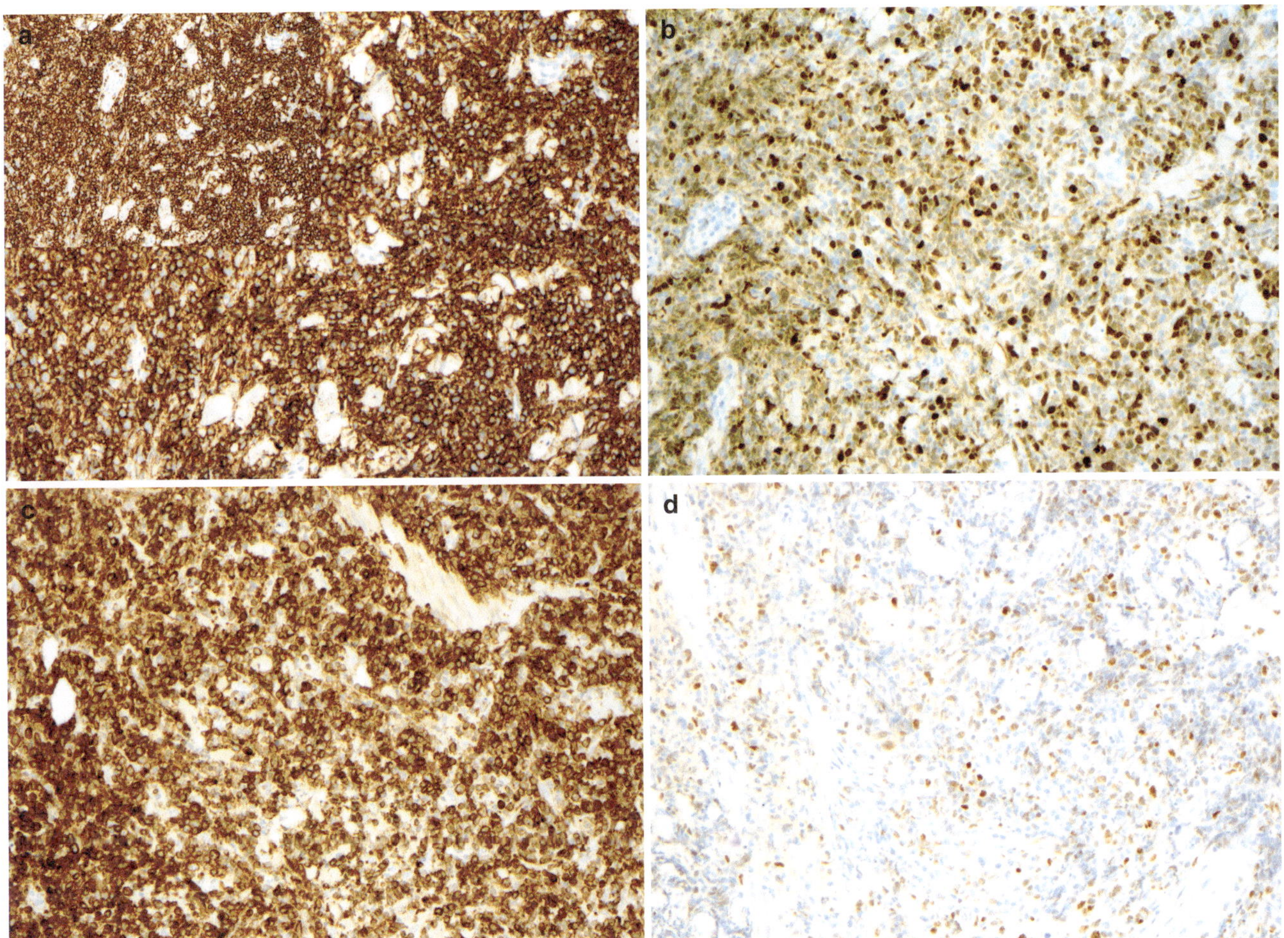

Fig. 18.6 Immunohistochemistry of pcDLBCL, LT from Case 18.1. (**a**) Large, atypical B cells stain strongly for CD20 on immunohistochemistry (CD20, 20×). (**b**) The neoplastic cells also express MUM1 (MUM1, 20×). (**c**) The atypical cells stain positively for Bcl2 (Bcl2, 20×). (**d**) Bcl6 is not expressed by the neoplastic B cells (Bcl6, 20×)

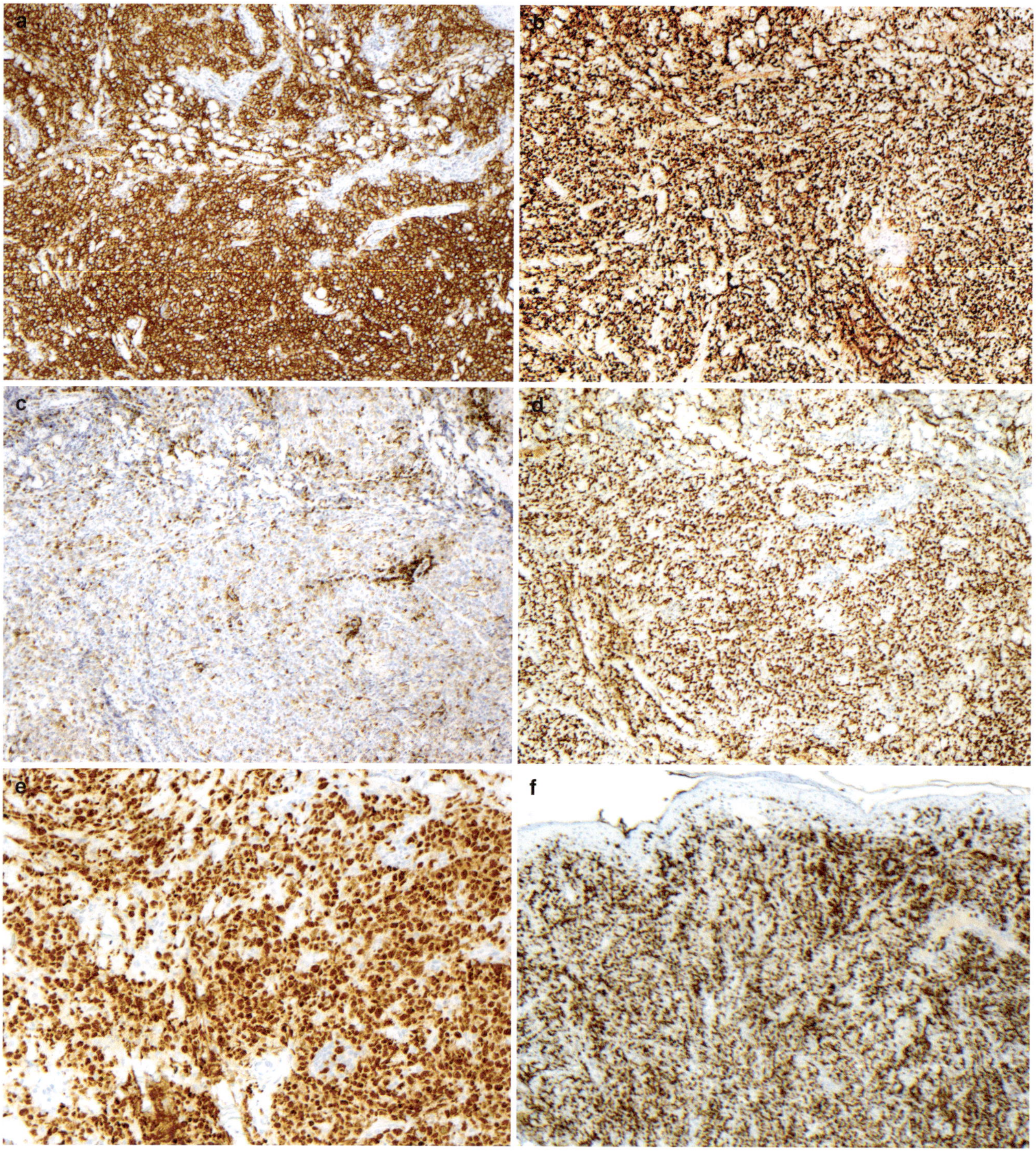

Fig. 18.7 Immunohistochemistry of pcDLBCL from Case 18.2. (**a**) The large, neoplastic B cells stain strongly for the B-cell marker CD20. (**b**) The neoplastic cells also stain positively for MUM1. (**c**) Rare cells stain positively for Bcl2. (**d**) Most atypical cells show staining for Bcl6. (**e**) Many of the neoplastic B cells demonstrate expression of Pax5. (**f**) This tumor has a very high proliferative index, with nearly 80 % of atypical cells staining positively for Ki67

18.3 Differential Diagnosis

18.3.1 Diagnostic Considerations

Although research to characterize the gene expression and molecular profile of pcDLBCL and other B-cell lymphomas has been quite fruitful, such studies are not yet used in clinical practice [20, 26]. Diagnosis of pcDLBCL rests on a synthesis of clinical presentation, histopathology, and immunohistochemistry. The differential diagnosis includes other lymphomas composed of large atypical cells, but most critical is that systemic lymphomas must be ruled out with appropriate staging studies, including full body PET-CT scanning, before a diagnosis of primary cutaneous lymphoma is made [18].

18.3.2 Differential Diagnosis

18.3.2.1 Systemic DLBCL

To make a diagnosis of pcDLBCL, systemic DLBCL with secondary cutaneous involvement must be excluded. Cutaneous involvement occurs in 7–10 % of cases of systemic B-cell lymphomas [27]. In addition, systemic DLBCL is far more common than pcDLBCL; it comprises 25 % of cases of non-Hodgkin's lymphoma overall [28]. Accurate differentiation between systemic DLBCL versus pcDLBCL can have a tremendous impact on treatment and prognosis. Clinical correlation and appropriate staging examinations are required to differentiate secondary cutaneous systemic DLBCL from pcDLBCL.

18.3.2.2 Testicular DLBCL

This form of systemic DLBCL is important enough to warrant separate discussion. Testicular DLBCL with secondary cutaneous involvement is indistinguishable from pcDLBCL, leg type, on the basis of pathology and phenotype: both lymphomas are histopathologically characterized by a diffuse infiltrate of centroblasts and immunoblasts with strong expression of Bcl2, MUM1, FoxP1, and pan–B-cell markers [29]. Clinical correlation and testicular ultrasound should be considered in all cases of pcDLBCL to rule out testicular involvement. Of note, one case of secondary testicular involvement of pcDLBCL has been reported [9].

18.3.2.3 Primary Cutaneous Follicle Center Lymphoma (pcFCL)

pcDLBCL and pcFCL can be particularly difficult to distinguish when they present on the lower leg. They may also mimic one another histopathologically when pcFCL shows a diffuse pattern. Histopathology can offer a clue as to the diagnosis: the presence of many admixed T cells, stromal reaction, and remnants of networks of follicular dendritic cells suggests a diagnosis of pcFCL [6]. Immunohistochemical studies are invaluable: pcFCL is typically Bcl2−, Bcl6+, FoxP1−, and IgM−, whereas pcDLBCL is typically Bcl2+, Bcl6+, FoxP1+, and IgM+ (Table 18.1) [30, 31]. MUM1 also serves as a primary differentiating factor: this marker is present in DLBCL but usually is absent in pcFCL. Finally, the deletion of the *CDKN2A* gene is common in DLBCL but rare in pcFCL [21].

18.3.2.4 Primary Cutaneous Marginal Zone Lymphoma (pcMZL)

When pcDLBCL presents on parts of the body other than the leg, it can be very difficult to distinguish clinically from pcMZL, but they are quite distinct on histopathology: pcDLBCL is characterized by a diffuse infiltrate of large B cells, but pcMZL present with a dense, nodular, dermal and subcutaneous lymphocytic infiltrate of small to medium-sized B cells with reactive lymphoid follicles. Immunohistochemistry also may be helpful: although pcMZL and pcDLBCL both express CD20, CD79a, MUM1, and Bcl2, pcMZL lack Bcl6 expression (see Table 18.1).

18.3.2.5 Intravascular Large B-Cell Lymphoma (IVLBCL)

IVLBCL is an extremely rare, highly aggressive lymphoma of large B cells. Its presentation may vary widely from isolated neurologic symptoms to hemophagocytic syndrome to cutaneous manifestations that include maculopapular eruptions, nodules with or without ulceration, violaceous infiltrated plaques, palpable purpura, and ulcers [32–34]. The histopathology of IVLBCL is quite distinctive, however: the neoplastic B cells are present only in small vessels and capillaries, with minimal to no extravascular extravasation. Although both neoplasms are composed of large, atypical B cells, cutaneous biopsy of pcDLBCL demonstrates a diffuse, monotonous dermal proliferation of neoplastic cells.

Table 18.1 Immunohistochemical markers for differentiation of pcDLBCL, pcFCL, and pcMZL

	CD20	CD79	CD10	Bcl6	MUM1	BCL2	FoxP1	IgM
pcMZL	+	+	−	−	+	+	±	±
pcFCL	+	+	±[a]	+	−	−	−	−
pcDLBCL	+	+	−	±[b]	+	+	+	+

Adapted from Jaffe et al. [35]

pcDLBCL primary cutaneous diffuse large B-cell lymphoma, *pcFCL* primary cutaneous follicle center lymphoma, *pcMZL* primary cutaneous marginal zone lymphoma

[a]CD10 positive in follicular, negative in diffuse

[b]Positive in most cases

18.4 Clinical Cases

Case 18.1 Patient 1

A 66-year-old woman presented with a 6-month history of new pruritic, dark pink nodules with some overlying scale on the right leg and faint pink plaques on both legs (see Fig. 18.2).

Biopsy revealed a perivascular and periadnexal infiltrate of CD20+, MUM1+, Bcl2+, Bcl6+ B cells with numerous admixed CD3+ T cells (see Figs. 18.4 and 18.5). The diagnosis was pcDLBCL, LT, located on the legs.

The patient underwent three rounds of R-CHOP chemoimmunotherapy, followed by involved-field radiation therapy, but several weeks after she completed chemotherapy and radiation, the lesions returned and biopsy revealed similar pathology. According to patient preference, she was treated with several courses of local radiation therapy. Although this treatment led to complete clearance of the nodules and plaques of pcDLBCL, she continues to develop new lesions. The patient otherwise remains free of systemic involvement.

Commentary This patient's pcDLBCL occurred on her legs, the most common site for this rare lymphoma. This patient was treated effectively with a combination of chemotherapy and radiation.

Case 18.2 Patient 2

A 35-year-old man presented with a 3-month history of a rapidly enlarging, soft, multilobulated, pink nodule at the vertex of his scalp (see Fig. 18.3). A biopsy of the nodule was performed at an outside institution a month after its appearance; although it resolved almost completely after the biopsy, it rapidly regrew to more than 4 cm.

A repeat biopsy of the lesion revealed a dense dermal infiltrate of large, atypical CD20+ B cells (see Figs. 18.6 and 18.7). These cells showed strong coexpression of Bcl6 and MUM1 but were negative for CD10 and Bcl2. A PET-CT scan revealed no evidence of systemic malignancy, and a testicular ultrasound was negative for lymphomatous involvement. The diagnosis was pcDLBCL, LT, located on the scalp. The patient was treated with six cycles of R-CHOP. Although the combination of radiation therapy and chemotherapy is known to improve local control in patients with limited-stage non-Hodgkin's lymphoma, radiation therapy was avoided in this patient to reduce the risk of permanent alopecia.

Commentary This case illustrates the important point that although pcDLBCL is called "leg-type," it can occur anywhere on the body, in this case, the scalp. As is expected in cases of pcDLBCL, the patient was treated with combination systemic chemotherapy, with good effect.

References

1. Meijer CJLM, Vergier B, Duncan LM, Willemze R. Primary cutaneous DLBCL, leg type. In: Swerdlow SH, Campo E, Harris NL, Jaffe ES, Pileri SA, Stein H, et al., editors. WHO classification of tumors of haematopoietic and lymphoid tissues. 4th ed. Lyon: International Agency for Research on Cancer; 2008. p. 242.
2. Bradford PT, Devesa SS, Anderson WF, Toro JR. Cutaneous lymphoma incidence patterns in the United States: a population-based study of 3884 cases. Blood. 2009;113:5064–73.
3. Paulli M, Viglio A, Vivenza D, Capello D, Rossi D, Riboni R, et al. Primary cutaneous large B-cell lymphoma of the leg: histogenetic analysis of a controversial clinicopathologic entity. Hum Pathol. 2002;33:937–43.
4. Bessell EM, Humber CE, O'Connor S, English JSE, Perkins W, Dickinson PD, et al. Primary cutaneous B-cell lymphoma in Nottinghamshire U.K.: prognosis of subtypes defined in the WHO-EORTC classification. Br J Dermatol. 2012;167:1118–23.
5. Kodama K, Massone C, Chott A, Metze D, Kerl H, Cerroni L. Primary cutaneous large B-cell lymphomas: clinicopathologic features, classification, and prognostic factors in a large series of patients. Blood. 2005;106:2491–7.
6. Senff NJ, Hoefnagel JJ, Jansen PM, Vermeer MH, van Baarlen J, Blokx WA, et al. Reclassification of 300 primary cutaneous B-cell lymphomas according to the new WHO-EORTC classification for cutaneous lymphomas: comparison with previous classifications and identification of prognostic markers. J Clin Oncol. 2007;25:1581–7.
7. Vermeer MH, Geelen F, van Haselen CW, van Voorst Vader PC, Geerts M-L, van Vloten WA, et al. Primary cutaneous large B-cell lymphoma of the leg. Arch Dermatol. 1996;132:1304–8.
8. Hamilton SN, Wai ES, Tan K, Alexander C, Gascoyne RD, Connors JM. Treatment and outcomes in patients with primary cutaneous B-cell lymphoma: the BC Cancer Agency experience. Int J Radiat Oncol Biol Phys. 2013;87:719–25.
9. Grange F, Beylot-Barry M, Courville P, Maubec E, Bagot M, Bergier B, et al. Primary cutaneous diffuse large B-cell lymphoma, leg type. Arch Dermatol. 2007;143:1144–50.
10. Kramer MH, Hermans J, Wijburg E, Philippo K, Geelen E, van Krieken JH, et al. Clinical relevance of BCL2, BCL6, and MYC rearrangements in diffuse large B-cell lymphoma. Blood. 1998;92:3152–62.
11. Brogan BL, Zic JA, Kinney MC, Hu JY, Hamilton KS, Greer JP. Large B-cell lymphoma of the leg: clinical and pathologic characteristics in a North American series. J Am Acad Dermatol. 2003;49:223–8.
12. Grange F, Maubec E, Bagot M, Beylot-Barry M, Joly P, Dalle S, et al. Treatment of cutaneous B-cell lymphoma, leg type, with age-adapted combinations of chemotherapies and rituximab. Arch Dermatol. 2009;145:329–30.
13. Senff NJ, Noordijk EM, Kim YH, Bagot M, Berti E, Cerroni L, et al. European Organization for Research and Treatment of Cancer and International Society for Cutaneous Lymphoma consensus recommendations for the management of cutaneous B-cell lymphomas. Blood. 2008;112:1600–9.
14. Persky DO, Unger JM, Spier CM, Stea B, LeBlanc M, McCarty MJ, et al. Phase II study of rituximab plus three cycles of CHOP and involved-field radiotherapy for patients with limited-stage

aggressive B-cell lymphoma: Southwest Oncology Group study 0014. J Clin Oncol. 2008;26:2258–63.

15. Miller TP, Dahlberg S, Cassady JR, Adelstein DJ, Spier CM, Grogan TM, et al. Chemotherapy alone compared with chemotherapy plus radiotherapy for localized intermediate- and high-grade non-Hodgkin's lymphoma. N Engl J Med. 1998;339:21–6.
16. Posada-Garcia C, Florez A, Pardavila R, Garcia-Cruz A, Amador L, Alvarez M, et al. Primary cutaneous large B-cell lymphoma, leg type, successfully treated with rituximab plus chemotherapy. Eur J Dermatol. 2009;19:393–4.
17. Hallermann C, Niermann C, Fischer R-J, Schulze H-J. New prognostic relevant factors in primary cutaneous diffuse large B-cell lymphomas. J Am Acad Dermatol. 2007;56:588–97.
18. Swerdlow SH, Quintanilla-Martinez L, Willemze R, Kinney MC. Cutaneous B-cell lymphoproliferative disorders: report of the 2011 Society for Hematopathology/European Association for Haematopathology workshop. Am J Clin Pathol. 2013;139:515–35.
19. Desouki MM, Post GR, Cherry D, Lazarchick J. PAX-5: a valuable immunohistochemical marker in the differential diagnosis of lymphoid neoplasms. Clin Med Res. 2010;8:84–8.
20. Hallermann C, Kaune KM, Gesk S, Martin-Subero JI, Gunawan B, Griesinger F, et al. Molecular cytogenetic analysis of chromosomal breakpoints in the IGH, MYC, BCL6, and MALT1 gene loci in primary cutaneous B-cell lymphomas. J Invest Dermatol. 2004;123:213–9.
21. Dijkman R, Tensen CP, Jordanova ES, Knijnenburg J, Hoefnagel JJ, Mulder AA, et al. Array-based comparative genomic hybridization analysis reveals recurrent chromosomal alterations and prognostic parameters in primary cutaneous large B-cell lymphoma. J Clin Oncol. 2006;24:296–305.
22. Senff NJ, Zoutman WH, Vermeer MH, Assaf C, Berti E, Cerroni L, et al. Fine-mapping chromosomal loss at 9p21: correlation with prognosis in primary cutaneous diffuse large B-cell lymphoma, leg type. J Invest Dermatol. 2009;129:1149–55.
23. Espinet B, García-Herrera A, Gallardo F, Baró C, Salgado R, Servitje O, et al. FOXP1 molecular cytogenetics and protein expression analyses in primary cutaneous large B cell lymphoma, leg-type. Histol Histopathol. 2011;26:213–21.
24. Grange F, Petrella T, Beylot-Barry M, Joly P, D'Incan M, Delaunay M, et al. Bcl-2 protein expression is the strongest independent prognostic factor of survival in primary cutaneous large B-cell lymphomas. Blood. 2004;103:3662–8.
25. Felcht M, Heck M, Weiss C, Becker JC, Dippel E, Müller CSL, et al. Expression of the T-cell regulatory marker FOXP3 in primary cutaneous large B-cell lymphoma tumour cells. Br J Dermatol. 2012;167:348–58.
26. Hoefnagel JJ, Dijkman R, Basso K, Jansen PM, Hallermann C, Willemze R, et al. Distinct types of primary cutaneous large B-cell lymphoma identified by gene expression profiling. Blood. 2005;105:3671–8.
27. Sterry W, Kruger GR, Steigelder G-K. Skin involvement in malignant B-cell lymphomas. J Dermatol Surg Oncol. 1984;10:276–7.
28. Morton LM, Wang SS, Devesa SS, Hartge P, Weisenburger DD, Linet MS. Lymphoma incidence patterns by WHO subtype in the United States, 1992–2001. Blood. 2006;107:265–76.
29. Muniesa C, Pujol RM, Estrach MT, Gallardo F, García-Muret MP, Climent J, et al. Primary cutaneous diffuse large B-cell lymphoma, leg type and secondary cutaneous involvement by testicular B-cell lymphoma share identical clinicopathological and immunophenotypical features. J Am Acad Dermatol. 2012;66:650–4.
30. Demirkesen C, Tüzüner N, Esen T, Lebe B, Ozkal S. The expression of IgM is helpful in the differentiation of primary cutaneous diffuse large B cell lymphoma and follicle center lymphoma. Leuk Res. 2011;35:1269–72.
31. Koens L, Vermeer MH, Willemze R, Jansen PM. IgM expression on paraffin sections distinguishes primary cutaneous large B-cell lymphoma, leg type from primary cutaneous follicle center lymphoma. Am J Surg Pathol. 2010;34:1043–8.
32. Shimada K, Kinoshita T, Naoe T, Nakamura S. Presentation and management of intravascular large B-cell lymphoma. Lancet Oncol. 2009;10:895–902.
33. Ferreri AJM, Campo E, Seymour JF, Willemze R, Ilariucci F, Ambrosetti A, et al. Intravascular lymphoma: clinical presentation, natural history, management and prognostic factors in a series of 38 cases, with special emphasis on the "cutaneous variant". Br J Haematol. 2004;127:173–83.
34. Orwat DE, Batalis NI. Intravascular large B-cell lymphoma. Arch Pathol Lab Med. 2012;136:333–8.
35. Jaffe ES, Harris NL, Stein H, Campo E, Pileri SA, Swerdlow SH. Introduction and overview of the classification of the lymphoid neoplasms. In: Swerdlow SH, Campo E, Harris NL, Jaffe ES, Pileri SA, Stein H, et al., editors. WHO classification of tumors of haematopoietic and lymphoid tissues. 4th ed. Lyon: International Agency for Research on Cancer; 2008. p. 158–66.

19 Intravascular Large B-Cell Lymphoma

Amrita Goyal, Joi B. Carter, Judith A. Ferry, and Lyn McDivitt Duncan

Intravascular large B-cell lymphoma (ivLBCL) is an aggressive form of diffuse large B-cell lymphoma with a markedly poor prognosis. It commonly presents with central nervous system (CNS) symptoms and a wide variety of cutaneous manifestations, including maculopapular eruptions, ulcerated nodules, and infiltrated indurated plaques. Because the tumor cells lodge in the vasculature, in cases without obvious cutaneous disease a biopsy of a small cutaneous hemangioma may yield the diagnosis. ivLBCL has had numerous names in the literature, including angiotropic lymphoma, malignant angioendotheliomatosis, and angioendotheliomatosis proliferans systemisata. These names reflect the incorrect initial belief that the neoplastic cells were of endothelial origin; they are in fact derived from post–germinal center B cells [1, 2]. This chapter discusses the clinical presentation, prognosis, treatment, histopathology, immunohistochemistry, molecular characteristics, and differential diagnosis of ivLBCL. The chapter closes with a clinical case featuring a patient with ivLBCL.

A. Goyal, M.D.
Harvard-MIT Division of Health Sciences and Technology, Harvard Medical School, Boston, MA, USA

J.B. Carter, M.D.
Department of Dermatology, Massachusetts General Hospital, Harvard Medical School, Boston, MA, USA

J.A. Ferry, M.D.
Hematopathology Service, Department of Pathology, Massachusetts General Hospital, Harvard Medical School, Boston, MA, USA

L.M. Duncan, M.D. (✉)
Dermatopathology Service, Department of Pathology, Massachusetts General Hospital, Harvard Medical School, Boston, MA, USA
e-mail: duncan@helix.mgh.harvard.edu

J.B. Carter et al. (eds.), *Atlas of Cutaneous Lymphomas: Classification and Differential Diagnosis*, DOI 10.1007/978-3-319-17217-0_19

19.1 Clinical Information

19.1.1 Clinical Presentation

Intravascular large B-cell lymphoma (ivLBCL) is a systemic lymphoma that commonly presents in the skin and is frequently diagnosed by means of a skin biopsy. This rare, aggressive form of diffuse large B-cell lymphoma (DLBCL) primarily strikes older individuals (median age of 67–70 years, range of 13–90 years) with poor performance status and a history of other malignancy [1, 3–5]. Less than one person per million is diagnosed with this disease each year, and there is no gender predilection [3, 4, 6]. Patients nearly always present with stage III or IV disease and have a very poor prognosis [2, 4].

ivLBCL is characterized by the growth of neoplastic B cells in the lumina of small vessels, likely caused by defects in cell homing and transvascular migration secondary to abnormalities in beta-1 integrin or ICAM-1 [3, 4, 7]. There are two major variants of ivLBCL: Asian and Western. Asian ivLBCL is much more likely to manifest with hemophagocytic syndrome, cytopenias, and hepatosplenomegaly but without cutaneous or CNS involvement [2, 8]. Western ivLBCL most often presents with cutaneous and CNS manifestations. There is also a subtype of Western ivLBCL that shows isolated cutaneous involvement and occurs almost exclusively in women, with a mean age of 59 years [4, 5].

Symptoms vary widely, depending on which vessels and capillary beds are involved. Most patients have widespread symptoms, including fever of unknown origin, night sweats, weight loss, and fatigue [2, 4]. When the CNS is involved, symptoms may include sensory and motor deficits, seizures, transient vision loss, or altered consciousness [4].

Cutaneous manifestations are present in 40 % of patients with Western ivLBCL and are most often found on the legs (35 %), thighs (41 %), and trunk (31 %) [9]. ivLBCL frequently is seen in the skin as violaceous nodules or plaques (49 %), blue or livid macules (22 %), and/or painful telangiectasias (20 %) [9]. Livedo-like reticular erythema, palpable purpura, ulcers, infiltrative peau d'orange changes, and cellulitis have also been observed [1, 2, 4, 9, 10]. Lower extremity edema is common (27 %) [9]. The cutaneous presentation of ivLBCL may be difficult to distinguish clinically from that of thrombophlebitis, erythema nodosum, and/or erysipelas [9].

19.1.2 Prognosis and Treatment

ivLBCL has a generally poor prognosis, with overall 3-year survival ranging from 30 %–80 %, with recent improvements in survival largely related to use of rituximab-based therapies [1, 2]. Cutaneous only disease has been reported as a favorable prognostic factor [2, 4]. Poor prognostic factors include poor performance status, advanced disease, elevated serum lactate dehydrogenase, and the presence of B symptoms (including fever, night sweats, weight loss) [8].

ivLBCL demonstrates a very poor response to multiagent chemotherapy [3]. The inclusion of rituximab with other multiagent chemotherapy regimens has been shown to improve the efficacy of response substantially [2]. Patients who undergo chemotherapy followed by a stem cell transplant have been documented to have significantly improved survival rates [1, 8], but because this cancer usually strikes older patients with poor health at baseline, few patients are candidates for transplants [4].

19.2 Pathology

19.2.1 Histopathology

The histopathology of ivLBCL is characterized by occlusion of the lumina of small- and medium-sized vessels by neoplastic cells. The tumor cells do not characteristically exit the vascular spaces to involve the surrounding tissue [4]. Angiodestruction is rare, given that the neoplastic B cells of ivLBCL are limited to within the vascular space and the vascular endothelia are rarely affected [4]. The involved vessels are nearly always capillaries or small venules, usually sparing the lymphatics (Fig. 19.1) [5]. Occasionally, there is associated hemorrhage, fibrin thrombi, and necrosis [3].

The intravascular tumor cells have large blastic nuclei with multiple nucleoli and coarse nuclear chromatin [2, 3]. Mitotic figures are typically easy to identify [2, 3]. Tumor cells may colonize cutaneous hemangiomas; therefore biopsy of a hemangioma may be helpful in making this diagnosis [10–12].

19.2.2 Immunophenotype and Molecular Findings

The neoplastic B cells express CD20, Bcl2, and MUM-1 with staining for CD5 and CD10 in 38 % and 13 % of cases, respectively [3]. Cases lacking CD10-expression are more likely to express MUM-1 [3]. It should be noted that CD20 may be absent in patients previously treated with rituximab [4].

Case studies have reported abnormalities or translocations of chromosomes 1, 6, 11, 14, 18, and 19 [2, 13–16]. The mixed lineage leukemia (*MLL*) gene has been implicated in several cases [17]. Clonal immunoglobulin rearrangement is often present [3]. Epstein-Barr virus infection has been rarely reported, and is typically absent in ivLBCL [4].

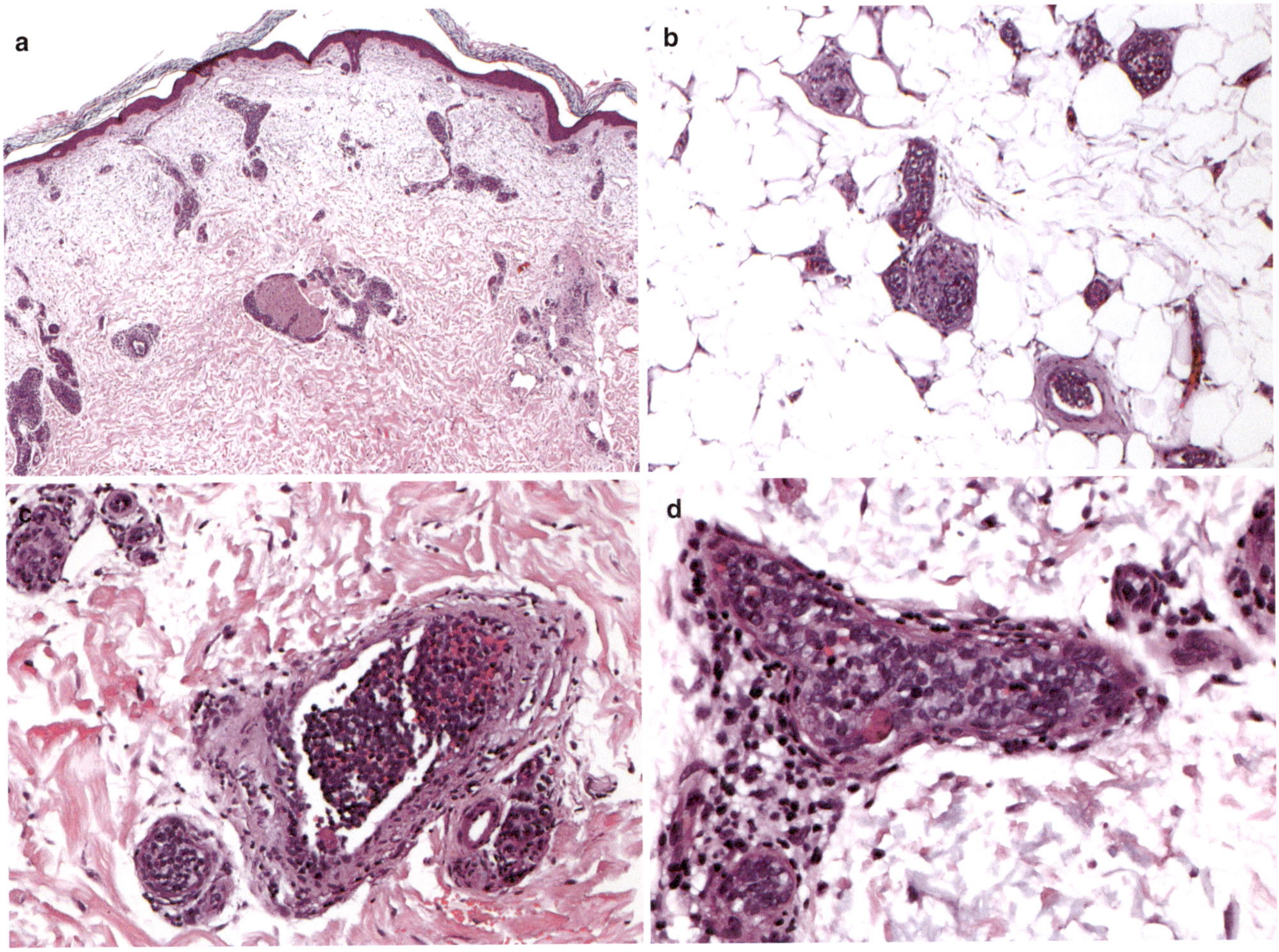

Fig. 19.1 Histopathology of ivLBCL. This patient's ivLBCL was diagnosed at autopsy. (**a**) Large atypical lymphocytes fill the lumina of superficial and deep dermal vessels. The vessels around the arrector pili muscle (*center*) are completely obstructed by lymphoma cells. There is no extravasation of neoplastic cells into the surrounding dermal tissue (H&E, 10×). (**b**) The vessels of the subcutaneous fat are similarly involved. (**c**) Aggregates of neoplastic large B cells fill the lumina of numerous vessels in the reticular dermis and adhere to the vascular endothelium (H&E, 20×). (**d**) Large atypical lymphocytes occlude the vascular lumina (H&E, 40×)

19.3 Diagnosis

19.3.1 Diagnostic Considerations

Diagnosis is often extremely delayed because of the heterogeneity of presentation, frequent absence of a mass lesion, strong tendency to mimic non-neoplastic conditions and the difficulty of obtaining a biopsy that contains a tumor specimen. Consequently, a quarter of patients are diagnosed postmortem [1, 3, 6]. Multiple skin biopsies and repeated bone marrow biopsies may be necessary [2]. Because patients typically lack mass lesions or lymphadenopathy, imaging scans were initially thought to offer minimal utility [1, 5, 8]; however, new case reports suggest that magnetic resonance imaging and/or positron emission tomography and computed tomography may be helpful in the setting of CNS [18, 19], uterine [20], and pulmonary involvement [21, 22].

Relevant and helpful laboratory findings may include elevated lactate dehydrogenase and beta-2-microglobulin levels, anemia, other cytopenias, and hemophagocytic syndrome [1, 4, 5]. The differential diagnosis includes other aggressive angiotropic B-cell lymphomas that manifest with systemic and/or neurologic findings, including lymphomatoid granulomatosis and primary DLBCL of the central nervous system [4].

19.3.2 Differential Diagnosis

19.3.2.1 Lymphomatoid Granulomatosis (LyG)

This aggressive systemic, Epstein-Barr virus–positive B-cell lymphoma frequently manifests in the skin as erythematous dermal and subcutaneous papules and nodules [23]. Both LyG and ivLBCL patients usually have systemic symptoms, including fever and weight loss. LyG commonly involves the lungs, and ivLBCL can involve any vascular bed [4, 23]. Histologically both involve the vasculature; however, LyG infiltrates the tissues surrounding the vessels with angiodestruction and angioinvasion, whereas ivLBCL is an intravascular embolic process [4, 5]. While LyG is typically Epstein-Barr virus–positive, ivLBCL has no clear association with the virus [4, 23]. Both diseases have a grave prognosis [23].

19.3.2.2 Primary Diffuse Large B Cell Lymphoma (DLBCL) of the CNS

CNS involvement by ivLBCL is common, occurring in nearly 30 % of patients [4]. Primary DLBCL of the CNS may also present with neurologic abnormalities and behavioral and personality changes [2, 4]. In ivLBCL the neurologic symptoms are secondary to ischemic changes resulting from capillary infiltration, and brain imaging typically demonstrates a pattern consistent with CNS vasculitis [24]. In primary DLBCL of the CNS, magnetic resonance imaging shows contrast-enhancing lesions [4]. Biopsy of DLBCL of the CNS typically shows a diffuse proliferation of large cells, often with a perivascular pattern at the periphery of the tumor. Also of significance is that multisystem involvement of ivLBCL is exceedingly common, whereas primary CNS lymphomas tend to remain confined to the CNS [4, 5].

19.4 Clinical Case

Case 19.1

A 64-year-old woman presented with one-and-one-half months of low grade fever, night sweats, weight loss, generalized weakness, dizziness, and dry cough. She had hepatosplenomegaly and rales but no cutaneous or neurologic findings. On admission to the hospital, she developed a coagulopathy, anemia, and thrombocytopenia. She died 1 month after admission with metabolic acidosis, hypotension, and respiratory failure. The diagnosis of ivLBCL was made on autopsy. Lymphoma was present in the skin, lymph nodes, bone marrow, liver, adrenal glands, kidneys, bladder, and uterus (Fig. 19.2).

Commentary This case highlights the point that many cases of ivLBCL are diagnosed post-mortem. Her lymphoma was widespread, evidence that this is a systemic disease with prominent cutaneous manifestations rather than a primary cutaneous lymphoma. In addition, this patient is in the age group most commonly afflicted by this disease. She ultimately developed symptoms consistent with hemophagocytic syndrome, as is often seen in ivLBCL.

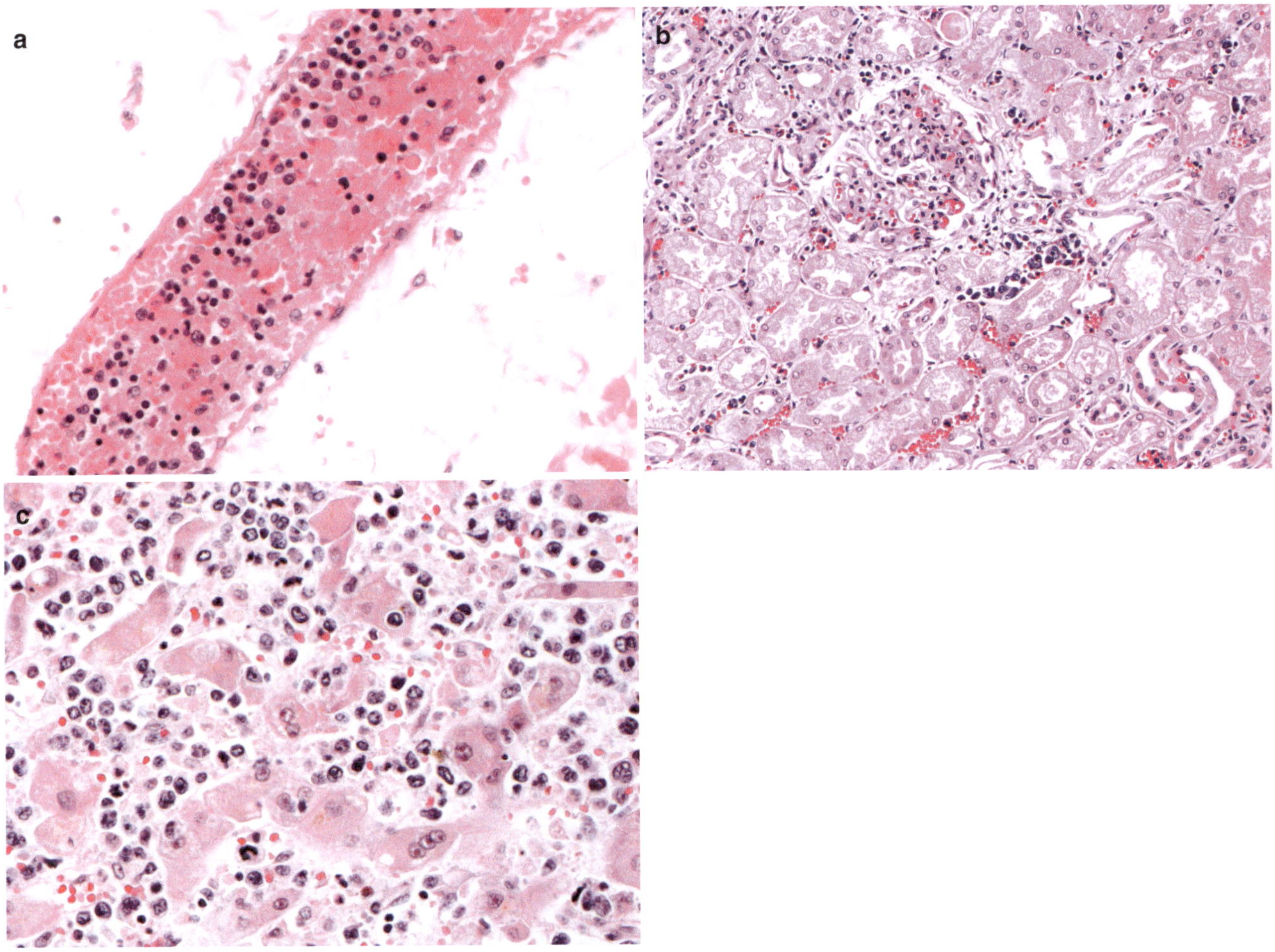

Fig. 19.2 Histopathology of ivLBCL, clinical case 19.1. (**a**) Skin. Aggregates of neoplastic large B cells fill the lumina of a vessel in the subcutaneous fat and adhere to the vascular endothelium (H&E, 40×). (**b**) Kidney. Neoplastic B cells fill the capillaries of the glomerulus (H&E, 20×). (**c**) Liver. Liver sinusoids are occupied by neoplastic B cells (H&E, 40×)

References

1. Ferreri AJM, Campo E, Seymour JF, Willemze R, Ilariucci F, Ambrosetti A, et al. Intravascular lymphoma: clinical presentation, natural history, management and prognostic factors in a series of 38 cases, with special emphasis on the "cutaneous variant". Br J Haematol. 2004;127:173–83.
2. Shimada K, Kinoshita T, Naoe T, Nakamura S. Presentation and management of intravascular large B-cell lymphoma. Lancet Oncol. 2009;10:895–902. Elsevier Ltd.
3. Nakamura S, Ponzoni M, Campo E. Intravascular large B-cell lymphoma. In: Swerdlow SH, Campo E, Harris NL, Jaffe ES, Pileri S, Stein H, et al., editors. WHO classification of tumors of haematopoietic and lymphoid tissues. Lyon: International Agency for Research On Cancer; 2008. p. 252–3.
4. Orwat DE, Batalis NI. Intravascular large B-cell lymphoma. Arch Pathol Lab Med. 2012;136:333–8.
5. Ponzoni M, Ferreri AJM, Campo E, Facchetti F, Mazzucchelli L, Yoshino T, et al. Definition, diagnosis, and management of intravascular large B-cell lymphoma: proposals and perspectives from an international consensus meeting. J Clin Oncol. 2007;25:3168–73.
6. Ferreri A, Dognini G. Variations in clinical presentation, frequency of hemophagocytosis and clinical behavior of intravascular lymphoma diagnosed in different geographical regions. Haematologica. 2007;92:486–92.
7. Ponzoni M, Arrigoni G, Gould VE, Del Curto B, Maggioni M, Scapinello A, et al. Lack of CD 29 (beta1 integrin) and CD 54 (ICAM-1) adhesion molecules in intravascular lymphomatosis. Hum Pathol. 2000;31:220–6.
8. Murase T, Yamaguchi M, Suzuki R, Okamoto M, Sato Y, Tamaru J, et al. Intravascular large B-cell lymphoma (IVLBCL): a clinicopathologic study of 96 cases with special reference to the immunophenotypic heterogeneity of CD5. Blood. 2007;109:478–85.
9. Röglin J, Böer A. Skin manifestations of intravascular lymphoma mimic inflammatory diseases of the skin. Br J Dermatol. 2007;157:16–25.
10. Kempf W, Kazakov DV, Mitteldorf C. Cutaneous lymphomas: an update. Part 2: B-cell lymphomas and related conditions. Am J Dermatopathol. 2014;36:197–210.
11. Krokowski M, Sellmann L, Feller AC. Intravascular large B-cell lymphoma within a subcutaneous cavernous haemangioma. Br J Haematol. 2010;151:2.
12. Ishida M, Hodohara K, Yoshida T, Okabe H. Intravascular large B-cell lymphoma colonizing in senile hemangioma: a case report and proposal of possible diagnostic strategy for intravascular lymphoma. Pathol Int. 2011;61:555–7.
13. Yamamoto K, Yakushijin K, Okamura A, Hayashi Y, Matsuoka H, Minami H. Gain of 11q by an additional ring chromosome 11 and trisomy 18 in CD5-positive intravascular large B-cell lymphoma. J Clin Exp Hematop. 2013;53:161–5.
14. Rashid R, Johnson RJ, Morris S, Dickinson H, Czyz J, O'Connor SJM, et al. Intravascular large B-cell lymphoma associated with a near-tetraploid karyotype, rearrangement of BCL6, and a t(11;14)(q13;q32). Cancer Genet Cytogenet. 2006;171:101–4.
15. Kobayashi T, Ohno H. Intravascular large B-cell lymphoma associated with t(14;19)(q32;q13) translocation. Intern Med. 2011;50:2007–10.
16. Cui J, Liu Q, Cheng Y, Chen S, Sun Q. An intravascular large B-cell lymphoma with a t(3;14)(q27;q32) translocation. J Clin Pathol. 2014;67:279–81.
17. Deisch J, Fuda FB, Chen W, Karandikar N, Arbini AA, Zhou XJ, et al. Segmental tandem triplication of the MLL gene in an intravascular large B-cell lymphoma with multisystem involvement: a comprehensive morphologic, immunophenotypic, cytogenetic, and molecular cytogenetic antemortem study. Arch Pathol Lab Med. 2009;133:1477–82.
18. Joshi PV, Lele VR, Shaikh I. Mortui vivos docent--the dead teach the living: 18-flurodeoxyglocose positron emission tomography-computed tomography findings in a case of intravascular B cell lymphoma. J Cancer Res Ther. 2013;9:141–4.
19. Yamamoto A, Kikuchi Y, Homma K, O'uchi T, Furui S. Characteristics of intravascular large B-cell lymphoma on cerebral MR imaging. AJNR Am J Neuroradiol. 2012;33:292–6.
20. Takeoka Y, Inaba A, Fujitani Y, Kosaka S, Yamamura R, Senzaki H, et al. Intravascular large B-cell lymphoma diagnosed by FDG-PET/CT and endometrial biopsy. Rinsho Ketsueki. 2011;52:1777–81.
21. Dasanu CA, Codreanu I, Mesologites T, Ali S, Sullivan P, Jethava A. Western variant of brain intravascular lymphoma displaying three distinct evolutive radiologic stages. Conn Med. 2014;78:73–6.
22. Yamashita H, Suzuki A, Takahashi Y, Kubota K, Kano T, Mimori A. Intravascular large B-cell lymphoma with diffuse FDG uptake in the lung by 18FDG-PET/CT without chest CT findings. Ann Nucl Med. 2012;26:515–21.
23. Beaty MW, Toro J, Sorbara L, Stern JB, Pittaluga S, Raffeld M, et al. Cutaneous lymphomatoid granulomatosis: correlation of clinical and biologic features. Am J Surg Pathol. 2001;25:1111–20.
24. Song DK, Boulis NM, Mckeever PE, Quint DJ. Angiotropic large cell lymphoma with imaging characteristics of CNS vasculitis. 2002;23:239–42.

20 Introduction to Precursor Neoplasms

Amrita Goyal, Joi B. Carter, and Lyn McDivitt Duncan

Blastic plasmacytoid dendritic cell neoplasm (BPDCN) is the only "precursor neoplasm" and only myeloid malignancy included in the WHO-EORTC classification of cutaneous lymphomas. This exceptionally rare and very aggressive lymphoma is derived from blastic plasmacytoid dendritic cells, an uncommon subtype of dendritic cells. In contrast to our detailed knowledge of T-cell and B-cell biology, very little is known about the biology and function of normal blastic plasmacytoid dendritic cells.

20.1 Blastic Plasmacytoid Dendritic Cell Neoplasm as a Precursor Neoplasm

The WHO-EORTC classification for primary cutaneous lymphoma includes a single non-T cell, non-B cell "precursor neoplasm:" blastic plasmacytoid dendritic cell neoplasm (BPDCN). This rare malignancy of blastic plasmacytoid dendritic cells is strongly associated with antecedent or subsequent myeloid malignancies. Because of the cellular immaturity of the blastic plasmacytoid dendritic cells, these neoplasms are grouped with precursor neoplasms rather than with true dendritic cell neoplasms in the WHO Classification of Tumours of Haematopoietic and Lymphoid Neoplasms [1].

A. Goyal, M.D.
Harvard-MIT Division of Health Sciences and Technology, Harvard Medical School, Boston, MA, USA

J.B. Carter, M.D.
Department of Dermatology, Massachusetts General Hospital, Harvard Medical School, Boston, MA, USA

L.M. Duncan, M.D. (✉)
Dermatopathology Service, Department of Pathology, Massachusetts General Hospital, Harvard Medical School, Boston, MA, USA
e-mail: duncan@helix.mgh.harvard.edu

20.2 Plasmacytoid Dendritic Cells

Blastic plasmacytoid dendritic cells, also known as "plasmacytoid monocytes" or "professional type-1 interferon producing cells," are a special subset of dendritic cells [2]. Although they account for only a tiny fraction of our immune cells (<0.1 % of peripheral blood mononuclear cells), they are the primary producers of interferon alpha in the human body [3]. By virtue of their production of type-1 interferons and other cytokines, they are critical to an array of immune functions, ranging from antiviral immunity to antitumor immunity to peripheral tolerance [3]. The mechanism of their derangement in BPDCN and other myeloid neoplasms is poorly understood. Ongoing research efforts will hopefully enhance our understanding of blastic plasmacytoid dendritic cell biology and in turn enlighten us about the pathobiology of BPDCN.

References

1. Swerdlow SH, Campo E, Harris NL, Jaffe ES, Pileri SA, Stein H, et al., editors. WHO classification of tumours of haematopoietic and lymphoid tissues. 4th ed. Lyon: International Agency for Research on Cancer; 2008.
2. Facchetti F, Jones D, Petrella T. Blastic plasmacytoid dendritic cell neoplasm. In: Swerdlow SH, Campo E, Harris NL, Jaffe ES, Pileri SA, Stein H, et al., editors. WHO classification of tumours of haematopoietic and lymphoid neoplasms 2. 4th ed. Lyon: International Agency for Research on Cancer; 2008. p. 145–7.
3. Jegalian AG, Facchetti F, Jaffe ES. Plasmacytoid dendritic cells: physiologic roles and pathologic states. Adv Anat Pathol. 2009;16:392–404.

J.B. Carter et al. (eds.), *Atlas of Cutaneous Lymphomas: Classification and Differential Diagnosis*,
DOI 10.1007/978-3-319-17217-0_20

21 Blastic Plasmacytoid Dendritic Cell Neoplasm

Amrita Goyal, Joi B. Carter, and Lyn McDivitt Duncan

Blastic plasmacytoid dendritic cell neoplasm (BPDCN) is a highly aggressive tumor of plasmacytoid dendritic cells that commonly presents with involvement of the skin, bone marrow, peripheral blood, and lymph nodes. This diagnosis portends a dismal prognosis. BPDCN has previously been referred to in the literature as blastic NK lymphoma, agranular CD4+ NK-cell leukemia, blastic NK leukemia/lymphoma, and CD4+ CD56+ hematodermic neoplasm, reflecting the initial incorrect belief that the neoplastic cells are derived from NK cells [1].

A. Goyal, M.D.
Harvard-MIT Division of Health Sciences and Technology,
Harvard Medical School, Boston, MA, USA

J.B. Carter, M.D.
Department of Dermatology, Massachusetts General Hospital,
Harvard Medical School, Boston, MA, USA

L.M. Duncan, M.D. (✉)
Dermatopathology Service, Department of Pathology,
Massachusetts General Hospital, Harvard Medical School,
Boston, MA, USA
e-mail: duncan@helix.mgh.harvard.edu

J.B. Carter et al. (eds.), *Atlas of Cutaneous Lymphomas: Classification and Differential Diagnosis*,
DOI 10.1007/978-3-319-17217-0_21

21.1 Clinical Information

21.1.1 Clinical Presentation

BPDCN is an aggressive tumor derived from plasmacytoid dendritic cells [1]. The neoplasm is incredibly rare, accounting for less than 0.8 % of all cutaneous lymphomas [2] and less than 1 % of all acute leukemias [3]. BPDCN is two to three times more common in men than in women [1, 4, 5]. The median age of onset is in the seventh decade of life, but reports include patients ranging in age from 3 months to 103 years [4–7]. There is no racial or ethnic preference for this disease [1].

Initial cutaneous manifestations of BPDCN can vary from a solitary bruiselike skin lesion to an asymptomatic violaceous nodule or plaque with a diameter spanning millimeters to 10 cm (Fig. 21.1) [3]. There are three major clinical presentations: 73 % of patients present with nodular lesions, 12 % with "bruiselike" patches (see Fig. 21.4), and 14 % with a combination of disseminated patches and nodules [5]. Men are more likely than women to present with bruise-like lesions (13 % *vs* 1 %, respectively). Mucosal involvement is rare but can occur [5]. Over time, patients often develop multiple lesions [1, 3, 6].

Although BPDCN begins in the skin, progression to leukemia with bone marrow involvement is the rule rather than the exception [8]. Leukemic dissemination may present before, during, or after the onset of cutaneous manifestations, and 50 % of patients have leukemic involvement at the time of diagnosis [5, 7]. Up to 20 % of patients initially present with regional lymphadenopathy, 20 % with massive lymphadenopathy [9], and 46 % with bone marrow involvement [1]. Up to 10–20 % of patients will develop associated secondary leukemias, including myelomonocytic leukemia or acute myelogenous leukemia (see Case 21.2) [1, 6, 10].

The blood is involved in 60–90 % of patients; the bone marrow, in 65–72 %; and lymph nodes, in 45 % [1, 4]. Organomegaly is common and can occur in up to 60 % of patients; involvement of the lungs, kidneys, muscles, and heart also has been reported [1, 4, 11]. Central nervous system involvement has been reported in 9–26 % of cases [5]. Cytopenias (thrombocytopenia in two thirds of cases, followed by anemia and neutropenia) are common in the setting of bone marrow involvement [3], and circulating blast cells can be seen in 60 % of patients; in these patients, between 1 and 90 % of their leukocyte count may be composed of neoplastic cells [6]. Nearly 60 % of patients will enter a fulminant leukemic phase resulting in death [1, 4, 6].

21.1.2 Prognosis and Treatment

This disease has a dismal prognosis, with a mean survival of 1 year [1, 3], a mean 2-year survival rate of 33 %, and a mean 5-year survival rate of 6 % [12]. Although many patients initially respond to chemotherapy, they almost universally relapse soon thereafter and progress rapidly [1]. Patients with isolated cutaneous lesions have a better prognosis than those who present with both cutaneous and extracutaneous manifestations, with a median survival of 21 months versus 12 months [12]. Age younger than 40 years is a positive prognostic factor [12]. Counterintuitively, a high proliferative index and expression of TdT are also associated with better survival [5, 12].

There is no established standard of care for this disease. Bone marrow transplantation offers the best chance of remission [5, 10]. Although 80–90 % of patients initially respond to multiagent therapy with CHOP or CHOP-like regimens [1, 11], most patients relapse and are resistant to chemotherapy within 3–18 months [6]. There have been sporadic cases of long-term remission in younger patients who underwent induction chemotherapy followed by an autologous or allogeneic bone marrow or stem cell transplant during their first remission [1, 11–13]. Bexarotene and interferon alpha have been used to induce partial remission [9].

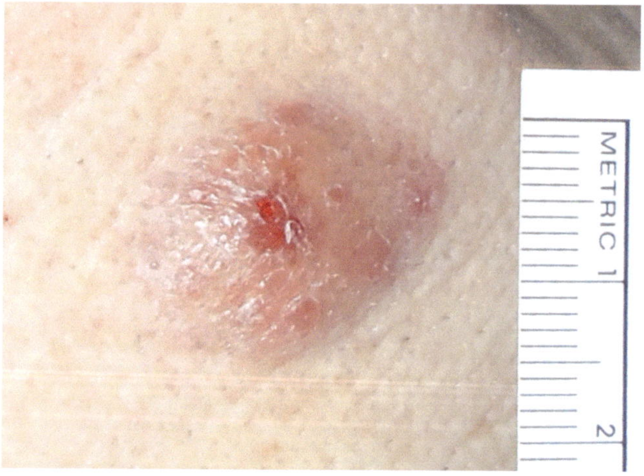

Fig. 21.1 Plasmacytoid dendritic cell neoplasm: a clinical image from Case 21.1. On the patient's jawline is a pink-to-violaceous tumor measuring 1.5×2 cm with a central ulceration. Similar nodules were present on his back and shoulders

21.2 Pathology

21.2.1 Histopathology

Skin biopsies in BPDCN demonstrate a diffuse, monomorphic infiltrate or large clusters of tumor cells in the dermis (Fig. 21.2; *see also* Fig. 21.5) [1, 6]. Infiltration of cutaneous appendages is common, and subcutaneous involvement may occur. The epidermis is generally spared [1, 3, 6]. There is no angiodestruction or coagulative necrosis; mitoses may be present, but they generally are not prominent [1, 6]. Red blood cell extravasation may be present [9].

The neoplastic cells have a varied cytopathological appearance; the nuclei are round or oval and occasionally cleaved with prominent small, basophilic nucleoli and fine nuclear chromatin. There is weakly basophilic, grey-blue cytoplasm without apparent cytoplasmic granules (see Fig. 21.2b) [1, 3, 6].

Involved lymph nodes demonstrate diffuse effacement. Bone marrow invasion by neoplastic cells can range from a mild infiltrate to complete replacement of the bone marrow; any remaining hematopoietic tissue is often dysplastic. Finally, smears of peripheral blood or bone marrow demonstrate cells with characteristic microvacuoles and pseudopods [1].

21.2.2 Immunophenotype and Molecular Findings

The neoplastic plasmacytoid dendritic cells of BPDCN are characterized by the absence of any specific myeloid, B-lymphoid, T-lymphoid, or NK markers (Tables 21.1 and 21.2) [3]. They are typically positive for CD4, CD56, and CD123 (Fig. 21.3; *see also* Fig. 21.6), similar to normal plasmacytoid dendritic cells [3, 6, 11, 15]. The tumor cells also usually stain positively for CD7, CD43, CD45RA, CD45, HLA-DR, TCL1, and CD303/BDCA2 [1, 6, 7, 11]. One-third of cases are TdT+ [1], and 50 % show CD68 staining in a cytoplasmic dot-like pattern [1, 6, 7].

A diagnosis of BPDCN is highly likely when four of the five markers are positive: CD4, CD56, CD123, CD303/BDCA2, and TCL1. There have been rare reports of cases negative for CD4, CD56, or both, however; this finding is likely to be attributable to immunophenotypic variation of neoplastic cells or lack of sensitivity of immunohistochemical staining (see Table 21.1) [7].

The neoplastic cells in skin biopsies are typically negative for nonspecific esterase, CD34, CD117, linker of activated T cells (LAT), lysozyme, myeloperoxidase (MPO), granzyme B, and T-cell intracellular antigen-1 (TIA-1). Although granzyme B is generally negative in skin biopsies, it may be positive in peripheral blood flow cytometry [1].

T-cell receptors are usually in their germline configuration [1]. Up to two thirds of patients demonstrate complex, abnormal karyotypes [1]. Although there are no consistent abnormalities, recurrent deletions of 12p13, 6q23, monosomy 9 and 15, and 5q abnormalities have been observed; deletions on chromosomes 4 and 13 may implicate tumor suppressor genes including *RB1* and *LATS2* [1, 11]. Loss of cell-cycle control genes, particularly *CDKN1B*, *CDKN2B*, and *TP53* may play a role in disease pathogenesis [5]. There is no association with Epstein-Barr virus (EBV) [1].

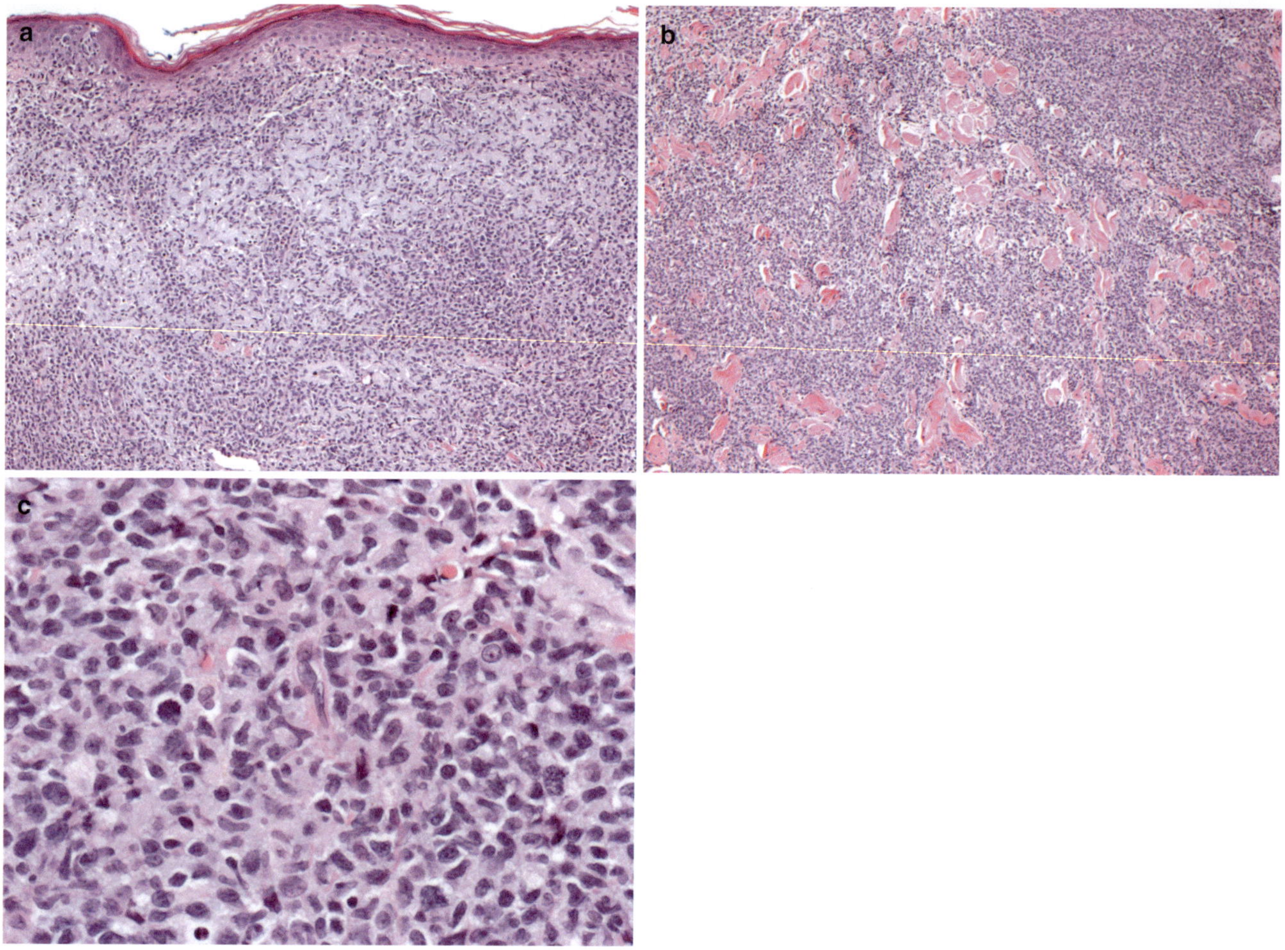

Fig. 21.2 Histopathology of blastic plasmacytoid dendritic cell neoplasm (BPDCN) from Case 21.1. (**a**) Diffuse sheets of atypical cells are present throughout the dermis with minimal involvement of the overlying epidermis (H&E, 10×). (**b**) Neoplastic plasmacytoid dendritic cells fill the deep dermis and disrupt the collagen bundles (H&E, 20×). (**c**) The medium-sized, atypical cells have dispersed chromatin, irregular nuclear borders, and small basophilic nucleoli (H&E, 20×)

Table 21.1 Antigens expressed in BPDCN, supporting a diagnosis

Antigen	Frequency (%)
CD4	94.6
CD56	96.5
CD123	95.3
TCL1	89.3
CD2AP	80.5
BDCA2/CD303	75.0

Adapted from Pagano et al. [14]
It is important to note that one or more of these markers may be negative in some cases of BPDCN; negativity does not rule out the diagnosis, but does make it less likely
BPDCN blastic plasmacytoid dendritic cell neoplasm

Table 21.2 Antigens usually absent in BPDCN

	Antigen
Pan–T-cell markers	CD3
Pan–B-cell markers	CD20
	CD79a
Myeloid markers	CD11c
	CD34
	CD163
	Lysozyme
	Myeloperoxidase

Adapted from Pagano et al. [14]
Positive staining of these antigens excludes a diagnosis of BPDCN
BPDCN blastic plasmacytoid dendritic cell neoplasm

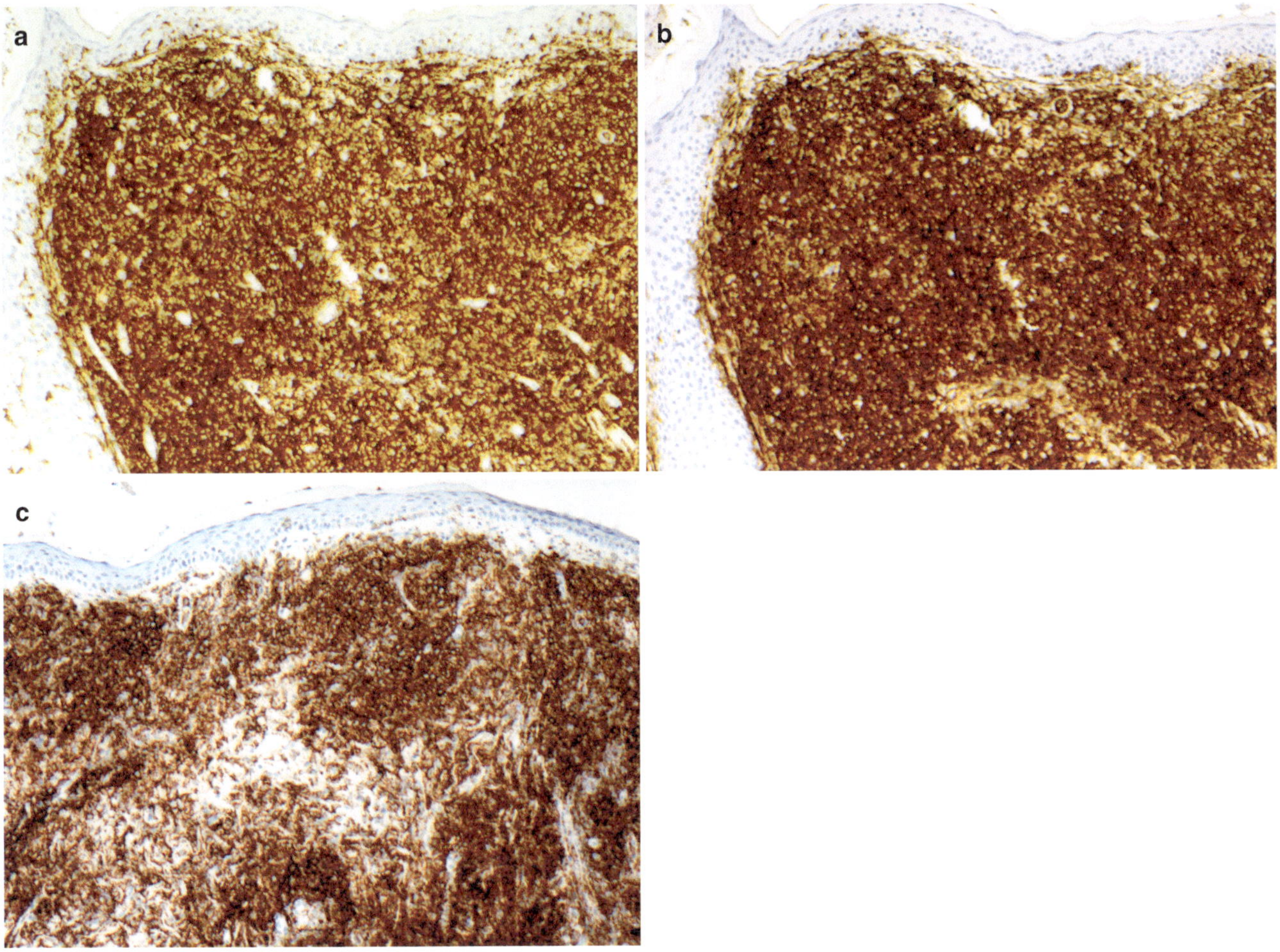

Fig. 21.3 Histopathology and immunohistochemistry of BPDCN from Case 21.1. (**a**) The atypical cells demonstrate expression of CD4 (CD4, 10×). The atypical cells also stain positively for CD123 (**b**) (CD123, 10×) and for CD56 (**c**), consistent with a plasmacytoid dendritic cell phenotype (CD56, 10×)

21.3 Differential Diagnosis

21.3.1 Diagnostic Considerations

Diagnosis is aided by clinical presentation and histopathologic analysis, but it ultimately rests on extensive immunohistochemical analysis to identify the plasmacytoid dendritic cell phenotype of the neoplastic cells. Diagnosis is frequently complicated by the fact that up to 20 % of BPDCN patients may develop additional hematologic neoplasms, especially acute myeloid leukemia (AML) and chronic myelomonocytic leukemia (CMML) [1, 6].

21.3.2 Differential Diagnosis

21.3.2.1 Acute Myeloid Leukemia (AML)

This leukemia of myeloid origin is the primary element on the differential for BPDCN. Unfortunately, AML also has a very poor prognosis. It can present with leukemia cutis (secondary cutaneous manifestations of the systemic lymphoma), and these cutaneous findings may present before, concurrently with, or after the discovery of leukemic involvement and portend an even worse prognosis [16]. Histopathologically, cutaneous lesions of AML present with nodular or diffuse infiltrates with perivascular and periadnexal accentuation [16]. The upper papillary dermis is often spared, and there is typically extension into the subcutaneous fat. Individual neoplastic cells may be present singly between collagen fibers [16]. Differentiating AML from BPDCN is further complicated by the fact that AML can also stain positively for CD123 [17], and 10–20 % of patients with BPDCN can develop associated systemic malignancies, including AML [1, 6, 10]. The neoplastic cells of AML will stain positively for myeloid markers including myeloperoxidase and lysozyme, however, and these markers by definition are negative in BPDCN [14].

21.3.2.2 Extranodal NK/T-Cell Lymphoma (eNK/TCL) [6, 11]

eNK/TCL presents with painful, commonly ulcerated, cutaneous nodules of neoplastic NK/T cells. The neoplastic cells of BPDCN are derived from blastic plasmacytoid dendritic cells and are strongly positive for both CD56 and CD123; in contrast, though the atypical cells of eNK/TCL stain positively for CD56, they are without staining for CD123 [18]. EBV positivity is one of the hallmarks of eNK/TCL, whereas the neoplastic cells in BPDCN are EBV negative. Finally, the cutaneous lesions of BPDCN lack the angiodestruction characteristic of eNK/TCL [6].

21.3.2.3 Mycosis Fungoides (MF)

Clinical findings usually allow the distinction of MF from BPDCN: MF typically goes through a classic patch-plaque-tumor progression, but BPDCN does not. On histopathology, MF is characterized by epidermotropism of neoplastic T cells with a CD3+ CD56− phenotype [6]. A clonal T-cell receptor (TCR) also favors a diagnosis of MF rather than BPDCN [4].

21.3.2.4 Chronic Myelomonocytic Leukemia (CMML)

The leukemic phase of BPDCN, which occurs in nearly 60 % of patients, can mimic CMML. In addition, cutaneous manifestations (leukemia cutis) may occur in between 10 and 50 % of cases of monocytic leukemia [19] and may include violaceous to red-brown papules and plaques, purpura, and ecchymoses, which can closely resemble the lesions of BPDCN [20, 21]. Immunohistochemical testing often yields the diagnosis: though both processes are CD56+, the plasmacytoid dendritic cells of BPDCN also stain for CD123 and CD4, whereas the cells of CMML are negative for CD123 and CD4 but stain positively for CD13, CD33, and CD68. [1]. This differential can be particularly challenging when the CMML presents with massive nodal involvement by plasmacytoid dendritic cells [22].

21.3.2.5 Aggressive NK-Cell Leukemia/Lymphoma (ANKCLL)

BPDCN can also be difficult to distinguish from ANKCLL, which shares the CD56+ immunophenotype. It may also present with fever, systemic symptoms, bone marrow and blood involvement (with resultant anemia, thrombocytopenia, and leukopenia), and occasional lymphadenopathy [23]. Although cutaneous involvement is rare, when it occurs, ANKCLL may present with numerous erythematous macules, papules, and plaques on the extremities and trunk [23]. They can be differentiated on the basis of immunohistochemistry: the tumor cells of BPDCN are CD56+, CD123+, CD4+, CD8−, and TIA-, whereas those of ANKCLL are CD4−, CD8+, and TIA+. In addition, the tumor cells of BPDCN are agranular but those of ANKCLL have cytoplasmic granules [6].

21.4 Clinical Cases

Case 21.1

A 71-year-old man presented with a 6-month history of fatigue and enlarging, pruritic nodules on his right cheek, back, and shoulders (see Fig. 21.1). Skin biopsy revealed diffuse sheets of atypical CD4+, CD56+, CD123+ cells throughout the dermis (see Fig. 21.2). Although a PET-CT scan demonstrated no lymphadenopathy, circulating tumor cells were present in peripheral blood. In spite of prednisone and chemotherapy, he died of complications of this disease 1 year after diagnosis.

Commentary The majority of patients with BPDCN present with multiple nodular lesions, as did this patient. He is in the classic demographic for this disease, a male in his 70s. His aggressive clinical course and lack of response to treatment are consistent with this diagnosis.

Case 21.2

A 66-year-old man presented with a 2-month history of numerous violaceous, indurated plaques on his forehead, cheeks, shoulders, chest, and legs, measuring 2–5 cm (Fig. 21.4). He experienced progressing fatigue and night sweats. A skin biopsy revealed sheets of atypical CD4+, CD56+, CD123+, MPO– cells permeating the dermis (Figs. 21.5 and 21.6). Peripheral blood flow cytometry revealed a marked monocytosis composed of atypical CD56+ monocytes with folded nuclei and variably condensed chromatin. Bone marrow biopsy demonstrated increased numbers of monocytes and 2 % blasts. The patient was diagnosed with cutaneous BPDCN with concomitant CMML-1.

Commentary This patient's case offers an example of BPDCN with concomitant CMML-1, which occurs in 10–20 % of patients. His clinical presentation differs significantly from that of the patient in case 1—this patient presented with plaques and ecchymoses, rather than nodules. Such lesions are found in 12 % of patients.

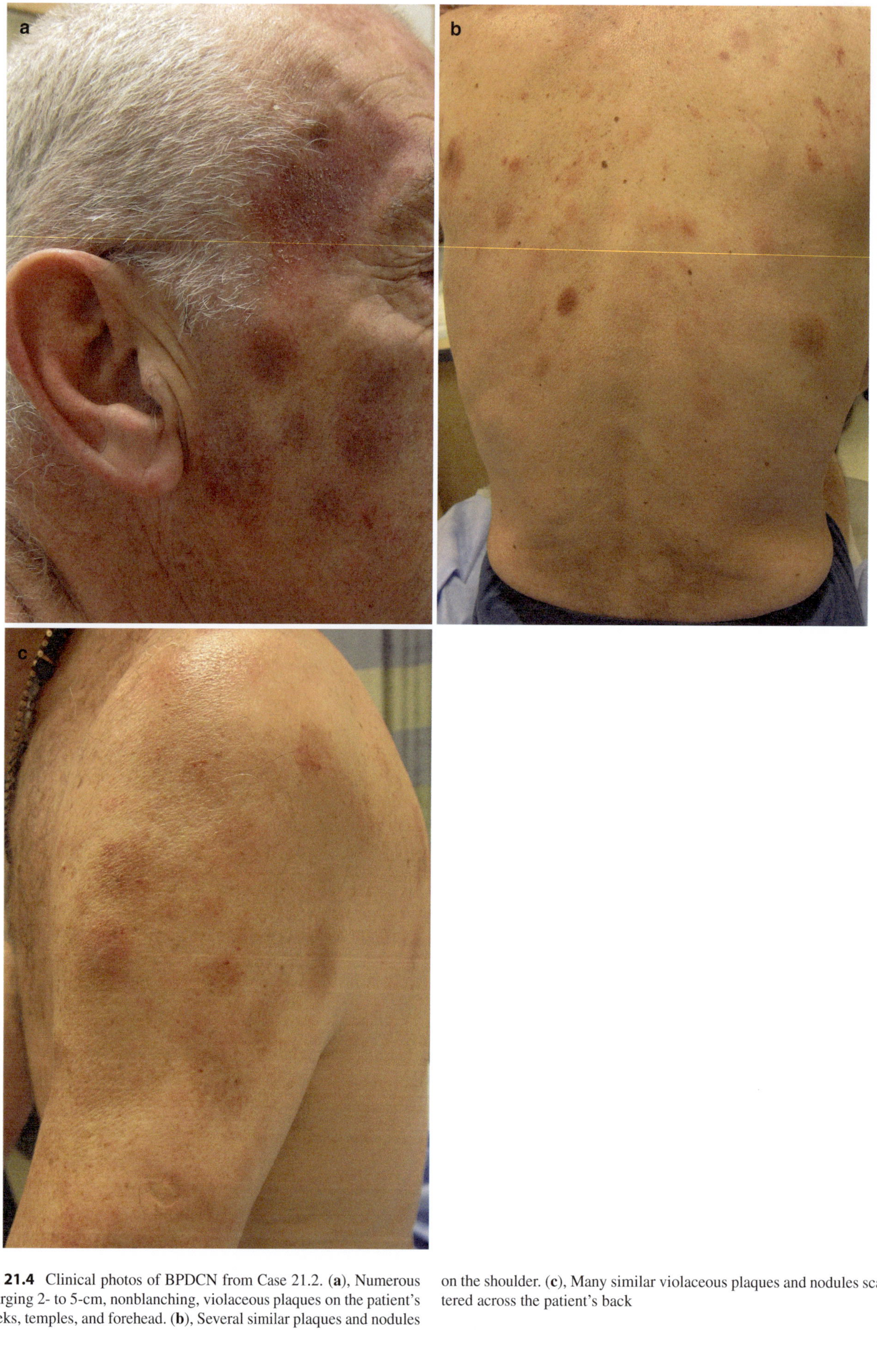

Fig. 21.4 Clinical photos of BPDCN from Case 21.2. (**a**), Numerous enlarging 2- to 5-cm, nonblanching, violaceous plaques on the patient's cheeks, temples, and forehead. (**b**), Several similar plaques and nodules on the shoulder. (**c**), Many similar violaceous plaques and nodules scattered across the patient's back

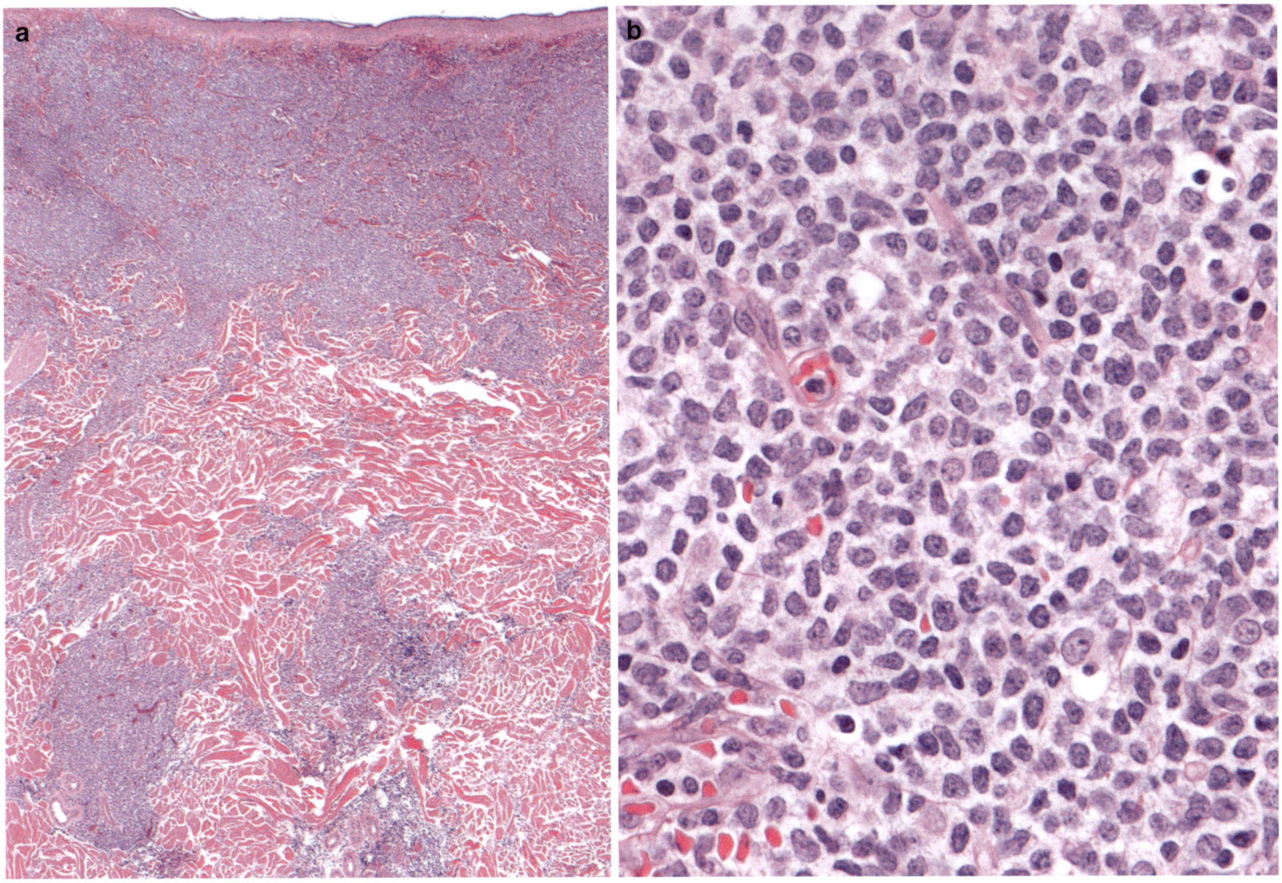

Fig. 21.5 Histopathology of BPDCN from Case 21.2. (**a**), Dense, superficial and deep dermal infiltrate of atypical blastic plasmacytoid dendritic cells (H&E, 4×). (**b**), The neoplastic cells demonstrate marked cytological atypia with large, irregularly shaped nuclei, prominent nucleoli, and fine nuclear chromatin. Many of the nuclei are cleaved (H&E, 63×)

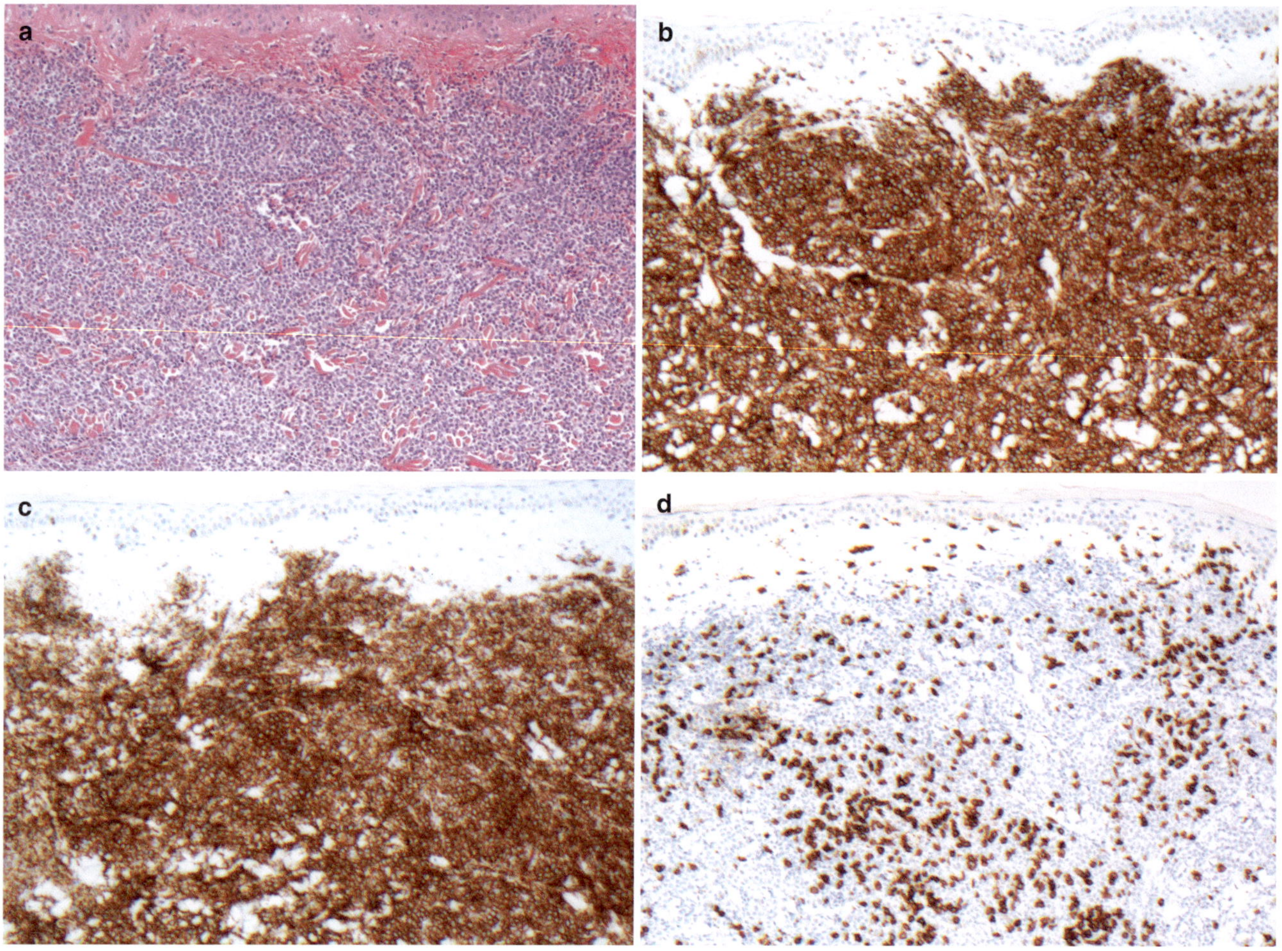

Fig. 21.6 Histopathology and immunohistochemistry of BPDCN from Case 21.2. (**a**) A dense, monomorphic dermal infiltrate of neoplastic cells (H&E, 10×). (**b**) Neoplastic cells stain strongly for CD4 (CD4, 10×). (**c**) Consistent with a blastic plasmacytoid dendritic cell phenotype, the neoplastic cells also express CD123 (CD123, 10×). (**d**) Although there are scattered CD3+ T cells within the neoplastic infiltrate, the tumor cells do not express CD3 (CD3, 10×)

References

1. Facchetti F, Jones D, Petrella T. Blastic plasmacytoid dendritic cell neoplasm. In: Swerdlow SH, Campo E, Harris NL, Jaffe ES, Pileri SA, Stein H, et al., editors. WHO classification of tumors of haematopoietic and lymphoid tissues. 4th ed. Lyon: International Agency for Research On Cancer; 2008. p. 145–7.
2. Petrella T, Facchetti F. Tumoral aspects of plasmacytoid dendritic cells: what do we know in 2009? Autoimmunity. 2010;43:210–4.
3. Garnache-Ottou F, Feuillard J, Saas P. Plasmacytoid dendritic cell leukaemia/lymphoma: towards a well defined entity? Br J Haematol. 2007;136:539–48.
4. Li Y, Li Z, Lin HL, Chen XH, Li B. Primary cutaneous blastic plasmacytoid dendritic cell neoplasm without extracutaneous manifestation: case report and review of the literature. Pathol Res Pract. 2011;207:55–9.
5. Julia F, Petrella T, Beylot-Barry M, Bagot M, Lipsker D, Machet L, et al. Blastic plasmacytoid dendritic cell neoplasm: clinical features in 90 patients. Br J Dermatol. 2013;169:579–86.
6. Naeim F, Rao PN, Song SX, Grody WW. Disorders of dendritic cells. In: Naeim F, Rao PN, Song SX, Grody WW, editors. Atlas of hematopathology: morphology, immunophenotype, cytogenetics, and molecular approaches. San Diego: Academic; 2013. p. 649–61.
7. Julia F, Dalle S, Duru G, Balme B, Vergier B, Ortonne N, et al. Blastic plasmacytoid dendritic cell neoplasms: clinico-immunohistochemical correlations in a series of 91 patients. Am J Surg Pathol. 2014;38:673–80.
8. Panwalkar AW, Armitage JO. T-cell/NK-cell lymphomas: a review. Cancer Lett. 2007;253:1–13.
9. Magro CM, Porcu P, Schaefer J, Erter JW, Furman RR, Shitabata PK, et al. Cutaneous CD4+ CD56+ hematologic malignancies. J Am Acad Dermatol. 2010;63:292–308.
10. Dietrich S, Andrulis M, Hegenbart U, Schmitt T, Bellos F, Martens UM, et al. Blastic plasmacytoid dendritic cell neoplasia (BPDC) in elderly patients: results of a treatment algorithm employing allogeneic stem cell transplantation with moderately reduced conditioning intensity. Biol Blood Marrow Transplant. 2011;17:1250–4.
11. Kharfan-Dabaja MA, Lazarus HM, Nishihori T, Mahfouz RA, Hamadani M. Diagnostic and therapeutic advances in blastic plasmacytoid dendritic cell neoplasm: a focus on hematopoietic cell transplantation. Biol Blood Marrow Transplant. 2013;19:1006–12.
12. Bekkenk MW, Jansen PM, Meijer CJLM, Willemze R. CD56+ hematological neoplasms presenting in the skin: a retrospective analysis of 23 new cases and 130 cases from the literature. Ann Oncol. 2004;15:1097–108.
13. Ferrándiz-Pulido C, López-Lerma I, Sábado C, Ferrer B, Pisa S, García-Patos V. Blastic plasmacytoid dendritic cell neoplasm in a child. J Am Acad Dermatol. 2012;66:e238–40.
14. Pagano L, Valentini CG, Pulsoni A, Fisogni S, Carluccio P, Mannelli F, et al. Blastic plasmacytoid dendritic cell neoplasm with leukemic presentation: an Italian multicenter study. Haematologica. 2013;98:239–46.
15. Dummer R, Asagoe K, Cozzio A, Burg G, Doebbeling U, Golling P, et al. Recent advances in cutaneous lymphomas. J Dermatol Sci. 2007;48:157–67.
16. Kaddu S, Zenahlik P, Beham-Schmid C, Kerl H, Cerroni L. Specific cutaneous infiltrates in patients with myelogenous leukemia: a clinicopathologic study of 26 patients with assessment of diagnostic criteria. J Am Acad Dermatol. 1999;40:966–78.
17. Rollins-Raval M, Pillai R, Warita K, Mitsuhashi-Warita T, Mehta R, Boyiadzis M, et al. CD123 immunohistochemical expression in acute myeloid leukemia is associated with underlying FLT3-ITD and NPM1 mutations. Appl Immunohistochem Mol Morphol. 2013;21:212–7.
18. Liang X, Graham DK. Natural killer cell neoplasms. Cancer. 2008;112:1425–36.
19. Pont V, Miquel FJ, Grau TC, Hernández F, Sánchez-Carazo JL, Aliaga A. Skin involvement in chronic myelomonocytic leukaemia as a predictor of transformation into acute myeloid leukaemia. J Eur Acad Dermatol Venereol. 2001;15:260–2.
20. Mathew RA, Bennett JM, Liu JJ, Komrokji RS, Lancet JE, Naghashpour M, et al. Cutaneous manifestations in CMML: indication of disease acceleration or transformation to AML and review of the literature. Leuk Res. 2012;36:72–80.
21. Braga D, Manganoni AM, Boccaletti V, Pancera C, Marocolo D, Facchetti F, et al. Specific skin infiltration as first sign of chronic myelomonocytic leukemia with an unusual phenotype. J Am Acad Dermatol. 1996;35:804–7.
22. Vermi W, Facchetti F, Rosati S, Vergoni F, Rossi E, Festa S, et al. Nodal and extranodal tumor-forming accumulation of plasmacytoid monocytes/interferon-producing cells associated with myeloid disorders. Am J Surg Pathol. 2004;28:585–95.
23. Radonich MA, Lazova R, Bolognia J. Cutaneous natural killer/T-cell lymphoma. J Am Acad Dermatol. 2002;46:451–6.

Glossary

Acanthosis Epidermal hyperplasia characterized by thickening of the stratum spinosum.

Adnexotropic With a tropism for cutaneous adnexal structures. *See* folliculotropic and syringotropic.

Anaplastic Atypical appearance of cell nuclei. Nuclei are often large, irregularly shaped, and hyperchromatic with prominent nucleoli.

Angiocentric Centered around or distributed around blood vessels.

Angioinvasion Invading the wall of the blood vessel with associated endothelial cell necrosis and dropout.

Angiotropic Describing an affinity for tumor cells to attach to the vascular surfaces, either the abluminal surface (in melanoma) or the luminal surface (as in intravascular large B-cell lymphoma).

Anthracyclines Family of cell-cycle nonspecific cancer chemotherapy agents derived from Streptomyces bacteria. These compounds inhibit DNA and RNA synthesis by intercalating between base pairs and also by inhibiting topoisomerase II. Examples include doxorubicin and daunorubicin.

B symptoms Fever (>38 °C), night sweats, and weight loss (>10 % body weight over <6 months). These are important prognostic factors in some lymphomas.

Bexarotene Retinoid antineoplastic agent used in the treatment of cutaneous T-cell lymphoma (CTCL). Bexarotene selectively activates the retinoid X receptors (RXRs), causing cell differentiation and apoptosis.

Blastic A cytologic descriptor of enlarged cells with round nuclei resembling stem cells.

Blastic plasmacytoid dendritic cell Also known as plasmacytoid monocytes or professional type 1 interferon-producing cells. Special subset of dendritic cells that produces the majority of interferon-alpha in the human body.

Borrelia burgdorferi Spirochete bacterium responsible for causing Lyme disease. Carried by the *Ixodes* tick.

Bulla Intraepidermal or subepidermal cavity greater than 5–10 mm in diameter and containing serous fluid and/or inflammatory debris.

Centroblast An intermediate cell in the process of B-cell differentiation. Centroblasts are B cells derived from antigen-stimulated B blasts and located in the dark zone of the germinal center; these undergo somatic hypermutation and proliferation.

Centrocyte An intermediate cell in the process of B-cell differentiation, centrocytes are B cells derived from centroblasts that have migrated to the light zone of the germinal center. They undergo selection.

Cerebriform Resembling the fissures and contours of the brain. Classically used to describe the nuclei of Sézary cells and the cells of mycosis fungoides.

CHOP Chemotherapy regimen commonly used for non-Hodgkin lymphoma, consisting of Cyclophosphamide (an alkylating agent), Hydroxydaunorubicin (an intercalating agent, also known as doxorubicin), Oncovin (a microtubule inhibitor, also known as vincristine), and Prednisone.

Colonized follicle Nonneoplastic lymphoid follicle overrun by neoplastic cells.

Constitutional symptoms Nonspecific, generalized symptoms including weight loss, fevers, fatigue, malaise, chills, night sweats, and decreased appetite.

Cutaneous Lymphocyte Antigen (CLA) A skin lymphocyte homing receptor. Typically present on Sezory cells.

Cutaneous lymphoid hyperplasia (CLH) A dense dermal reactive lymphoid infiltrate that mimics cutaneous lymphoma (*see* pseudolymphoma).

Dendritic cell (DC) Antigen-presenting cell that acts as an intermediate between the innate and adaptive immune systems. DCs are present in the skin, mucosal epithelium, bloodstream, and lymph nodes.

Disseminated intravascular coagulation (DIC) Widespread activation of the clotting cascade, resulting in formation of thrombi in small vessels throughout the body, causing tissue ischemia and necrosis. A consumptive coagulopathy that also depletes clotting factors and platelets, simultaneously resulting in severe bleeding.

Doxorubicin Anthracycline chemotherapy agent. *See* anthracycline.

J.B. Carter et al. (eds.), *Atlas of Cutaneous Lymphomas: Classification and Differential Diagnosis*,
DOI 10.1007/978-3-319-17217-0

Epidermotropism The presence of cytologically atypical lymphocytes in the epidermis usually with minimal to no accompanying spongiosis. Cells may either be present singly, surrounded by a clear halo, or in groups, as in the Pautrier microabscesses of mycosis fungoides. The cytologic atypia of the lymphocytes distinguishes epidermotropism from exocytosis. *See* Pautrier microabscess.

Epstein-Barr virus (EBV) Also known as human herpes virus-4 (HHV-4); one of the most common human viral pathogens. Enveloped DNA virus responsible for causing infectious mononucleosis and associated with an array of malignancies, including extranodal natural killer/T-cell lymphoma (eNK/TCL), Hodgkin lymphoma, Burkitt lymphoma, and nasopharyngeal carcinoma.

Erosion Incomplete loss of epidermis without damage to the basement membrane. Typically heals without scarring.

Erythroderma Also called exfoliative dermatitis; characterized by diffuse erythema and scaling involving most, if not all, of the skin (>80–90 % of body surface area).

Etoposide Cytotoxic antineoplastic agent in the class of topoisomerase II inhibitors. Prevents religation of DNA strands after unwinding and causes the formation of double-stranded breaks; DNA damage then promotes apoptosis. Used to treat a variety of hematologic and solid malignancies.

Exocytosis The presence of mononuclear cells in the epidermis with or without accompanying spongiosis. Typically seen in inflammatory conditions. The lack of significant lymphocytic atypia distinguishes exocytosis from epidermotropism.

Extranodal lymphoma Lymphoma arising in sites other than the lymph nodes, most commonly the skin and gastrointestinal tract.

Flow cytometry Biophysical technique that permits assessment of the size, granularity, and expression of cell-surface markers for individual cells. Cells are treated with fluorescently labeled antibodies and suspended in liquid. Suspended cells flow one by one through an exciting light (a laser), and light scatter and emission spectra are recorded, allowing the phenotype of individual cells to be assessed.

Flower cell Characteristic cellular morphology of cells in adult T-cell leukemia/lymphoma (ATLL).

Follicle center cells Centrocyte and centroblast B cells located in the follicle center of a lymphoid follicle. Typically CD10+ Bcl6+ Bcl2−.

Follicular dendritic cells (FDC) CD21+ CD23+ dendritic cells of mesenchymal origin found in primary and secondary lymphoid follicles. These cells form the meshwork that supports the B cells of the follicle center; FDC meshworks may be disrupted in neoplastic or colonized lymphoid follicles.

Follicular mucinosis Accumulation of dermal mucin in the pilosebaceous unit.

Folliculotropic With a tropism for the hair follicle.

Grenz zone Area of uninvolved dermis between the basement membrane zone and the underlying dermal infiltrate or neoplasm.

Hematopoietic stem cell transplantation (HSCT) The transfer of multipotent hematopoietic stem cells from the bone marrow, peripheral blood, or cord blood. These transplants may be autologous (from the recipient) or allogeneic (from another individual).

Hemophagocytic syndrome (HPS) Also known as hemophagocytic lymphohistiocytosis (HLH). Characterized by macrophage phagocytosis of erythrocytes, leukocytes, platelets, and precursors in the bone marrow. It can be associated with a variety of conditions, including malignancy, infection, immunodeficiency, and autoimmune diseases. In cutaneous lymphoma, HPS may be seen in gamma-delta T-cell lymphoma and rarely in subcutaneous panniculitis-like T-cell lymphoma.

Histiocyte Tissue macrophage. Histiocytes have large, elongated, lightly staining nuclei with visible nuclear borders.

HTLV-1 Human T-lymphotropic virus-1, the delta retrovirus responsible for adult T-cell leukemia/lymphoma. The lymphomagenic effect of this virus is likely secondary to random integration into the host cell genome.

Imiquimod Toll-like receptor 7 agonist, used as a topical chemotherapeutic agent. Works as an immune modifier, causing cancer cell death by enhancing the local immune response.

Immunoglobulin heavy chain (IgH) The large polypeptide subunit of an immunoglobulin. An antibody is composed of one IgH chain and two Ig light chains.

Immunophenotype Immunohistochemical characteristics of a cell or group of cells. In dermatopathology, typically assayed using immunohistochemical stains.

Inside-out follicle Large neoplastic follicle center cells may surround aggregates of small T and B cells.

Langerhans cell CD1a+, langerin+, CD4+ dendritic cell present in the upper layers of the stratum basale and spinosum.

Leukemia cutis Infiltration of the epidermis, dermis, and/or subcutis by neoplastic leukocytes or precursors, manifesting as clinically apparent cutaneous lesions.

Lichenoid Characterized by a band-like inflammatory infiltrate in the superficial dermis. Typically parallel to the epidermis but may abut and obscure the dermal-epidermal junction.

Lymphoid follicle Aggregate of lymphoid cells composed of a central area of large B cells and a surrounding area of smaller T cells and B cells.

Macrophage Monocyte-derived phagocytic and antigen-presenting cell. Macrophages play an important role in both innate and adaptive immunities.

Macule Circumscribed flat area less than 5–10 mm in its largest dimension, without elevation or depression relative to the surrounding skin.

Marginal zone cell B cell located in the marginal zone of a germinal follicle or having a cytologic phenotype similar to that of cells in the marginal zone (also termed monocytoid B cell).

Methotrexate Commonly used antimetabolite and antifolate drug to treat malignancies and autoimmune conditions. Used either alone or in combination with other chemotherapeutic agents.

Microabscess Small accumulation of cells in the epidermis. They may also be present in the subepidermal papillae.

Monoclonal Group of cells derived from the same ancestral cell by repeated cellular replication.

Monomorphic No variation in the appearance of nuclei of cells of the same type (e.g., monomorphic appearance of B cells in chronic lymphocytic leukemia/lymphoma).

Monomorphous Homogeneous population of cells (e.g., a monomorphous infiltrate of lymphocytes without histiocytes, plasma cells, or granulocytes).

Mucin In the dermis, mucin usually refers to hyaluronic acid; dermal mucin is a major component of the ground substance of tissue. Dermal mucin stains with Alcian blue, colloidal iron, and toluidine blue but is PAS-negative. Epidermal mucin is composed of neutral and acid mucopolysaccharides. It is PAS-positive, mucicarmine-positive, and diastase-resistant.

Multiagent chemotherapy Use of a combination of chemotherapeutic drugs to treat a neoplasm.

Munro microabscess Small aggregate of disintegrated neutrophils in the parakeratotic stratum corneum of psoriasis.

Naked follicle Collections of neoplastic follicle center cells apposed to the reticular dermal collagen without an intervening mantle zone of small lymphocytes.

Narrowband UV-B (NBUVB) Type of phototherapy using a specific wavelength of ultraviolet radiation (311–312 nm). Used in a variety of benign skin conditions such as psoriasis, atopic eczema, vitiligo, and lichen planus as well as in cutaneous T-cell lymphoma. Referred to as "narrowband" because it uses a single wavelength of light compared with its precursor treatment, broadband UVB therapy (290–320 nm).

Natural killer (NK) cell Cytotoxic lymphocyte of the humoral immune system, analogous to the cytotoxic T cell of the adaptive immune system. Involved in host response to viral infection and tumors.

Neutrophil Also known as polymorphonuclear cells, these granulocytes are a key component of the humoral immune system and are responsible for phagocytosis.

Nodule Palpable, nonfluctuant lesion, often in the dermis or subcutis, greater than 5–10 mm in width and depth.

Oligoclonal Group of cells derived from a few ancestral cells by repeated replication.

Pan T-cell markers Immunohistochemical markers found on the majority of T-cell subtypes. These include CD2, CD3, CD5, and CD7.

Papule Well-circumscribed, firm elevation of the skin without visible fluid; less than 5–10 mm.

Parakeratosis Incomplete keratinization with retention of nuclei in the stratum corneum, often associated with attenuated or absent granular layer.

Parapsoriasis Patches of erythema greater than 6 cm in diameter with overlying adherent scale. Frequently accompanied by atrophy and poikiloderma. The patches of parapsoriasis often occur in a bathing suit distribution and are considered by some to be a patch-stage mycosis fungoides (MF).

Patch A large macule (area of change in surface color) greater than 5–10 mm in its widest dimension.

Pautrier microabscess Intraepidermal accumulation of three or more atypical T cells within the stratum spinosum of the epidermis; seen in mycosis fungoides.

Plaque Circumscribed thickened, indurated, or elevated plateau-like lesion greater than or equal to 1 cm in diameter.

Pleomorphic Variation in appearance of nuclei of cells of the same type.

Poikiloderma Combination of telangiectasia, hyper- and hypopigmentation, and atrophy of the epidermis, yielding a mottled appearance.

Polyclonal Group of cells derived from numerous different ancestral cells.

Polymorphous Heterogeneous population of cells.

Positron emission tomography (PET) scan Nuclear medicine scan that produces a three-dimensional image of the body, indicating areas of increased metabolic activity. Patients receive a bolus of a biologically active tracer, most commonly fluorodeoxyglucose (FDG), which is taken up in larger quantities by metabolically active tissue and then imaged.

Prednisone Synthetic corticosteroid used for immune suppression. Used in chemotherapy, autoimmune diseases, rheumatic disorders, allergic disorders, and for the treatment and prevention of posttransplant rejection.

Proliferative index Immunohistochemically based measurement of tumor cell proliferative rate using markers of cellular proliferation, most commonly Ki-67.

Provirus Viral genomic material integrated into host cell DNA. In many cases, this integration can be oncogenic.

Pseudoepitheliomatous hyperplasia Histopathologic reaction pattern characterized by a benign hyperplasia of epidermal and adnexal epithelia resembling squamous cell carcinoma.

Pseudolymphoma Benign lymphocytic proliferation that clinically and histopathologically may resemble a lymphoma (*see* cutaneous lymphoid hyperplasia).

Psoralen + UVA (PUVA) treatment A form of phototherapy using oral or topical psoralen, a photosensitizing agent derived from plants that intercalates into DNA in combination with light in the UV-A spectrum. Has been used successfully in mycosis fungoides and other cutaneous T-cell lymphomas as well as in benign conditions, including psoriasis, eczema, and vitiligo.

Pustule Intraepidermal or subepidermal fluid-filled space containing inflammatory cells, typically neutrophils.

R-CHOP CHOP chemotherapy with the addition of rituximab. *See* CHOP.

Reactive follicle Benign lymphoid hyperplasia resulting in follicle formation.

Retinoid Class of compounds derived from vitamin A. Common examples include bexarotene, isotretinoin, and tazarotene.

Rituximab Chimeric monoclonal antibody against the B-cell cell-surface protein CD20, commonly used in the treatment of B-cell-derived hematologic malignancies.

Sézary cell Characteristic cell of Sézary syndrome, a T cell with a convoluted/cerebriform nucleus. Typically found in the circulation but occasionally may be found in skin biopsies.

Somatic hypermutation Diversification of B-cell receptors via mutation of variable regions of immunoglobulin genes.

Spongiform pustule of Kogoj Multilocular pustule in the upper stratum spinosum composed of neutrophils in a sponge-like network of degenerated keratinocytes. These are suggestive of psoriasis but can be seen in a variety of other conditions.

Spongiosis Intercellular edema between keratinocytes of the epidermis (with increased space between the keratinocytes) and visible intercellular junctions. Severe spongiosis may result in spongiotic intraepidermal vesicle formation.

Syringotropic With a tropism for eccrine structures.

T cell Lymphocyte that is the primary affecter of cell-mediated immunity. T cells derive their name from the fact that they mature in the thymus. Subsets of T cells include CD4+ helper T cells, CD8+ cytotoxic T cells, follicular helper T cells, and more.

Tagging In mycosis fungoides, tagging refers to the presence of atypical cells with cerebriform nuclei arrayed along the dermal-epidermal junction, either singly or lined up in a row.

T-cell receptor (TCR) Molecule on the surface of T cells responsible for binding antigens presented by major histocompatibility complex (MHC). In 95 % of T cells this receptor is composed of alpha and beta chains, while 5 % are composed of gamma and delta chains.

Telangiectasia Visible dilation of small superficial blood vessels.

Tumor Neoplastic proliferation in the epidermis, dermis, or subcutis forming a solid mass greater than 10 mm in diameter.

Ulcer Discontinuity of the epidermis caused by complete loss of epidermis and basement membrane zone. Parts of the dermis and subcutaneous fat may also be lost. Typically associated with granulation tissue and healing with scarring.

Vesicle Well-circumscribed, fluid containing cavity less than 5–10 mm in diameter.

Vincristine Vinca alkaloid, used in chemotherapy. A mitotic inhibitor that prevents microtubule assembly by binding to tubulin, thus killing rapidly dividing cells. Also called Oncovin, it is the "O" in CHOP chemotherapy regimens. *See* CHOP.

Zidovudine An antiretroviral drug used to treat HIV/AIDS. A member of the class of nucleoside analog reverse-transcriptase inhibitors (NRTIs).

Index

J.B. Carter et al. (eds.), *Atlas of Cutaneous Lymphomas: Classification and Differential Diagnosis*,
DOI 10.1007/978-3-319-17217-0

MIX
Papier aus verantwortungsvollen Quellen
Paper from responsible sources
FSC® C105338

If you have any concerns about our products,
you can contact us on
ProductSafety@springernature.com

In case Publisher is established outside the EU,
the EU authorized representative is:
Springer Nature Customer Service Center GmbH
Europaplatz 3, 69115 Heidelberg, Germany

Printed by Libri Plureos GmbH
in Hamburg, Germany